NATURAL REMEDIES

FROM AROUND THE WORLD

CURES FOR 300 COMMON AILMENTS
from Arthritis to Varicose Veins

DR. JOHN HEINERMAN

MAGNI

Printed in the United States of America

10 9 8 7 6 5 4 3 2 1

This book is a reference work based on research by the author. This book is intended as an education devise to keep you informed of the latest medical knowledge. It is not intended to serve as a substitute for changing the treatment advice of your doctor. You should never make a medical change without first consulting with your doctor.

ISBN 1-882330-88-9

Published by:
The Magni Company
PO Box 849
McKinney, TX 75070
E-mail: info@magnico.com

Lovingly dedicated to
Frederick William Sohn (1902–1999)
and Rodney Turner (born 1922),
modest men of light and truth who have been acquainted with each other, followed principles of natural health, and have lived exceptional lives in the service of God and their fellow human beings

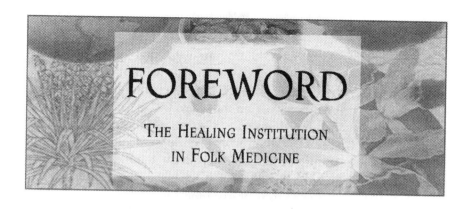

FOREWORD

THE HEALING INSTITUTION
IN FOLK MEDICINE

A while back a colleague of mine, a prominent medical doctor with a large university hospital, upon learning from a discussion we had what the theme of this book would be, asked a proper question: "How will consumers buying your book know whether or not the remedies mentioned in it are safe and effective?" Coming from an obvious "let's-test-it-in-the-laboratory-first-to-see-if-it-works" mentality, his question was only natural and to be expected.

I gave my reply in two parts: an oral explanation followed up several weeks later with a written response. The verbal part dealt with the "healing-intuition" aspect of folk medicine, while my correspondence drew upon a number of scientific (and expensive) reference works on the subject in my research-center library, which are typical of the books I sometimes consulted.

I told my physician friend that the majority of the folk remedies I intended to include in this book came from shamans, witch doctors, medicine people, herbalists, grandparents, immigrants, and just plain common folks from a number of different countries I had visited or cultures I had come in contact with Stateside or abroad. Many of these remedies had already been "time-tested" over many generations to prove some validity, otherwise they would have been discarded a long time ago. "Why keep something around that doesn't work or isn't safe?" I reasoned; he had to admit to the good logic in my reasoning.

Folk-Healing Intuition

But the thing that really fascinated him and obviously occupied a good part of our conversation when we were together at a medical conference was the topic of folk-healing intuition, which he found both curious and inspiring. My explanation to him was much longer and more detailed, yet here I compare it to the proverbial "woman's intuition." A woman can tell if her man has been lying to her though he may look her straight in the eye and swear on a stack of Bibles that what he said was the absolute, unvarnished truth. By the same gut instincts, she knows if something is troubling one of her adolescent children, though that teenage son or daughter may deny it and claim with presumed happiness that everything is okay.

The world's greatest and most complete lexicon, the definitive *Oxford English Dictionary* (2nd Ed.) (Oxford, England: Oxford University Press, 1991) defines "intuition" this way in Volume 8 of its massive 20-volume set:

> **intuition.** 1. Looking upon or into by contemplation. 2. Mentally looking at (something) by consideration. 3. An action of thoughtful perception. 4. Spiritual intuitiveness or immediate knowledge ascribed to supernatural means. 5. An immediate apprehension of an object by the mind without the intervention of any reasoning process. 6. Immediate apprehension by the intellect alone. 7. Immediate apprehension by sense.
>
> 1864 BOWEN *Logic*. In receiving Intuitions, the mind exerts no conscious activity. Derived from processes of observations or hunches. In a more general sense, direct or immediate insight.

This "sixth sense of healing," as I prefer to call it, is almost universally shared by folk healers everywhere; at least the ones I've had the good fortune of meeting, interviewing, and working closely with all had it. So did my dad's mom, Grandmother Barbara Liebhardt Heinerman, who was an eigth-generation folk healer from the former Hungarian city of Temesvar (after World War I boundary lines changed and it became part of Romania and was renamed Timisoara). Her peasant background afforded her no chance for a formal education as we know it now. But her uncanny ability to know what to do or what to use in times of sickness more than compensated for the lack of the other.

I still can remember her telling me when I was a young boy of five, "John, your grandmother is able to help others who become ill because of what she has here [pointing to her head] and also here [laying her hand over heart]." She always gave Providence the credit for being as astute as she was in the healing arts. She used no magic in any of her curative methods, but did swear by a full moon for planting the best herbs with the strongest healing virtues in them. She once said that "no cure can ever be affected if the healer isn't at peace and in touch with nature at all times."

Her "healer's intuition" leapfrogged over my father Jacob and by-passed my brother Joseph to find a place in me. I always knew, even as a small child, that doing certain things for minor problems was the right way, even though no one could really confirm such methods would actually work. For example, my first dog, a German shepherd, became strangely ill all of a sudden. Grandmother had since passed on, and my parents were beside themselves as to what should be done. They considered taking the animal to a vet, but in a matter-of-fact tone this precocious eight-year-old boy informed them not to worry and that he would take care of the matter himself.

I took some scissors and a paper bag and went outside and proceeded to clip some lawn grass. I don't remember how much I gathered that day or even knew *why* it would work but I brought the material into the kitchen and set it on a countertop. I filled a large cooking pot half full of water, put it on the stove, turned the gas burner on, and waited a while until the water started bubbling. I then pushed a kitchen chair in front of the oven door, climbed on top with my sack of grass, and emptied the contents into the pot. I stirred everything with a large meat fork (I probably couldn't find any spoons at the time to do this with), turned the burner off, and covered the pot with a lid.

Later, when everything had pretty much cooled down, I asked my father to strain the liquid out for me. I then put some into my dog's empty water dish and finally coaxed him long enough to where he started slowly drinking it. I gave him more of this "lawn-grass tea" for the next couple of days until I noticed an improvement in his condition. His appetite returned, and he looked and felt 100 percent better. Now if anybody had asked me to give the particulars on why I chose lawn grass instead of something else, I would have shrugged my shoulders and said, "I dunno." But *within* my being I *knew* this was the material to use and that somehow it would make my pet better. *That* is the clearest example of the "folk-healing intuition" that I inherited from my grandmother, God rest her soul.

The Science Behind the Folklore

Later, when I grew to manhood and decided upon medical anthropology as my scholastic vocation in life, I went to school and acquired the necessary discipline, determination, and investigative training that comes with the pursuit of higher learning. Yet in spite of a lettered degree after my name to legitimize my study of folk medicine, the *real force* behind my ultimate success in this field has always been my peasant grandmother's "healing intuition," which she inherited from some of her ancestors and which was eventually bequeathed to me, one of eight grandchildren.

My doctor friend was awestruck by the simple narration of my earliest childhood experience with this gift. But he truly felt that there were some things in life that science itself was incapable of explaining. He certainly valued this gift I had and mentioned something similar within himself, though nowhere near as profound or spectacular. He also felt more comfortable in learning that I had applied a certain amount of science to my folk remedies, because he felt that by doing so I had "legitimized" them more and taken them out of their superstitious origins.

In my follow-up letter to him sometime later I cited some of the reference works I frequently drew upon for this and previous books, though most of the remedies mentioned in each of them were from my own field research in more than 32 different nations. For instance, for some of the remedies coming out of the African continent, I turn to five specific works for further validation of the primary plant ingredients in each of them:

Loutfy Boulous, *Medicinal Plants of North Africa* (Algonac, MI: Reference Publications, Inc., 1983).

Bep Oliver-Bever, *Medicinal Plants in Tropical West Africa* (Cambridge University Press, 1986).

J. M. Watt and M. G. Breyer-Brandwijk, *The Medicinal and Poisonous Plants of Southern and Eastern Africa* (2nd Ed.) (London: E. & S. Livingstone Ltd., 1962).

As for African remedies that were brought over by slaves and popularized in the United States, I relied on William Grimé's *Ethnobotany of the Black American* (Algonac, MI: Reference Publications, Inc., 1979).

Since some of my informants have been Chinese, I have basically trusted two books for the necessary scientific support:

D. Bensky and A. Gamble (Compilers & Translators), *Chinese Herbal Medicine Material Medica* (Seattle: Eastland Press, 1992).

Kee Chang Huang, *The Pharmacology of Chinese Herbs* (Boca Raton: CRC Press, Inc., 1993).

With regard to Native American traditional medicine, there are local, regional, and general scientific works from which to choose:

S. L. Orellana, *Indian Medicine in Highland Guatemala* (Albuquerque: University of New Mexico Press, 1987).

Julia F. Morton, *Atlas of Medicinal Plants of Middle America* (Springfield, IL: Charles C Thomas, 1981).

Virgil J. Vogel, *American Indian Medicine* (Norman: University of Oklahoma Press, 1982).

References of equal scholarly value for *real* Indian remedies from faraway India also constitute a part of my huge book inventory, and several titles were given to the good doctor as proof of this.

Furthermore, some works come from the most unlikely sources. Take Eduardo Qusiumbing's *Medicinal Plants of the Philippines*, which was printed in Manila in 1951 as Technical Bulletin 16 by the Department of Agriculture and Natural Resources. This, coupled with my own trip there a few years ago, gave me both the science as well as the folk side of things that were necessary for the remedies I obtained from there. The same holds true of repeated trips made to the Malay archipelago. The Massachusetts Institute of Technology (MIT) Press in Cambridge put out a rather definitive work in 1980 compiled by Lily M. Perry and Judith Metzger, *Medicinal Plants of East and Southeast Asia: Attributed Properties and Uses*. I've used this innumerable times for the scientific corroboration of many remedies gathered from Burma, Malaysia, Singapore, New Guinea, and Indonesia.

My letter was long and occupied a fair number of pages. But with the many references I cited (far more than the few I've mentioned in these couple of pages), my doctor friend soon became convinced that I did, indeed, have more than adequate science behind the medical folklore used. In his own reply received a while after this, he stated: "Your letter truly astonished me! I never knew there were that many reliable guides to folk medicine. You certainly made your point with me in this respect."

America, the Melting Pot

But you, the reader, may be surprised to learn that a good percentage of the folk remedies contained herein, while obviously from foreign lands, came by way of their immigrants who have relocated to our shores. America, is, indeed, the great "melting pot" for many different types of ethnic cultures as I've found in my travels across our nation. I'm always on the prowl for meaningful medical lore and find it in the least expected places. Sometimes, though, what may be relevant and actually works can't always be used in a book like this.

Take the recent encounter I had with an Indian diplomat and his wife in the staff-operated elevators of the old but posh Pierre Hotel close by Central Park in New York City. He was impeccably dressed in a white shirt, tie, and gray business suit. Except for the turban atop his head, he would have passed for any corporate executive here. His wife was attired in the traditional *sari*, a principal outer garment consisting of embroidered silk that was about as long as I am tall (6-foot 5-inches). She wore it wrapped around her body with the end left hanging over her head as a makeshift hood to keep the sun off. On her forehead was the *binbi* marking, applied every morning with the forefinger using a lead-derived substance *(sindhur)* to indicate she was a married woman. (This *binbi* sign is the equivalent of a wedding ring in the Western world.)

As our glances met for the first time, he nodded and she smiled. Then, seeing a copy of my *Nature's Super Seven Medicines* (Paramus: Prentice Hall, 1997) in my hand, she inquired in pretty good English if I was an author of health books. I answered in the affirmative and showed them the chapter in that book devoted to turmeric. I explained I was a scientist who gathered folk remedies from all over the globe.

Upon hearing this, the gentleman responded by giving me a common cure for earaches popular in his native land. He said that if a little warm animal or human urine were dropped into the ear (with the head in a tilted position), it would quickly relieve the most painful earache imaginable. "Maybe you can use this, perhaps?" he politely offered.

I managed a smile and sincere expression of gratitude. But as we parted company on the ground floor, I made a mental note for future reference: "Undoubtedly a very effective remedy, but cannot use in any of my health books—just too gross and disgusting for sensitive readers to tolerate!"

Fortunately, though, the many things I've gleaned from people of all walks of life and occupations have been more sophisticated than this. And their inclusions in this volume will prove extremely helpful to those seeking simple health solutions to sometimes relatively complex problems.

The "Inner Knowing" in Each of Us

I conclude this foreword with the way it began by reiterating the importance of intuition in whatever skills we utilize. Just about everyone has some of it in him or her to a certain extent. And unlocking that hidden wisdom, or what London-based Christine Page, M.D., terms "an inner *knowing*" isn't that difficult. She has been giving three-day workshops on this subject all over Europe and throughout North America. "Intuition is a potent tool," she told me in an overseas phone conversation we had in early July 1999, "but it has been neglected in deference to the wonderful advances made in technology, as well as our need to have a rational explanation for most daily experiences."

I was blessed to have inherited the "healer's intuition" that my grandmother possessed. But for many people this "inner knowing" usually remains fairly latent and is rarely, if ever, fully utilized. Dr. Page passed on some of the more valuable tips for developing personal intuition, for which eager seminar participants shell out big bucks, pounds, francs, or marks. To my knowledge this is the *only* alternative health book in which you'll ever find such information. I've deliberately placed it here in the beginning so that readers can avail themselves of it and start to enhance the power of their own unused intuitive skills.

FIRST: *Always* empty the mind and heart of negative thoughts and emotions. This is absolutely *critical* in order to allow the unseen "stillness of fact" within us to gently flow forth in *undisturbed* fashion.

SECOND: "Contemplate but don't meditate." Go back to the dictionary definitions given for the word "intuition" and reread them. You will notice the obvious absence of meditation. Now, most dictionaries draw no particular distinction between either word; in fact, as a rule it is a very fine line between the two. But that shade of difference, however thin, is a significant one that cannot be ignored here. The *Oxford English Dictionary* (2nd Ed.) cited earlier provides that slender but profound interpretation. It notes that meditation is the "continuous revolving in the mind for the purpose of conceiving, planning or designing something mentally." By contrast, contemplation is the "thoughtful observation or purposeful consideration of something BUT *usually with* A MIXTURE of *sense.*" (Capitals and italicization are mine.) To be entirely meditative is to be so focused that there is hardly any room for hunches. But the contemplative individual also operates by instinct or "gut feeling." *This* then is the subtle but important difference between the two.

THIRD: Compassion for others *must be* present in the heart before any intuitive instincts can be unlocked. Dr. Page believes "love for others" overwhelms "love of self" and that such "*selfless* sacrifice" brings out personal intuition more clearly. For myself, I know this to be true. Whenever a desire to help others with their health problems is present, my intuitive healing skills work like a charm. But when I do it with an attitude of *detachment* and am somewhat nonemotional toward those being assisted, then it works very weakly and I'm left only with the knowledge learned as a scientist, but nothing more.

FOUR: "Intuition is *a way of being,*" Dr. Page points out. "You learn to listen with an open mind but to judge from the soul. Cultivating inner peace releases the special *sensing* capabilities with which we were all endowed at the time of our births. Going with *gut feelings* in addition to mental review enables us to see the broader picture and get more of a correct overview." You need it with you at all times to avoid making serious and costly mistakes.

FIVE: Mormon scriptures *(Doctrine & Covenants* 6:36) admonish us to "doubt not, fear not." Dr. Page gives her own spin on this beautiful injunction by describing how fears and anxieties can "paralyze the intuitive skills of even the best of us." Being somewhat of a daydreamer or engaging in a little imaginative storytelling helps to dispel such negative moods.

A Personal Invitation

Whenever I sit down to write another health book, I try to make the contents different from the previously published ones. Ultimately, though, all of my books are intended solely for one purpose and that is to help readers regain good health. As I sit behind this typewriter and punch out on the keyboard the words and thoughts that flow into my soul, I can usually imagine in a general way a significantly huge crowd of people who will benefit from what is transcribed.

But in taking on this particular project, something unique occurred during the course of the manuscript's development. There was much more of a *personal touch* included than had been the case with other books. It's as though I were writing this book for *y-o-u*, the reader, rather than for a segment of society at large. This is to say that there is an "aura of care" about the contents that seems to be manifested more strongly here than in some of my other works.

Therefore, in keeping with this delightful spirit, I would like to extend to you a *personal* invitation to carefully examine the contents of this book in a studious fashion. And certainly try some of the remedies in order to see their value. This informal request comes from the heart. It is genuine and sincere—nothing phony about it at all!

I wrote the book *with you in mind!* We've never officially met, and I don't know your name or anything about you. But you are the direct handiwork of Providence. And as such the imprint of the Almighty is clearly stamped in your features. It is to that basic goodness and need for help for which this volume was prepared. You may be one of many readers, it is true, but by the same token there is *only one* of YOU. And while perusing these pages, know this, my dear friend, that our personalities are reaching out to touch each other through the medium of this book in a special way that only the human soul could ever savor.

—John Heinerman
March 2000

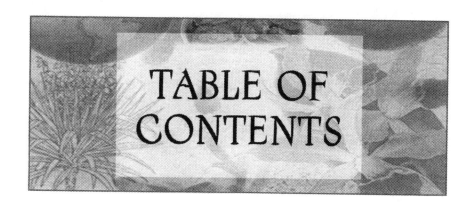

TABLE OF CONTENTS

FOREWORD: The Healing Intuition in Folk Medicine. v

Symptoms

A

Abscesses. 1
Abdominal Cramps, Distress, and Pain 2
Abrasions 3
Acne 4
Addiction. 5
Age Spots. 7
Aggressive Behavior 7
AIDS (see Cancer) 12
Airplane Ears 12
Alcoholic Hangover 13
Allergies 14
Alzheimer's Disease 16
Amebiasis (see Diarrhea) 23
Anal Bleeding, Burning, Itching, and Pain 23
Anemia 24
Aneurysm 26
Angina 28

Animal Bites 29

Ankle Pain 29

Anorexia Nervosa 30

Anxiety 31

Appendicitis 34

Appetite Loss 35

Arm Pain 36

Arthritis 37

Ascites (see Fluid Retention) 39

Asthma 39

Athlete's Foot 40

Atrophic Vaginitis 41

Autism 41

B

Back Pain (Upper and Lower) 45

Bacterial Vaginosis 45

Bad Breath 46

Bags Under the Eyes 47

Bed Sores 47

Bedwetting 49

Benign Prostatic Hyperplasia 50

Bladder Infection 51

Bleeding 54

Bleeding Gums 56

Blisters 57

Blood Clots 58

Blood Poisoning 60

Body Odor 62

Body Piercing 63

Boils and Carbuncles 64

Brain Stress 65

Breast Cancer 66
Breast Pain 69
Breast Swelling 72
Broken Bones 73
Bronchitis. 76
Bruises 77
Bulimia 78
Bunions. 80
Burns. 82
Bursitis 83

C

Caffeinism 84
Cancer 89
Cardiac Arrest 106
Carpal Tunnel Syndrome. 107
Cataracts 109
Celiac Disease 109
Cerebral Palsy 110
Chapped Hands and Lips 111
Charley Horse 111
Chest Pain 112
Chickenpox 112
Chlamydia 113
Choking 115
Chronic-Fatigue Syndrome. 121
Cirrhosis of the Liver. 124
Cockroach Infestation 125
Cold Hands and Feet 126
Cold Sores 126
Colic. 128
Colitis 128

Colon Cancer 129

Color Blindness 130

Coma 131

Common Cold 133

Compulsions 134

"Computer-Screen" Eyes 134

Concussion 136

Conjestive Heart Failure 136

Conjunctivitis 138

Constipation 138

Contact-Lens Problems 139

Cough 139

Crabs 140

Cracked Heel 141

Crohn's Disease 142

Croup 143

Crow's Feet Around Eyes 143

Cuts 144

Cystic Fibrosis 144

Cystitis (see Bladder Infection) 145

Cysts 145

D

Dandruff 147

Deep-Vein Thrombosis 148

Delirium 150

Dementia 150

Dental Cavities 152

Depression 153

Dermatitis, Diabetes, Diaper Rash 153

Diarrhea 154

Difficult Urination 155

Diverticular Disease 155
Dizziness. 155
Double Vision 155
Drug Abuse by the Elderly 155
Drug Addiction 155
Drug and Alcohol Withdrawal 155
Dry Skin. 155
Dyslexia 155

E

Earache, Ear Infection, Ear Pain, Earwax Buildup 160
Eating Disorders 164
Eczema 164
Elbow Pain. 164
Emphysema 165
Encephalitis 165
Endometriosis 165
Epilepsy 166
Erection Problems 166
Erysipelas 166
Eye Floaters 166
Eyestrain 167

F

Facial Paralysis 168
Fainting 169
Fear 169
Fever 172
Fibromyalgia. 172
Finger Injury 173
Flatulence 174

Flu 174
Fluid Retention 175
Food and Drug Interactions 177
Food Poisoning 180
Foot Pain 182
Fractures 183
Frostbite 183

G

Gallstones 185
Gastritis, Gastroenteritis, Giardiasis 186
Glaucoma 190
Glue Ear 191
Gonorrhea 192
Gout 193
Gray Hair 193
Gum Inflammation 193

H

Hair Loss 194
Hallucinations 195
Hand Pain 196
Hangover (see Alcoholism) 197
Hay Fever 197
Headache 198
Hearing Loss 199
Heart Attack 199
Heartburn, Heatstroke 201
Heel Pain 201
Hemorrhoids 202
Hepatitis 203
Hernia 203
Herpes 205

Hiatal Hernia (see Heartburn/Heatstroke) 206
Hiccups 206
High Blood Pressure 206
High Cholesterol 207
Hip Pain 208
Hives 208
Hoarseness and Laryngitis 208
Hodgkin's Disease 209
Hot Flashes 210
Hypoglycemia 211
Hypothermia 214
Hypothyroidism 216

I

Impetigo 217
Impotency 217
Indigestion 219
Infection 220
Infertility 222
Influenza (see Flu) 223
Ingrown Toenails 223
Insect Bites and Stings 224
Insomnia 225
Intestinal Parasites 225
Irritable Bowel Syndrome 226
Irritation 226
Itching 227

J

Jaundice 229
Jet Lag 230
Jock Itch 231

K

Kidney Failure/Kidney Stones 233
Knee Pain 234

L

Labor and Delivery Problems 236
Lactose Intolerance 240
Learning Disabilities 240
Leg Pain 241
Leukemia (also see Cancer) 241
Lice 241
Light Sensitivity 241
Liver Disease 241
Loss of Sexual Interest (also see Erection Problems
    and Impotency) 242
Low Blood Pressure 242
Lupus Erythematosus 242
Lung Cancer (also see Cancer) 242
Lyme Disease 243

M

Macular Degeneration 244
Malaria 245
Manic Depression 245
Measles 246
Melanoma 246
Meningitis 247
Menopause 247
Menstruation Difficulties 248
Mental Illness 249
Mexican-Restaurant Syndrome 250
Migraine 250
Miscarriage 253

Moles 254
Mononucleosis. 254
Mood Changes 255
Motion Sickness 256
Multiple Personalities 256
Multiple Sclerosis 256
Mumps 257
Muscle Cramps 257
Muscle-Tone Loss 257
Muscular Dystrophy 258

N

Nail Problems 259
Nausea 260
Neck Pain 260
Nerve Pain. 261
Nervous Stomach 262
Nervousness. 262
Neuralgia 263
Night Blindness 264
Nosebleeds. 265

O

Osteoarthritis 266
Osteoporosis 267
Overweight 268

P

Paget's Disease. 274
Pain 275
Painful Breathing 275
Painful Intercourse 276

Palsy 277

Pancreatitis 278

Paralysis 278

Parkinson's Disease 279

Peptic Ulcer 280

Pinkeye (see "Conjunctivitis") 281

Pinworms (see "Intestinal Parasites") 281

Pneumonia (see "Common Cold," "Flu,"
  and "'Walking' Pneumonia") 281

Poison-Plant Contact (see "Rash") 281

Poisoning 281

Postnasal Drip 282

Premenstrual Syndrome 283

Prostate Cancer/Prostatitis 285

Psoriasis 285

R

Rabies 288

Rash 289

Red Eyes 291

Respiratory-Distress Syndrome 292

Restless-Legs Syndrome 292

Ringworm 293

S

Sciatica Nerve Pain (see "Pain") 294

Shingles (see "Herpes," "Itching," "Rash,"
  and "Skin Problems") 294

Shock 294

Shortness of Breath 296

Shoulder Pain (see "Pain") 298

Sinus Infection (see "Infection") 298

Skin Cancer (see "Cancer")..................... 298

Smoking.. 298

Snoring 299

Sores 300

Sore Throat 301

Spider Bites (see "Insect Bites and Stings"
and "Poisoning") 302

Sprains (see "Swelling") 302

Stomachache 302

Strep Throat (see "Sore Throat") 302

Stress 302

Stroke 305

Stuffy Nose 306

Sunburn.. 307

Sweating Excessively............................. 308

Swelling.. 309

Syphilis (see "Gonorrhea")....................... 311

T

Tapeworm (see "Intestinal Parasites") 312

Teething.. 312

Tendinitis (see "Swelling") 313

Thumbsucking.................................... 313

Thrush (see "Yeast Infection") 314

Tics and Twitches 314

Toe Pain (see "Gout" and "Pain")................. 315

Tonsillitis (see "Sore Throat").................... 315

Toothache 315

Torn Ligament.................................... 317

Tuberculosis (TB) 319

U

Ulcerative Colitis 321

Ulcers 322

Urinary-Tract Infection (see "Bladder Infection") 323

V

Vaginal Problems 324

Varicose Veins 325

Vomiting. 326

W

"Walking" Pneumonia 327

Warts 328

Wheezing (see "Asthma," "Emphysema," and "Hay Fever") . . . 329

Whooping Cough (see "Cough" and "Infection") 329

Worms (see "Intestinal Parasites") 329

Wounds 330

Wrinkles. 334

Wrist Pain (see Pain) 336

Y

Yawning Excessively 337

Yeast Infection 338

IN TOUCH WITH NATURE'S CURES 339

TESTIMONIALS 345

PRODUCT APPENDIX 350

INDEX 353

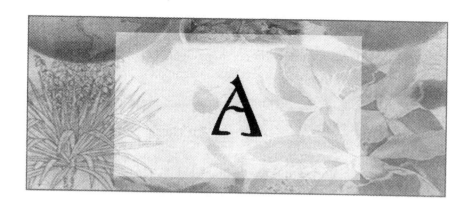

ABSCESSES

A Greek Remedy

Frequently I am in the Big Apple as a speaking guest at different alternative health conventions. One of these, the NewLife Expo, is held regularly several times a year at the Hotel New Yorker adjacent to Penn Station. On the evening of Friday, May 7, 1999, I was part of a five-member Nutritional Panel in the Murray Hill Room of said hotel. A crowd of about 50 or so people had assembled and were waiting for the rest of the panel members to appear.

Since I was early and the only one seated at the head table, several people approached me and said they couldn't find my name or picture listed with the other panelists. One Greek fellow, in particular, declared outright, "If you are not pictured here in the printed program, then why are you up there?"

I politely explained that the Smiley Face depicted in the first black square represented me. I then slid my chair over in front of a mobile blackboard and remarked good-naturedly, "Can't you tell the resemblance?" as I did a mock pose of the drawn Smiley Face. The joke took well and cracked up the other guy. After that, he became warmer, and we chatted amiably until the other panelists arrived about ten minutes later.

He asked me what I did, and I told him that I wrote health books for a living. Whereupon George Papanopoulos (for that was his name) told me the following story.

When he was a boy and lived in Athens he developed a large boil on the back of his neck. He thinks it may have been due to some kind of bacterial infection. It continued to grow, and a pus cavity formed beneath the skin. His mother became alarmed by this development and grew nervous.

But her aged mother, who lived with the family at the time, told her daughter not to worry. George remembers his grandmother seating him on a stool and having him remove his shirt. She then scrubbed the area around the boil with some soap and water. After this, she took a large sewing needle and held it over the open flame of a burning candle for 30 seconds to sterilize it. She then lanced the boil in several places and pressed with her thumbs to push the purulent matter out. After this she poured some vinegar over the area and wiped the skin dry. He never again had a problem with this and grew to manhood free of it.

He said that one of his own sons, a boy Stefan, aged 11, came down with a similar condition just last year. His wife wanted to take their son to the pediatrician, but George tended to the matter himself in the same manner his grandmother had done, with satisfying results.

ABDOMINAL CRAMPS, DISTRESS, AND PAIN

Herbal Relief from the Isle of Crete

This same NewLife Expo in New York City attracted close to 3,000 people in early May of 1999. On Saturday evening, May 8, I stepped into the Central Park Room for a few minutes to listen to a psychic healer by the name of Starr Fuentes. The room was packed to hear this woman speak on such diverse topics as channeling, hands-on healing, psychic readings, and so forth.

After a while I left and was followed by a middle-aged gentleman who asked me if I was Dr. Heinerman. Upon discovering that I was, he said he had several of my health books and was (in his words), "a devoted fan" of mine. In the course of our remarks, he asked what my next book would be and I told him the name of this volume. My mentioning this elicited from him a brief but effective treatment for "any kind of abdominal spasm or pain" that he insisted "really works."

He told me it came from the Isle of Crete, the largest of the Greek islands and the original site of one of the world's earliest great civilizations, the Minoan Civilization, named after King Minos, the presumed author of Cretan institutions. He noted that folk healers in the island's largest city of Iráklion frequently used it for such conditions with good success.

Half of a handful (or the equivalent of one tablespoonful) of poppy seeds, such as those used to sprinkle over poppy-seed bread before it is baked, are crushed in a mortar with a stone pestle. If these aren't available, place the seeds in a zippered plastic bag and then gently crush them with a rolling pin or pound them with a hammer. Next, boil a pint of wine and then pour the seeds into the pan. Cover with a lid, lower the heat, and simmer for several minutes. Then set aside and steep for an additional 20 minutes. Strain and drink one cup of the warm brew.

My informant assured me that this would bring relief to the worst abdominal distress imaginable. But I would hastily add that any such condition as this, if prolonged and excessive and not due to intestinal gas, should be immediately looked at by a doctor, for it may warrant prompt medical attention!

ABRASIONS

Cocklebur Tea

In ancient times abrasions were routinely treated with honey. Modern research shows just how correct the physicians were in using this. Honey has antibacterial properties and doesn't induce allergic reactions, which are always likely with antibiotics.

Early Indian tribes inhabiting the Rocky Mountains of North America had an even better remedy. According to *A History of Box Elder County* (Salt Lake City: Utah State Historical Society, 1999, p. 20) by Frederick M. Huchel, "cocklebur leaves were boiled to a tea" and then used to frequently bathe abrasions with. Also "cocklebur seeds, when crushed, were used as an antiseptic for skin abrasions," the author noted.

Cockleburs are found on such persistent weeds as burdock and yellow dock; the two-seeded oval burrs are especially troublesome to sheep growers and anyone hiking in the wilderness. In fact, the idea for Velcro® came from the cocklebur's knack of attaching itself to clothing.

ACNE

A Blemish-Free Face

An estimated 85 percent of adolescents suffer the heartbreak of "zits," the pimples, blackheads, cysts, and nodules of acne. Acne incidence peaks at around 18 years of age, but many people suffer pimples on the face, chest, and back well into their forties. Acne tends to run in families.

Medical experts have been puzzled for years over the actual cause of acne, but most point to a combination of enlarged oil glands, excess oil, bacteria, and enzymes or hormones. But this is only part of the story. Teens' favorite foods—soft drinks, French fries, greasy burgers, and chocolate of any kind—also produce acne, though doctors won't admit to it. Dermatologists think that poor skin hygiene may also be a contributing factor.

In a rare, long-out-of-print book by Charles A. Eastman entitled *Indian Boyhood* (Garden City, NY: Doubleday, Page & Company, 1911), the author mentioned a number of his boyhood impressions and experiences, up to the age of 15 years, with some Native American tribes. One thing that caught my eye as I read this fascinating account was his remark concerning the "near absence of facial acne among the Indian youth I knew."

His curiosity got the best of him, and he inquired as to the reason for this. His young Indian friends told him that their parents made them wash their faces regularly with a *warm* tea made from sagebrush leaves. Now the most common sagebrush is a silvery-gray low shrub with a pungent odor of sage, although it is unrelated to the actual culinary sage cooks know best. Sagebrush is one of the most common shrubs of the West, where it serves as an important forage plant on many cattle ranges and is usually indicative of good soil.

Eastman related that the young Indians' parents would heat up a large pot of water and then throw in an unspecified amount of sagebrush leaves and twigs and cook them for a while uncovered. The amount needed would then be strained while still warm and their sons and daughters would then wash their faces with this solution morning and evening. He also stated they would drink a little of it as well; Eastman tried some of it and found it to be quite bitter. However, when a little acne started appearing on his own skin, young Eastman resorted to this simple Indian remedy himself and happily discovered that he, too, soon had a blemish-free complexion just like his Indian friends enjoyed *all the time!*

Other "tried-and-true remedies" include wiping his face down several times every day with cotton balls soaked in apple-cider vinegar or making a smooth paste from kaolin or Fuller's earth (available in most pharmacies or health-food stores) by mixing a teaspoon of the clay with enough water and then applying it over the face and letting it set for ten minutes before rinsing off with cold water.

A young or older person afflicted with acne should also try giving his or her face an herbal steam bath. Boil two cups of water with one half cup of either chamomile or fennel. Reduce heat and simmer. Set the pot aside and place your face over the steamy liquid, but not so close as to injure yourself from the heat. Drape a towel over your head to form a tent. Remain in this position for ten minutes before rinsing with cool water.

ADDICTION

A Priest's Confession

Over the years I've had a number of different opportunities to visit the Province of Quebec in eastern Canada. In fact, at one time I was betrothed to a woman named Louise from Sherbrooke, but the marriage never took place because of our sharp differences regarding birth control (she was for it, and I was very much opposed to it).

During one particular trip to Montreal, I visited in the company of a Quebecois friend of mine at the Catholic parochial school, Our Lady of Pompeii Elementary on the city's north side. I can still recall the numerous crucifixes on the wall of every classroom and the statues of the patron saint in the corridors. When the principal entered a classroom with my friend and me, every student would stand and bid us good morning in unison (in French, of course). Twice a week, we were informed, homeroom teachers, all of them good Catholics, set aside multiplication tables and the study of vertebrates and turned their attention to Matthew, Mark, Luke, and John.

Father Jean-Pierre Morin, the priest who then presided over this private parochial school, was an amiable host and quite friendly. We took lunch with him in the school cafeteria and visited in his private office for several hours afterwards. Ever on the prowl for useful and effective remedies, I asked him at some point in our lengthy conversations if he knew of anything on this subject.

The good father folded his hands out of habit (probably from frequent praying) and soberly mused on the subject for a minute or two before responding. "Yes," he finally said with a soft smile, "I have one for you that is very personal and that I know, for a fact, *works!*" He then proceeded to share with us the following story.

"When I was a young man I became addicted to some very bad substances, which I found myself unable of shaking." He wouldn't say what they were. "When I would try to quit them for a few days or even a week, it just seemed as if my body gave in to these wicked appetites and I went right back to using them again.

"About this time I determined to enter the priesthood, take my vows with the church, and live the rest of my life serving God. I went down to the Immaculate Conception Church in the heart of this city and there knelt before statues of the Virgin Mary and Christ and pleaded for their assistance. It seemed as if the Virgin Mother spoke to my mind, for I heard a female voice say ever so quietly in my head, 'Go use catnip and you will be cured of this affliction.'

"To be honest with you, I didn't even know at the time what this was. But upon making some inquiries, I soon learned it was an herb. But I was faced with another dilemma. Even though I knew which herb was right for my problem, I didn't know how to use it. Was I to eat it raw? Was I to make a tea out of it? Was I to soak it in alcohol and use it as a tincture that way? Or were gelatin capsules of the dried powder the way to go?

"I tried each and every possibility and soon discovered that the hot tea was the best course to follow. In about a quart of boiling water I would put one good-sized handful of the cut *fresh* catnip herb and let it simmer for a few minutes before setting it aside to steep a while. I would then pour myself a couple of cups of this brew while it was still quite warm and sip it down whenever the craving came over me for more of these addictive substances.

"I was amazed, quite frankly, at just how well this tea worked. My withdrawal symptoms were nowhere near what they used to be before. I sincerely believe that the good Virgin Mother used this common herb to help me overcome my addiction. I then entered the priesthood, where I've served with honor and distinction ever since," he concluded.

I looked up at him from my note-taking and asked with a smile, "I believe this is the *first* time I've ever heard a priest confess to a commoner and non-Catholic." All three of us enjoyed a hearty laugh following this remark.

AGE SPOTS

Grandpa Walton Knew Better

Some years ago, the late actor Will Greer, who played Grandpa Walton in the television series *The Waltons*, appeared on a late-night TV talk show (probably Johnny Carson's) and informed his host and the viewing audience that the sappy or milky latex from old dandelions or milkweed was a "sure-proof" way of getting rid of age spots. He recommended rubbing some of the white juice on the backs of the hands every day until they faded away.

AGGRESSIVE BEHAVIOR

Solutions from Covered-Wagon Days

Aggressive behavior in measured amounts can be a good thing. It enables individuals to excel in life and achieve what they've previously determined to accomplish. But in excessive amounts, aggression can be an unhealthy thing for a person and certainly quite unpleasant for those exposed to it. And, if left totally unattended, aggressive behavior can lead to dangerous, if not life-threatening situations.

Sometime in the summer of 1998 I happened to be in Canada in Vancouver, British Columbia, on health-related business and took time to visit an antiquarian bookstore near the university campus. Amid my browsing, I found a small but curious and rare piece of Western Americana entitled *The Ox Team or The Old Oregon Trail 1852–1906* published by the author, one Ezra Meeker. Finding an envelope filled with some newspaper clippings and personal writings about the author, I decided to purchase the book for my own large library.

Ezra Meeker was born in Huntsville, Butler County, Ohio (25 miles northeast of Cincinnati), on December 29, 1830, and died at the Frye Hotel in Seattle, Washington, at 4:05 A.M. on the morning of December 3, 1928, being just 26 days shy of his ninety-eighth birthday. The copy of his book I bought was not only inscribed by him, but also must have belonged to a journalist at one time, for a number of press clippings and handwritten reporter's notes concerning this old gentleman came with it. These additional materials together with the book itself helped to flush out more of Meeker's illustrious pioneer career.

The subject of aggressive behavior first surfaced in Ezra's early schoolboy days, "of which I had so few. I was certainly not five years old when a drunken, brutal school teacher undertook to spank me while holding me on his knees because I did not speak a word plainly. That was the first fight I have any recollection of, and hardly know whether I remember that but for the witnesses, one of them my oldest brother, who saw the struggle, where my teeth did such excellent work as to draw blood quite freely. What a spectacle that, of a half drunken teacher maltreating his scholars! But then that was a time before a free school system. . . ." In the reporter Richard G. Baldwin's notes, Meeker mentioned what happened after that. "I went home mad as a wet hen and vowed I'd never go back to school again. But my mother, a reasonable and easy-going woman, sat me down and told me that I should let this thing pass and get over my anger of it. She then proceeded to sing me several lullabyes, which had the desired effect of calming my feisty young soul down a great deal." So, *soothing music* is one way of curbing aggressive behavior.

The next method that Ezra successfully employed when a bit older involved fanciful imagination at times when "my boyish anger tended to boil over" on account of working with oxen. He was then seven years of age and walked most of the way from Ohio to Indiana behind the family's covered wagon, where he soon learned the delicate "art of driving four yoke of oxen to a breaking plow, without swearing." Hardly anyone today is acquainted with oxen or know something of their temperament, but they sometimes tend to have "a mind of their own" and can be even *more* stubborn than the worst mules!

So, it was common in his time to find men who worked with oxen a lot habitually swear at their cattle, whip them mercilessly on occasion, and then curse them to high heaven some more if these animals didn't obey their wishes. He tells of an experience one time near Bridgeport, Indiana, where he happened to be hauling a heavy cider-press beam to the home of an ardent Quaker with the assistance of three yoke of oxen. The cattle refused to go through the front gate, but "kept doubling back, first on one side and then on the other." But the youthful Ezra kept his cool and continued working with them until they finally went through the front gate as desired.

The ardent Quaker, "a good old soul named Uncle John Kinworthy, noticed I did not swear at the cattle . . . like a good many others; he thought oxen could not be driven without swearing at them. But I told him all it took was some patience. Out of curiosity he then asked me how I came by so much of this virtue when most other men couldn't. I told him that whenever oxen made me frustrated or angry, I would simply begin building 'castles in the air' and let my mind wander off into a little harmless fantasy. I found that this stayed my anger and then I was better equipped to deal more kindly with my animals and help them overcome their periodic stubbornness." Thus, a little *mental diversion* for a few minutes away from the cause of sudden aggression seems to be helpful in coping with vexing problems with a clearer head.

On the dietary front, Ezra wrote in his book that cornmeal mush and whole, raw milk "kept my attitude right and feelings pretty sound most of the time." "Our diet was so simple, the mere relation may create a smile with the casual reader. The mush pot was a great factor in our home life; a great heavy iron pot that hung on the crane in the chimney corner where the mush would slowly bubble and splutter over or near a bed of oak coals for half the afternoon. And such mush it was, ever nourishing and tasty, and always made from yellow corn meal and cooked three hours or more. This, eaten with plenty of fresh, rich milk, and some cheap molasses comprised the supper for our family.

"Sugar? It was too expensive—cost fifteen to eighteen cents a pound. Meat was pretty scarce too, but we had eggs in abundance." It is interesting to observe that in his later remarks made to reporter Baldwin, Meeker stated that "sugar is bad for you . . . made me feel kind of crazy the few times I used it so I left it alone after that." He also seldom ate much meat in his life, undoubtedly stemming from the scarcity of it in his early childhood.

Some of Meeker's little-known dietary philosophy has since received scientific validation. The information is equally divided between three classic works: Michio Kushi's *Crime & Diet* (New York: Japan Publications, Inc., 1987); Richard J. and Judith J. Wurtman's *Physiological & Behavioral Effects of Food Constituents* (Chicago: Raven Press, 1983); and Judith Wurtman's *Managing Your Mind and Mood Through Food* (Lebanon, NH: HarperCollins, 1988).

This trio of books examine the food–mood connection in depth. Abundant proof is given to show that when red meat and sugar are severely curtailed and replaced instead with cereal grains, dairy products, eggs, and fresh fruits and vegetables, aggressive behavior virtually disappears overnight. The work of former probation officer Barbara Reed in Cuyahoga Falls, Ohio, and social researcher Alexander Schauss at the Morris County Jail Rehabilitation Center in New Jersey are profiled, among other things. They were some of the first ones to show that when probationers or inmates were given better food to eat, they behaved in a totally different, more responsible and mature way. Thus, Meeker's suggestion that *wholesome foods* contribute to *less* aggression makes perfect sense today. Ironically, he never said anything about coffee, though, which if moderately used shouldn't promote aggressive behavior.

Dealing with Adult Anger

Ezra had a few more things to say about aggressive behavior when he turned 77. The year was 1907, and he challenged the attention of our nation to the cause of reblazing the old Oregon Trail by retracing this historic highway from the Pacific Northwest to the Mississippi with ox team and prairie schooner, of all things! But wait . . . there's MORE! After reaching the "Mighty Mississippi," he figured, "Why stop here?" and continued over the National Pike and the Mohawk Trail and into—are you ready for this?—the throbbing heart of the Big Apple itself. There he was stuck in the middle of a big traffic jam on Wall Street with his plodding oxen and covered wagon.

It took half of the police force to extricate him from that terrible situation. Street-car operators and vintage-car and truck drivers were understandably angry with him. The police chief was so upset at Meeker he had him promptly arrested once the traffic snarl was unraveled. But newspaper reporters all over the city, smelling a front-page story of considerable human interest, quickly came to his rescue, and Mayor Mitchell had no choice but to give the old geezer his freedom.

Upon his release, when questioned at length concerning his overnight incarceration by a battery of eager reporters, he truthfully stated, "Of course, I was angry; wouldn't you be if you were falsely arrested?" But then he went on to tell them this: "After sitting in my cell for a little while, I began reflecting on my unhappy circumstances. And decided to not let these things get the best of me. I went over to the barred window of my cell and started to breathe in some air from the outside. I did this very slowly and then let it out the same way. I stayed with this for some time until I was relaxed. I learned this technique from an old Cheyenne medicine man, who taught it to me many years before. He said the Great Spirit was in the air and that if a man in anger would just spend some time breathing deeply in and out, enough of the Great Spirit would come into your body to drive all of the anger out. I believe he was right."

Ezra also admitted that he found ample time to "build myself more 'castles in the air' while sitting in the city pokey." So *deep-breathing exercises* and some fanciful meditation of sorts helped this elderly gentleman to get over his hostility and accept the surroundings until set free a short time later.

Nutritional Assistance

There are some nutrients that can be helpful in restoring composure to an agitated state of mind. Vitamins A, B-complex, C, and E offer positive nutritional support to brain, nerves, heart, adrenal glands, and other organs that have been whipped into an agitated frenzy. But rather than taking these nutrients individually it is best to take them in a balanced formula, such as the Total Care nutritional packet offered by Earth's Pharmacy. The company also makes a wonderful herbal blend called Repose that helps to restore harmony to a body put out of sync with anger and aggression. (See Product Appendix for more information.)

Sipping warm herbal teas such as chamomile, hops, lavender, or peppermint are equally useful.

AIDS
(See "CANCER")

AIRPLANE EARS

The Flight from Hell

I have logged nearly *one million* miles in the air in some 27 years of worldwide travel. Just about all of those flights have been tolerably comfortable. Only a few were what I would consider to have been extremely miserable. I've always characterized them as my "flights from hell." The flight attendants, pilots, and fellow passengers have nothing whatsoever to do with them. I alone have been responsible for each of these dreaded trips.

They invariably come about those few times in my life that I've caught a bad head cold and its accompanying middle-ear infection. Anyone who's experienced this will know exactly what I'm writing about. Rapid changes in aircraft-cabin pressure cause immediate middle-ear pain, which is excruciating. Sometimes it can reach the point where you feel as if you're about to faint from the sheer agony of the ordeal.

But some years ago when I was in Cairo, Egypt, on folk-medicine-research business, I learned a nifty trick from one Mohammed Al-Azawar, a purveyor of fine Persian rugs. He told me something rather remarkable, which went beyond the conventional swallowing, yawning, gum chewing, or nose blowing with mouth closed that probably everyone knows about. My friend said that whenever he had to fly somewhere on carpet business and had a nasty cold, he would take along some eucalyptus cough drops *and* a small bottle of eucalyptus oil, together with some sticks of cinnamon chewing gum.

He would commence sucking on a couple of these eucalyptus drops at least one hour *before* take-off to give it time to work. Then just *before* the plane was due to actually take off, he would remove from his coat pocket the eucalyptus oil and unwrap a stick of chewing gum. He would then carefully apply *only* one drop at each end of the gum, and then insert it into his mouth and begin chewing, after carefully putting the bottle of herbal oil away. He warned me to *never use* more than two drops of the oil at any time on a stick of gum, owing to the extreme potency of the oil itself. He said that as the plane gradually climbed higher into the air, his pace of chewing would similarly increase. He claimed that by doing this a person would hardly feel any pain.

Well, there have been a few occasions since then when I've had the chance to put this simple method into practice. And I can personally vouch for its surprisingly quick efficacy within a matter of minutes following take-off or landing.

ALCOHOLIC HANGOVER

Some Russian Cures

Years ago, when the Soviet empire was still intact and before all of the democracy nonsense set in to now make conditions much worse in the Russian Republic, I had an opportunity to visit there in the summer of 1979 with a group of other specially invited doctors and scientists to learn more about their culture and their antiquated health-care system.

Alcoholism was a problem then and since has mushroomed into an epidemic of enormous proportions. Several *babuska* (grandmother) remedies for treating a full-blown hangover have proven effective for those who've tried them.

1. Get plenty of rest.
2. Drink warm willow-bark tea (2 cups) or take willow-bark capsules with plenty of water (3 capsules with an 8-ounce glass).
3. Place some ice cubes in a plastic bag, then wrap the bag in clean cloth and apply to the forehead for 30 minutes, then remove it for 15 minutes before reapplying.
4. Drink several cups of *warm* mint tea to which has been added a pinch of powdered ginger root *or* cayenne pepper (but not both).
5. In an 8-ounce glass of *hot* water add 2 tablespoons of honey and a pinch of black pepper. Stir and slowly sip through a plastic straw. You'll be astonished at just how well this works!

ALLERGIES

Let's Cut to the Chase

Numerous books and articles have been written about allergies over the years. Those suffering from allergies of some kind typically have to wade through many pages of personal philosophy, nutritional counseling, and medical jargon to find out what they can do for themselves. So, for the sake of brevity and out of respect for my readers, I'll disperse with all of that and just "cut to the chase," as they say.

European Allergy Recovery Program

Note: Follow this regime for one week and see if you don't feel 100 percent better!

A. Eliminate ALL foods containing white sugar or white flour from the diet—NO EXCEPTIONS!

B. Drink only mineral or spring water plus permitted fruit juices.

C. These fruits are permitted and can be consumed whole or juiced in a Vita-Mix food preparation unit (see Product Appendix): apples (only organic), apricots, bananas, berries (organic), cantaloupe, cherries (organic), coconuts, figs, grapes (only organic), kiwis, mangos, papayas, peaches, pears, persimmons, plus (organic), pomegranates.

D. These vegetables are permitted and may be consumed raw (where advantageous to do so), lightly cooked (preferably steamed or baked), or juiced (if feasible): artichokes, asparagus, avocados, beet greens, beets, broccoli, Brussels sprouts, cabbage, carrots, cauliflower, celery, collard greens, cucumbers, kale, mustard greens, okra, olives, parsley, parsnips, pumpkins, radishes, rutabaga, spinach, squashes, sweet potatoes, turnips, and watercress. (*Note:* Try to use organic vegetables wherever possible; wash and peel those that are nonorganic.)

E. Stay away from dairy products (milk, butter, and cheese), ALL soy foods, eggs, and wheat (including wheat grass).

F. Protein needs should come from the following acceptable meat, fish, nuts, and seeds: almonds, Brazil nuts, butternuts, cashews, chestnuts, deer, duck, filberts, game hen, goose, hazelnuts, hickory nuts, lamb, macadamia nuts, pheasant, pistachios, pumpkin seeds, quail, rabbit, sesame seeds, sunflower seeds, tahini, water chestnuts, and water-packed fish (mackerel, tuna, salmon, sardines). (*Note:* Nuts should be eaten raw and not cooked. Meat and fish can be seasoned with powdered kelp, a seaweed, and some sea salt. And if used moderately, neither should upset blood-pressure levels in those suffering from hypertension.)

G. These additional things may also be fully utilized without a problem: bay leaves, buckwheat kasha, buckwheat grits, buckwheat groats, caraway, celery seed, cumin, dill, millet, and vinegar (apple cider, pear, or plum; absolutely NO white vinegar).

H. Stay away from ALL condiments: catsup, mustard, pickles, and mayonnaise.

I. Have NOTHING fried or deep-fried.

J. At the conclusion of this one-week program, your symptoms will most likely have disappeared. If a few still linger, you may wish to carry this program over into a second week. By then, all of them should have disappeared for good.

K. After this, slowly start adding back some of your former foods to the diet, but ONLY ONE FOOD EVERY OTHER DAY! Give strict heed to how you feel toward each newly introduced item. Write in a daily food diary any symptoms and the items responsible for such.

L. Try adding back foods only in their most basic form. For instance, when adding wheat, begin with shredded-wheat cereal (but only with goat's milk) rather than with bread. When adding eggs, try eating hard-boiled.

M. Midway during this one-week European Allergy Recovery Program, elect to take an enema or colonic to really clean out your intestines!

There is no real mystery or magic to this plan. It is simple and highly effective when faithfully adhered to. Some determination, of course, on your part is needed in order to make this work effectively. But I *guarantee* that you will feel *a lot better* than you did before, even if some minor allergic symptoms linger and require a second-week continuance of the same regimen. The nice thing is that you don't even need a physician to follow it, although you should feel free to consult one for your own peace of mind if that proves necessary.

Bear in mind that this program is in some part an experimentation on yourself and your body. You're the proverbial laboratory guinea pig in such a thing and will obviously meet with some expected frustrations along the way. But the overall program is quite sound. I spent many years canvassing Europe in search of the best natural-treatment advice for allergies from holistic-minded doctors. Some of the information came from the United Kingdom countries, while other portions of the data originated by way of France, Belgium, Luxembourg, Switzerland, Germany, and the Netherlands.

The only individuals who may wish to have their physical conditions monitored by doctors while on this program would be pregnant women, those with respiratory diseases, and individuals with long histories of blood-sugar problems (hypoglycemia). Also, anyone experiencing anaphylactic shock MUST GO TO A HOSPITAL EMERGENCY ROOM IMMEDIATELY, as such an allergic reaction can definitely be life-threatening.

Now, some readers may wonder where all the nutritional-supplement suggestions are. Well, I have a piece of surprising news for them: There aren't any in this section! As strange as it may seem, NONE of my European informants recommended so much as a vitamin pill or mineral tablet. In fact, if one has been around Europe long enough, as I've been, that person will quickly find out that attitudes regarding health-food supplements are different over there from what they are here in America. Europeans aren't in the habit of supplementing themselves very much nor are their doctors so likely to recommend it. For these reasons, data on such are noticeably absent.

ALZHEIMER'S DISEASE

A German Named It

In 1907 a German neurologist named Alois Alzheimer, M.D., gave senility a new, more clinical-sounding name—Alzheimer's disease—and we've been seeing more of it ever since. It affects an estimated 15 percent of the U.S. population over age 65 and about 50 percent of those older than 85. And now it costs America about $100 billion in annual medical care.

But doctors still wrestle with the diagnostic dilemma of whether this is a disease or merely an unfortunate function of aging itself. For the most part, physicians still don't know which it may be. However, they do talk about age-associated cognitive decline, a mild dwindling of mental abilities that presumably accompanies aging. Medical statistics indicate that this condition of cognitive decline converts into Alzheimer's at the rate of about 15 percent of cases per year and within the span of about two years.

Help for Victims of AD

For many families with victims of Alzheimer's disease (AD), it seems almost as if the end of their perfect and tidy little world has arrived. The psychological impact is usually more profound on family members than it is on AD sufferers themselves. However, there need not be feelings of despair, for AD can be successfully managed *without drugs* and AD victims can be returned to a reasonably normal life in many instances.

A number of important European studies point to food therapy, folk medicine, and megavitamin supplementation as being highly effective in reversing some or much of the dementia that this dreaded geriatric disease induces in many elderly people. Also a startling report from an American dentist may offer additional preventive assistance to many *potential* AD victims.

The Wine Is Always Better in France

Medical statistics show that the people of France have very low incidence of AD as compared with surrounding nations. Until recently no one could explain a logical reason for this medical phenomena. However, according to a report from the University of Bordeaux that was published in the *British Medical Journal* (314:997) in 1997, wine may be the answer. Researchers there discovered that people who drink wine are five times more likely than others to develop AD. They tracked almost 4,000 men and women over age 65 for a three-year period, during which AD developed in 0.9 percent of moderate drinkers as compared with 4.9 percent of nondrinkers. Surprisingly, those who drank heavily were even more likely to develop AD (5.1 percent) than were the nondrinkers.

These findings strongly suggest that wine drinking protects people from AD, but only when taken in moderation.

Something Fishy Here

As men and women become older they may want to think about increasing their intake of fresh- and saltwater fish. It may just be the critical key to keeping them from losing their minds and memories. At least that's what research out of two Scandinavian countries and the Netherlands suggests.

Medical researchers have been aware of the fact that Finland and Sweden have much lower AD-prevalence rates than do England and Italy. But until just a short while back no one really knew what to attribute the difference to. It now turns out that the fish consumption that Scandinavia is famous for separates the brilliant from the less than memorable. Scientists believe that the omega 3-6-9 fatty acids common to fish prevent the brain tangling and significant neural loss typically found in aged brains.

A similar study conducted in Rotterdam in the Netherlands found additional support for the "fish theory"; it appears in the *Annals of Neurology* (42:776–82; 1997). All 10,275 residents of that Dutch city over the age of 55 were invited to participate, and 7,983 agreed to do so, with 5,386 completing their dietary surveys properly. Follow-up surveys found that 58 of the subjects became demented during the approximately 2.1-year interval. Those who did become demented were found to have a caloric intake 6.2 percent higher than controls, 4.7 percent greater fat intake, and 31 percent less fish intake. The risk ratios calculated were as follows: 2.4 for total fat, 1.9 for saturated fat, and 0.4 for fish. Clearly, fish is an extremely significant dietary factor in the prevention of AD in those past middle-age.

A Case for Megavitamin Therapy

The following true-life medical case was contributed by Abram Hoffer, M.D., to the June 1998 edition of the *Townsend Letter for Doctors & Patients*. Dr. Hoffer practices orthomolecular medicine in Victoria, British Columbia, Canada, and is one of the pioneers in the use of megavitamin therapy for the treatment and prevention of many major illnesses.

A 76-year-old female patient whom he identifies only as Mrs. S. was brought to his clinic by her husband because he was really "worried about her failing memory and poor balance." Dr. Hoffer notes in his medical report the following symptoms suggestive of AD: "Her memory was very poor especially for recent events, she was confused, and her concentration was greatly diminished. She was not depressed but she was tired and napped four hours or more each day."

He put her on niacin 500 mg. TID (medical Latin for *ter in die* or three times a day), vitamin C 500 mg. TID, and folic acid 5 mg. daily. "Ten months after I first saw her," he writes, "she was perhaps 10% better. She was more alert . . . She had gained four pounds and her balance was better. In addition, she was more sociable." One year after her initial visit "she was brighter, needed less sleep, and had again started doing her crossword puzzles," a previous favorite pastime. Dr. Hoffer then added thiamine 500 mg. TID to her program.

At 21 months, he added the herb ginkgo biloba, 40 mg. TID, and reports the following: "After two years she was significantly better. She was able to help her husband with crossword puzzles [and] participated more in conversation. For the first time since I had seen her I was able to talk to her, and she was able to respond without turning to her husband for his response."

Is Ginkgo Biloba Good for AD?

German scientists have been in the forefront of using natural substances for treating serious diseases. Based on empirical folklore associated with the herb ginkgo biloba for improved mental clarity and function, German doctors decided to put this old wives' tale to the test. In one significant study published in *Pharmacopsychiatry* (29:47–56; 1996) it is shown that a special concentrated extract of ginkgo biloba was, indeed, of some definite benefit in outpatients suffering from mild to moderate primary degenerative dementia of the Alzheimer type or multiinfact dementia. A follow-up study published in the *Journal of the American Medical Association* a year later had similar results.

Several German scientific monographs have confirmed a number of pharmacological actions for a standardized extract of ginkgo biloba leaves that seem to be useful in the management of AD. These include:

- Improving the ability of tissues, especially brain tissues, to withstand insufficient oxygen
- Inhibiting the development of a traumatically or toxically produced brain swelling and acceleration of decongestion
- Increasing memory performance and learning capacity
- Improving compensation of disturbed equilibrium due to impaired blood flow to the brain and inner ear
- Improving circulatory flow, particularly in the small vessels
- Inactivating toxic oxygen radicals (i.e., it's a good free radical scavenger)
- Producing a general neuroprotective effect

Consumers should be aware, however, that not all ginkgo biloba products are the same; many, in fact, are pretty worthless. Look for those that have the words "standardized extract" somewhere on the label. A Utah company, Earth's Pharmacy, has an excellent ginkgo biloba extract of superior quality, as well as several other natural products (Intellect and Memorzine) for plugging in a person's brain power and helping the individual to mentally focus better (see Product Appendix for more information).

Can Mercury Fillings Contribute to Alzheimer's?

Mercury that oozes from dental fillings and is assimilated into the body can produce symptoms similar to those associated with AD. According to patient studies in America, Canada, and Sweden, these symptoms may include a surly disposition, depression, loss of energy and stamina, lack of mental focus, and some memory loss.

Some interesting research from Hal Huggins, D.D.S., of Colorado Springs, Colorado, suggests that once even minute amounts of mercury enter the brain, this can seriously damage nerve cells and produce the physical and structural damage of brain tissue now linked with AD. Brain biochemistry is extremely complex. However, mercury damages a key substance needed for the brain's energy processes called creatine kinase. This is an enzyme (made from proteins) that accelerates chemical reactions involving energy release. Autopsies show that the brain of a healthy person contains a whopping 2,300 percent *more* creatine kinase than the brain of a person with AD.

In a recent Canadian study, rats were made to inhale a small amount of mercury vapor (comparable to that emitted by dental fillings, over time, in a human mouth) for four hours each day. After 14 days, their brains had formed the same neurofibrillary tangles so common to Alzheimer brains. Dr. Huggins believes that "the result of this process is the eventual loss of brain cells and brain function."

In one incredible case, he managed to reverse AD in a 50-year-old female patient who had three mercury fillings and a nickel hip replacement (prosthesis). At the time of treatment, she had been completely incommunicative with the external world. "She could handle the fillings," he reported, and even the prosthesis, but *not* both at the same time. The two together literally shoved her over into a classic Alzheimer's situation. When he removed the mercury fillings and detoxified the patient's body of all residual mercury, her Alzheimer's symptoms receded and she resumed normal talking and living again.

The reader should be cautioned, however, with regard to the removal of his or her own amalgam fillings. Sometimes, the old adage of "letting sleeping dogs lay," or in this case keeping old fillings in place, may be applicable here. Not everyone who has been subjected to amalgam fillings in past years is going to contract AD. In fact, my own father, Jacob Heinerman, who still retains some very old mercury fillings at the age of 86, has never once exhibited *any* signs of mental erosion. His mind is, to borrow an old phrase, "sharp as a tack"!

So what's going on here anyway? Simply this: Not everyone appears to react to mercury leakage in the same way. Believe it or not, a great deal depends upon your diet. My father, for example, is very careful in what he eats. His relatively limited diet (on account of borderline noninsulin-dependent diabetes and hypoglycemia) consists of cereal grains (cooked oatmeal and shredded wheat), soy milk, wholegrain bread, some meat and vegetables (usually in a stew), lots of avocados (he loves them and can't seem to get enough), tomato or V-8 (low-sodium) juice, raw nuts (shelled, of course), some fish (either baked or canned), baked and cooked squash (when in season), and very little fresh fruit (due to the natural sugars). This relatively simple diet, I feel, enables his system to adequately cope with mercury leaching so that it doesn't cross the blood–brain barrier where it could cause significant damage.

On the other hand, I know of several personal cases where older individuals experiencing unexplained memory loss and mood swings, acting on my advice, had their mercury fillings removed and reported afterwards "a return to normal" in their cognitive functions and general behavior. Before you elect to undertake such a procedure, discuss your concerns with your family dentist and certainly get a second or even a third opinion from someone who practices holistic dentistry.

Folic Acid Staves Off Dementia

In 1999 roughly four million Americans suffered from Alzheimer's disease. But many of them may have more than just their lucky stars to thank with regard to the discovery of the B-vitamin folate as a strong preventive against this degenerative brain disorder.

Accolades should go to epidemiologist David Snowdon of the University of Kentucky and a group of Roman Catholic nuns, the School Sisters of Notre Dame. Snowdon has been studying AD for quite a while now. And the nuns cheerfully volunteered to give their bodies—and, after death, their brains—to medical science to assist him in his research.

The nuns and their carefully preserved brains have proven to be an Alzheimer's treasure trove for scientists such as Snowdon. From it, he has already discovered that tiny strokes may be the switch that flips a mildly deteriorating brain into full-fledged dementia, as well as noting that the density of ideas expressed in the writings of a 20-year-old novice could be, for still unexplained reasons, a predictor of AD at age 80.

In 1998 Snowdon discovered that those nuns who had the highest blood-serum levels of folic acid also had the *least* amount of brain atrophy (this observation being made through autopsies after some of them died of old age). I briefly spoke with Dr. Snowdon by phone recently and he insisted that his evidence for folate delaying the onset of AD was "sound and good science, too!"

Folic acid controls the amino acid homocysteine, which has already been implicated in a broad range of diseases, as well as in certain neurological birth defects: heart disease and stroke, cancer, and spina bifida. A daily dose of 800 mcg. is recommended for the average person. Folic acid is found in dark leafy greens, such as romaine lettuce, parsley, spinach, turnip greens, mustard greens, beet greens, and Swiss chard, as well as in liver and legumes.

AMEBIASIS
(See "DIARRHEA")

ANAL BLEEDING, BURNING, ITCHING, AND PAIN

Training Bees to Find Land Mines

Several times a year I visit some of my Hutterite friends at different colonies located near Great Falls and Harlowton in Montana. In April 1999 I took such a "spiritual vacation" to get away from everything and give my soul a badly needed rest from the materialism of this world. (The Hutterites are Anabaptist in belief just as are the Amish and Mennonites, but live in communal orders that the former do not. The Hutterites live separate from the world and have no radios, televisions, videos, audiotapes, newspapers, magazines, or books that the rest of us have easy access to.)

While traveling some distance between two different colonies, I chanced to meet up with an entomologist (insect scientist) who was doing an unlikely piece of research: seeing if bees can be trained to find land mines! As nutty as it sounds, there is a great deal of scientific logic behind it. Here's how the idea works: Bees are always charged with static electricity. As such, their little bodies are like flying dust mops, picking up bits of dust, pollen, and other particles and bringing them home to the hive. Chemicals from buried land mines tend to leak into the soil and ground water after a while. They are soaked up by plant roots and then distributed elsewhere in stems and flowers.

Bees are capable of detecting such chemical odors and with some patience and perseverance can be programmed by scientists to seek out and smell for those particular chemicals common to land mines. Upon their return to a specifically located hive, researchers can then analyze the dust and flower pollens brought back for chemical content. As my informant told me, "Bees are incredibly powerful tools for seeking out and finding things." In fact, they could be the insect equivalent of the miner's canary and the king's food taster.

Witch Hazel for Anal Discomforts

After listening to his fascinating discourse on bee recruitment for land-mine locations, I made a few comments that shifted the course of our conversation more into the health realm. I started taking notes when he volunteered his own simple remedy for anal discomforts. But as soon as he saw me start to write, he paused and asked that neither his name, college affiliation, nor community of residence be identified, which I hastily agreed to do.

He admitted that for some years he had been bothered with anal bleeding, itching, burning, and pain at different times, but never thought to attribute it to diet. I raised the point that his affection for catsup, mustard, mayonnaise, black pepper, hot dogs, pickles and pickle relish, baloney, ham, and potato chips probably had quite a bit to do with it. He shrugged his shoulders in a "could-be,-but-don't-care" sort of manner and continued talking.

This entomologist said that the best relief he ever found for these problems was available in any drugstore or supermarket pharmacy section. It is tincture of witch hazel and "does a first-rate job" of stopping anal bleeding and greatly relieving any burning or itching sensation. What he would usually do is to lightly soak four or five cotton balls with some tincture of witch hazel, gently press out any excess liquid, and then insert them into his rectum one by one and leave them there for a while. "This remedy has never failed to relieve the pain," he swore with a profanity for emphasis.

ANEMIA

"O Give Me a Home, Where the T. rex Roams . . ."

South Dakota's badlands is an area so rich in *Tyrannosaurus rex* fossils that some paleontologists (dinosaur hunters) happily forget themselves in moments of joyful discoveries and are apt to sing instead the revised words "where the T. rex roams" to the all-familiar tune of "O Give Me a Home."

In August 1990 a field paleontologist for the Black Hills Institute of Geological Research uncovered the largest flesh-eating dinosaur skeleton of this particular species on the eroded badlands of the Cheyenne River Indian Reservation north of Faith, South Dakota. The fossil was found on land ranched by Maurice Williams, who is a member of the Cheyenne River Sioux. At more than 40 feet long, standing some 13 feet tall at the hip, and with an estimated live weight of somewhere between 6 to 8 tons, Sue (as it was aptly named) turned out to be one very B-I-G carnivore with an equally huge appetite to match.

But while Sue lived in the age of dinosaurs some 67 million years ago, its fossilized remains were unearthed during the nasty epoch of lawyers. (Remember the nice touch that Steven Spielberg gave his thrilling film *Jurassic Park*, in which a rampaging T. rex swallows whole in one gulp a trembling lawyer sitting on a toilet in a demolished public restroom with his pants down around his legs and begging pitifully for his life—"*Please* don't eat me!"). Convoluted custody battles ensued as to who really owned this dino's remains. Eventually, the Indian tribe and particularly Williams won out and a U.S. District Court ruled that Sue could be sold. In 1996 Sotheby's auction gallery in New York City acquired this gigantic fossil and had it inventoried, photographed, and catalogued before a gaggle of potential Sue buyers came forward.

When the sale began—with Sue's partly prepared skull placed near the auctioneer's podium for inspiration—a fierce bidding war, almost as vicious as Sue must have been in real life, commenced. The opening price was $500,000, then climbed to $1.2 million in seconds. At $5.3 million the renowned Field Museum in Chicago joined the chase and eventually outbid everyone else to get Sue at $7.6 million ($8.3 million with Sotheby's usual commission).

Where the Iron Is

Besides knowing where other T. rex fossils might be buried, Williams is pretty savvy at knowing where good sources for mineral iron are located. "See that plant over there," he said, pointing to a lone stinging nettle. "Well, that has more iron in it than anything you'd find in a drugstore," he snorted with disdain. "And see this little feller over here," he continued, digging his boot tip into the ground to uproot a pair of dandelions. "Just as much here as in that over there." We walked a little ways further before pausing near some yarrow. "And that right there," he said with deliberate spitting action, "is just as good for iron needs as them other two back yonder."

Williams doesn't consider himself an herbalist by a long shot, let alone lay any claim to being a shaman. "I leave those things up to the women," he confided. "I'm better at ranching than doctoring any day." But his grandmother, mother, and wife have used all three of these herbs for treating anemia in their families and among other tribal friends and relatives.

Nettle leaves and the tops and leaves of dandelion and yarrow are used in different forms at various times, but always for the same problem of iron-deficiency anemia. Sometimes the fresh flowers and leaves may be picked in the spring, lightly boiled, and then served as a cooked side dish or else mixed with a little vinegar and oil and eaten as salad greens. The herbs may also be juiced in a Vita-Mix with a little water added, but Williams and his people aren't into that method of preparation at all.

A respectable amount of iron is also present in the dried powders of each of these herbs. And it is possible to mix equal parts of all three together in a dish and then fill empty 00-size gelatin capsules and take them that way—four capsules daily with a meal. All of these are fairly common herbs and can be found in a number of places, such as fields, pastures, parks, lawns, backyards, woods, and even waste places. When gathering, be sure they haven't been previously sprayed with weed killers of some kind. Health-food stores will have them available in the bulk powders or individual capsules.

ANEURYSM

What Is It?

An aneurysm is a weak spot in the wall of the aorta, the primary artery that carries blood from the heart to the head and extremities. There are three common types: Two of them are balloonlike swellings of the arterial wall that can occur in the portion of the aorta within the chest or, more frequently, just below the kidney in the abdomen; the third is a longitudinal, blood-filled split in the lining of the artery, usually happening in the aortic arch near the heart.

Almost 95 percent of aneurysms are brought about by hardening of the arteries due to the buildup of fatty plaque. Hypertension intensifies the force of blood on the walls of the arteries and contributes to the development of aneurysms.

What to Look For

In most cases, there are no direct warning signals for an impending aneurysm; only an X-ray during a routine physical exam can pick it up.

Sometimes hoarseness, difficulty in swallowing, or persistent coughing may indicate the presence of an aneurysm in the chest area.

A throbbing lump in the abdominal area, severe backache, leg pain or a feeling of coldness in the leg, or severe abdominal pain could mean an aneurysm is in the abdominal area.

Severe chest pain that could be mistaken for a heart attack may signal the presence of an aneurysm.

What to Do

Prevention is the first key, by all means. Watch your cholesterol and triglyceride levels at all times. Remember that eating a low-cholesterol diet isn't everything—the body also produces its own cholesterol and could, therefore, be contributing to a higher reading irrespective of what you're eating. In that event, eat more garlic and onion or take Kyolic garlic (three capsules daily). Also, supplement your diet with more ginger and cayenne pepper in food form or capsules (one of each daily with a meal).

Keep a sharp watch on your blood pressure and take prompt action to treat it naturally if it commences to rise at all. Potassium is the real key here to keeping it down. The highest foods containing this mineral are powdered cocoa and carob, which can be made into delicious beverages; one tablespoon of either in a glass of soy or goat's milk will yield about 1,500 mgs. of potassium. Other high food sources include apricots, avocado, banana, blackstrap molasses, brown rice, dried fruit, garlic, nuts, onions, potatoes, wheat bran, winter squash, and yams. Medium food sources for potassium are beef liver (baked), beans and lentils, carrots, celery, green snap beans, and hard-boiled eggs.

Magnesium is another mineral you should be looking at to take for the prevention/treatment of an aneurysm. Food sources rich in this mineral consist of dairy products, fish, red meat, seafood, apples, apricots, avocado, banana, black-eyed peas, cantaloupe, leafy green vegetables, lentils, lima beans, millet, various nuts, seaweeds, sunflower and sesame seeds, watercress, wheat, millet, rye, and oats (in the form of cooked oatmeal).

Supplementation of both minerals may also be necessary. An average daily intake of 1,400 mgs. potassium and 800 mgs. magnesium is ideal for this.

ANGINA

Frederick's Story

Frederick Wilhelm, aged 57, is a very successful German banker in the city of Düsseldorf. He started experiencing recurrent chest pains that radiated down into his left arm. He consulted a medical herbalist in his city, who prescribed some things for him. Each morning he would take a ten-minute walk, then skip rope for five minutes. He would take 15 drops of fluid extract of hawthorn berry twice daily. He reduced his business stress by learning to meditate for ten minutes every two hours. He took up gardening as a hobby in the summer and volunteered to do youth counseling for troubled teens in the winter.

He started eating more root vegetables such as carrots, parsnips, potatoes, radishes, and turnips. He eliminated all sausage and other fatty meats from his diet and instead started eating more fish, rabbit, and deer. He cut out most alcohol except for a bottle of dark Löwenbrau (a brand of German beer) or dark ale (made from herbs and plant roots) every other day.

And instead of two or three big meals a day, he switched to four or five lighter ones spread across the day, making sure his last two contained no heavy foods. Instead of *fressen wie ein Vieh* ("eating like a beast"), he took up to 45 minutes for some meals, chewing slowly and enjoying each bite or, in other words, *essen wie ein Mann* ("eating like a human"). His pains completely disappeared, and he declared to a journalist reporting his story in a 1998 issue of *Bild Zeitung* (Düsseldorf's largest newspaper), "*Ich fühle mich wie ein neuer Mann*" ("I feel like a new man").

ANIMAL BITES

A Curandera Helps Out

An archaeologist buddy of mine from Harvard University was doing some excavation work at the ancient Maya site of Seibal in Petén in 1969. Its ruins rise above the right bank of the Rio de la Pasión, a tributary of the Usumacinta River in Guatemala.

One day a dog belonging to one of the local Maya laborers assisting him got in his way as he was carrying a heavy artifact to a table to examine it more closely. He accidentally tripped over the dog and fell down but not before the animal had bitten him. My friend became worried that the injury might become infected or, worse still, that he might get rabies.

But in a village close by the site, an old Maya female folk healer offered to tend his wound at no charge. She mixed some crushed red-pepper pods and squeezed lime juice in a half-full bottle of Mexican tequila, shook the contents well, and then thoroughly washed the area of the bite. She had him drink some of the fiery liquid, too, and he suffered no ill effects after that.

ANKLE PAIN

A Hungarian Grandmother's Remedy

My dad's mother, Barbara Liebhardt Heinerman, was a great folk healer in the city of Temevár, Hungary (since renamed Timisoara in western Romania). She emigrated to America in 1906 with her husband Jacob Heinerman I. They briefly lived in Baltimore before finally settling in Salt Lake City, where she continued her folk-healing ways until permanently falling asleep one night at a very advanced age still in relatively good health and without any pain or suffering.

Her remedy for ankle or foot pain of any kind was quite simple. She would get two round enamel pans and set them on the floor. One would be filled about eight inches high with hot water to which was added a generous handful of Epsom salts and then mixed in by hand. The other pan was filled with cold water to about the same depth and a little chipped ice thrown in to keep the temperature constant.

The suffering individual was then instructed to remove both shoe and stockings and keep pant legs rolled up or dress pulled up toward the knee. The person would then place his or her injured foot first into the hot water for about 30 seconds before lifting it and transferring it over to the pan containing the ice water and retaining it there for about the same length of time. This back-and-forth procedure between both pans continued for roughly 30 minutes or until the hot water turned lukewarm and the ice water became mildly cool.

It took between only two and five of these treatments every seven hours to reduce any swelling or inflammation in the tender area of affliction. After that the person could walk normally without any more pain. Through the years I've relied on this simple method myself to take care of many such limb and body pains with very good success.

ANOREXIA NERVOSA

One Woman's Recovery Story

During the early 1990s, the ABC television comedy sitcom *Growing Pains* was immensely popular. Actress Tracey Gold, who played the part of Carol Seaver for seven years, suffered from a serious malady that no one on the set wanted to discuss with the media. Tracey had been battling anorexia on and off since the age of 12. She had a morbid image of food making her presumably "fat" and so refused to hardly eat anything until she approached nearly the point of starvation. This see-sawing between hating food and absolutely loving it occurred periodically throughout her teenage years and early-to-midtwenties.

Finally, after word leaked out what her true condition was, and the letters of sympathy and support for her started pouring in from thousands of her loyal fans, Tracey decided finally to do something serious about her problem. She checked herself into an eating-disorders clinic, where under the watchful guidance of a psychotherapist and nutritionist she at last came to grips with this private demon. *Admitting* to herself that she really had a problem was the first step toward recovery. *Recognition* for the lovely and talented person she was came next. After that came some behavior modification to *change eating patterns:* small snacks of just *one food item* throughout the day instead of the typical three meals consisting of different things. *Getting closer* with family and friends and becoming less isolated followed next.

Tracey starting taking St. Johnswort for her depression long before it became the popular herbal fad that it now is for this particular disorder. She drank warm chamomile tea to help her relax and warm peppermint tea with most of her snacks to assist in their digestion. She *reoriented her perception of good,* convincing herself over and over again that everything she was consuming was only to help *make her more beautiful* by filling out her emaciated body. Gone was the dread of even a single soda cracker making her look "fat"!

She took a high-potency B-complex every day as well as vitamins A, C, and E. Her mineral intake included potassium, magnesium, calcium, iron, sulfur, and phosphorus, in that order. Some amino acids were added to the program as well.

Tracey attributed some of her recovery to *meditation and soothing music.* She claimed that both of these "helped me to relax my body and mind a lot so that I could get a clearer perspective of myself and see where my life was headed." With the constant *encouragement* of so many around her who truly loved the woman and felt deeply for her dire straits, as well as her own *persistence and determination,* she eventually regained control of her life, filled her body out nicely, and won the battle that almost did her in for good!

ANXIETY

Two Cups of Ginseng—and Many Deep Breaths

The weekend of May 7–9, 1999, found me at the NewLife Expo at the Hotel New Yorker in Manhattan near Penn Station. I gave a lecture and was on two separate health panels. At one of these engagements, I met a 34-year-old Lithuanian woman named Tamara who spoke impeccable English. She worked at the United Nations as a translator for Russian diplomats. She shared the following true story with me.

A certain Russian diplomat whom she identified only as Mr. X often met in conferences with other foreign delegates where world issues of pressing importance were discussed. Being of visceral temperament, he could become highly animated in these heated debates. This, of course, would pump larger amounts of adrenaline into his system.

As a result he began experiencing some of the common symptoms of high anxiety: lightheadedness, headaches, backache, dry mouth, queasy stomach, sweating hands, weak legs, and hints of faintness. His level of anxiety had proceeded well beyond the former nail-biting and lip-chewing stages to these, which had him worried about his personal health. Knowing of Tamara's interest in holistic health, he desperately sought her out for badly needed advice.

I now quote her direct instructions to him from her narrative. "I informed Mr. X of some things he could do for himself to bring down his anxiety. I told him to drink a cup of hot ginseng-root tea before he went to his UN office in the morning and another cup in the afternoon with his lunch. I use ginseng myself and it helps me to relax a lot.

"I also showed him a breathing technique I learned at one of the NewLife workshops. I always noticed that whenever Mr. X was experiencing a lot of anxiety, he would take shallow 'chest' breaths. He used only his chest muscles to inhale rather than his diaphragm [the muscle found at the bottom of the lungs]. Therefore only the top part of his lungs was filling with air and oxygen. To help him increase his oxygen intake, I suggested doing this simple exercise at least once a day for a whole month.

"First, I instructed him to sit in a chair without armrests, with his feet flat on the floor and his thighs parallel to the floor. His back was to be held straight, either supported or unsupported by the chair. I had him lay one hand over the other or else place his palms in a comfortable position on his thighs. He then was told to inhale through his nose and breathe deeply, without forcing it, and to let his belly expand. I suggested that he imagine that the breath was filling his belly.

"Then, in a continuous breath, he was to imagine filling his chest and lungs. 'Feel your chest expand fully and your shoulders rise slightly,' I told him as he did this. 'Imagine the air expanding your abdomen and chest in all directions,' I advised. Next, I said he should slowly exhale through his nose and to make sure that his exhalation took longer than his inhalation did.

"He was to do this for at least two minutes. I recommended doing it in a comfortable rhythm and not straining himself; also to stay focused on keeping his breathing deep and full and his body completely relaxed. After trying this for a few days he told me he felt less tension in dramatic debates."

Why There Is No Anxiety in Polynesia

The Polynesian islands cover a vast triangular area in the Pacific with Hawaii, Easter Island, and New Zealand as its apices and with a scattering of outlying islands westward into Melanesia and Micronesia. All the islands are tropical or subtropical except New Zealand and its outlying islands and groups, which are temperate or even cold.

I have found little anxiety among Polynesians. As a whole the natives on the many different, widely dispersed islands seldom feel the tension that tens of millions of others feel elsewhere in the world. This is because of a traditional beverage that is consumed in nearly all Pacific societies. Melanesians, Micronesians, and Polynesians alike grind the fresh or dry roots of the *Piper methysticum* shrub to make their favorite and relaxing drink. It is called *kava* (the common name also given to the plant) and is just as much a part of Oceania culture as wine has been to southern Europe.

Although kava isn't classified as a drug, it exhibits psychoactive properties but curiously isn't hallucinogenic or a stupefacient. A group of active compounds called kavalactones demonstrate enough anesthetic qualities to classify kava as a narcotic and a hypnotic, although its consumption has never led to addiction or dependency. It truly is a most amazing relaxant, to say the least!

In the early history of Polynesia the various island chiefs or people of high social rank would drink kava, but never commoners. Today, however, it is drunk by all social classes. In the nineteenth century it was prepared in a rather gross manner: Kava roots were first ground on a stone, then well masticated by village natives before being expectorated into a vessel to which water was added; the fermented mixture was eventually filtered through coconut leaves and then passed around in a formal ceremony to be drunk by everyone.

But today kava is prepared in a more conventional way: The dried, coarsely chopped root is simmered for a while on low heat in double the amount of water needed to cover it. When half that amount remains the brew is set aside and covered to steep longer. As a beverage of great social importance, kava is popular during feasts and as a sign of hospitality and for pleasure. Hawaiian *kahuna* (native shamans) still imbide in it for ritual and esoteric purposes.

Among the underprivileged classes, though, kava finds merit for well-deserved relaxation after work. It creates "a serene state of mind," as one French horticulturist with the University of Hawaii aptly put it.

In the marvelous book, *Islands, Plants, and Polynesians* (Portland, ME: Dioscorides Press, 1991), Vincent Lebot describes the composure that was discernibly felt by kava drinkers. "When the beverage is not too concentrated drinkers attain a state of happy unconcern, well-being and contentment. They feel relaxed and free of any physical or psychological excitement. At the beginning, conversation flows gently and easily; hearing and vision are also improved, allowing subtle sounds and shades to be perceived. Drinkers remain masters of their conscience and reason because kava is not a central nervous system depressant but acts on the spinal system. The beverage soothes temperaments and drinkers never become angry, unpleasant, noisy or quarrelsome. Kava is considered as a means of easing moral discomfort and killing anxiety. In many cases, it helps thought processes and solves the problems of everyday life as drinkers can talk to each other without any nervous tension. The following day, drinkers awaken in excellent shape, having fully recovered their physical and mental capacities."

Kava is best employed in beverage form, although different brands of the encapsulated powder work reasonably well for milder anxiety but not for as long.

APPENDICITIS

A Cuban Approach

Marie Lizette is Quebecois and proud of her heritage. And like so many other French Canadians, she enjoys vacationing in Cuba every so often. Unlike the United States, which places restrictions on its citizens to visit there, Canada permits anyone who wishes to go to Cuba to do so.

I met Ms. Lizette in October 1998 at a Canadian Health Food Association convention in Toronto, where I was a keynote speaker. She had spent some time in Havana and described it as "that magnificent but crumbling city," which holds a little over two million residents. She claimed that there were really two Havanas: One represents the old Communist ways and the other the new ways.

She reported going down a narrow street filled with people, potholes, carts, voices, music, dogs, laundry fluttering from balconies, a mattress being lowered by rope from an upper floor, and men on top of an old decaying building attempting to fix a leaky roof. She went to

Obrapia No. 511 to meet the local general practitioners who served the medical needs of that entire block.

Dr. Emilio Sanchez, a state employee in a socialized medical system, was at work in a small, hot, humid room. As patients came in from a dark passage outside, he would listen attentively, take blood pressure, draw urine samples, look at tongues, and so forth. In seven hours he saw 32 people. Ms. Lizette, who speaks Cuban Spanish quite fluently, said she freely conversed with him on a number of different health-related issues.

He told her that due to the shortage of medical supplies and the lack of necessary equipment, he often had to improvise in lieu of prescription drugs and surgery. A young man, age 27, had visited him that morning and had complained of abdominal pains atypical for appendicitis. But since it didn't seem lifethreatening at the moment, Dr. Sanchez recommended herbs instead of an operation.

He gave the young man some coarsely cut dried bark of *cascara de salamo* with written instructions for preparation and taking. The patient was to boil a pint of water, then add just one-half teaspoon of the bark. He was verbally admonished by the good doctor not to use any more than this when making a pot of tea on account of its extreme potency. After stirring the contents with a spoon, he was to reduce the heat to a much lower setting, cover the pot with a lid, and simmer for a few minutes longer. The patient was told to take four ounces or one-half glass of the strained tea morning, noon, and night, always on an empty stomach and before a meal.

My informant told me that this was a fairly common remedy that other doctors besides Sanchez often prescribed for problems of this sort. But he pointed out that it worked for appendicitis only if the condition was caught early enough; if too far advanced and lifethreatening, then surgery was the only other option. (*Note:* Cascara sagrada bark, dried and coarsely cut, may be substituted for the other if it cannot be found. The *powdered* bark *won't* work as well as the whole cut pieces will.)

APPETITE LOSS

An Old Havana Method

Marie Lizette, the French Canadian woman who visits Cuba often, told me of an interesting remedy she learned about while visiting a *curan-*

dera in Old Havana some years ago. The herb lady she went to see introduced her to a broth made from boiled-potato peelings, yam skins, and a tablespoon of basil leaves. The broth was administered in one-half cupsful every three hours to those who didn't feel like eating anything. The folk healer claimed that in every case, people who drank this several times a day would find their appetites returning soon and then become hungry for food again.

I've had a few occasions since hearing this to recommend it to others with reasonably good success. It's safe and cost-effective.

ARM PAIN

Peppermint by Any Other Name

David is the third largest city in the republic of Panama, the country that connects Central and South America. In the *mercado,* or open marketplace, one may find on any given day numerous vendors hawking everything from dried fish and shrimp to sugar, coffee beans, fabric, manufactured goods, and, of course, *hierbas medicinales.*

One of the plants sold there is *hierba buena de olor.* A visitor such as myself can stroll through the bustling mercado and see bunches of this fresh plant tied together with strong or brightly colored yarn and hanging from nails or pegs. Several of the herb vendors with whom I spoke about it told me how they used it for relieving arm, hand, or leg pain.

Two bunches of peppermint leaves, or what I would judge to fill two cups, are put into one and a half pints of boiling water, covered, and then allowed to cook on a much lower heat setting for ten minutes or until one-half pint of the water has evaporated away. A clean cloth or small towel of some kind is soaked in this hot tea and some of the excess liquid gently wrung out. It is then folded over once or twice and promptly applied to the afflicted area. Another piece of *dry* cloth material is put over the hot pack to retain the heat as long as possible.

Several continuing applications of this will greatly diminish even the most severe pain and bring relief to the limbs. A few drops of peppermint oil may also be put on a hot, wet, folded washcloth and then that placed on the point of pain with the same good results. However, be forewarned that peppermint oil is extremely potent and may not be well tolerated by some sensitive skins; also, just a few drops are needed at any time.

ARTHRITIS

Bill Clinton's Book of Virtues

A fellow I know by the name of Raymond Wong is a stand-up comic on the West Coast and works a number of small nightclubs on the weekend, when he isn't busy working as a high-school shop teacher in his local community. I went to watch his comedy routine one time and ended up with my rib cage hurting due to so much side-splitting laughter.

Knowing I was a great book collector, he created a little skit that night just for my benefit. "Here are some of the shortest titles ever written," he deadpanned. *"My Plan to Find the Real Killers* by O. J. Simpson. Or wait, how about this one? *All the Men I've Loved Before* by Ellen DeGeneres." Then momentarily pausing and rubbing his chin with one hand, he moodily reflected, "Hmmm! *Human Rights Advances in China* . . . now there's a winning title for a lost cause!

"Say, does anyone here like to travel very much?" A number of hands went up. "Well, here's a nifty little volume you might want to catch at your local Barnes & Noble: *Amelia Earhart's Guide to the Pacific Ocean.* Or if you've got some attorney buddies you'd like to do a little something for to show them your appreciation, this next volume would be right up their alley—*America's Most Popular Lawyers.*

"Any morticians in the house?" No hands were raised. "Oh well, I guess I'll pass on *Dr. Kevorkian's Collection of Motivational Speeches.* And for all of you gourmet cooks out there, may I suggest *Spotted Owl Recipes* put out by the Environmental Protection Agency (EPA). Have trouble finding the perfect gifts for really b-o-r-i-n-g people in your life? Well then consider getting them *Staple Your Way to Success* or *The Amish Phone Directory.*"

Guggul and Hot Stuff to Tame the Pain

The only thing that Raymond didn't find much of a laughing matter was the arthritic pain that would flare up in his joints every so often, especially in his shop classes. Something as simple as grabbing a hammer or holding the end of a board as it was put through a planer could hurt his hands and wrists quite a bit. He asked me what could be done for his situation.

A short time before our visit I had attended a health food industry seminar in Anaheim, California. There I listened to several speakers address the issue of Nutritional Support for Arthritis. An herbalist cited half a dozen effective remedies from different cultures: Salai *(Boswellia serrata)* and guggul *(Commiphora mukul)*, two potent Ayurvedic tree gums from India; black pepper and cayenne pepper from China; and spinach and yarrow from Europe.

The Ayurvedic herbs can be obtained from any health-food store and come in capsules (three a day) or fluid extracts (15 drops beneath the tongue twice daily). A nice liniment can be made at home from the two peppers. Melt down in a small stainless-steel saucepan enough Vaseline to equal one-half cup. Add to it one-quarter teaspoon each of black pepper and capsicum. Stir thoroughly and cool until the mixture congeals. Apply topically to swollen joints twice daily. Or, an easier way would be to purchase any commercial ointment already containing the capsaicin, which makes cayenne pepper so hot to the taste buds. Spinach and yarrow can be cooked together (equal parts) in some water for about 20 minutes and then the liquid drained off and a six-ounce glass drunk morning and evening.

The speaker who followed was a nutritionist and spoke at some length on the virtues of glucosamine and its salts, chondroitin, shark cartilage, and sea cucumber. He showed how each of these things helped independently to relieve joint inflammation, but worked even better when used together. Although he never mentioned it, one product that I've found extremely beneficial for rheumatoid arthritis is Arth-X Plus from Trace Minerals Research of Roy, Utah (see Product Appendix). The combination of ionic mineral salts, glucosamine, chondroitin, and certain anti-inflammatory herbs make this an excellent choice for this problem.

The nutritionist also encouraged the use of methylsulfonylmethane, otherwise known as MSM. This he labeled the "latest nutriceutical superstar" and claimed it was good for rheumatoid arthritis as well as for osteoarthritis. (See page 351 of my *Encyclopedia of Nature's Vitamins & Minerals* for more on MSM.)

I presented all of this information to Raymond and said he could pick and choose from several of these and see which ones worked best for him. A couple of weeks passed by before I heard from him. And when he called me by phone, he was ecstatic about the relief he had experienced. He happily exclaimed, "You wouldn't believe how much stronger my grip is in my shop classes at school. I can grab and lift and hold things now without any pain, whereas before I'd have to grit my teeth and endure the suffering. Thanks a million!"

He was in a rush and so I didn't have a chance to ask him which specific things had worked best for him. But knowing the guy I presumed he tried them all or nearly most until he got the relief desired. Before hanging up, he gave me several more new titles that I was to look for in my local bookstore: *The Wild Years* by Al Gore, *Different Ways to Spell Bob*, and *My Guide to Dating Etiquette* by boxer Mike Tyson.

ASCITES
(See "FLUID RETENTION")

ASTHMA

A Turkish Oil That Does the Trick

Cass Ingram, D.O., an Illinois physician and surgeon, is the author of a dozen books on health-related topics. Some years ago he became concerned about the routine use of standard asthma medications such as cromolyn sodium (Intal), ipratropium (Atrovent), beta-adrenergics, theophylline, and corticosteroids, many of which are available in oral inhalers. He felt there had to be a better way with natural substances that were safer.

His worldwide search eventually took him to a remote Turkish village located high in the Taurus mountains. From their vantage point, both he and his guide/interpreter had a magnificent view of the Southern Mediterranean at a height of some 5,000 feet above sea level.

In the home of one of their hosts, they happened to meet the aged mother who was, at that particular moment, suffering from a severe asthma attack. According to Dr. Ingram's faxed message to me on the night of May 24, 1999: "Her attack was one of the worst I'd ever seen. Her chest heaved in great motions and the muscles on her neck were visibly tightened. The son walked over and had the old woman tilt her head back and open her mouth a little ways. He then placed three drops of oil of oregano under her tongue every one and a half minutes. Within five minutes (by my wristwatch) the asthma was remarkably under control and within 15 minutes the symptoms had completely disappeared!"

Such quick recovery led Dr. Ingram to investigate oregano further. What he soon found out, though, was that *not* just *any* oregano would work. The particular type growing wild in the high mountainous regions of Turkey seemed to have within it those important medical constituents that could deliver the kind of action he was looking for. This particular oil is available in some but not all health-food stores.

ATHLETE'S FOOT

The Cure Is in the Cupboard

Dr. Cass Ingram has been a proponent of wild-grown oregano oil from Turkey for quite a while. In a little book on the subject, he wrote the following, which he kindly permitted me to excerpt here. "Athlete's foot is perhaps the most common fungal infection of humans, afflicting untold millions of individuals. When the fungus grows, it produces toxins, which are responsible for itching and irritation. At times the itching is so extreme that excoriation occurs. When this happens, the raw wound may become secondarily infected by bacteria. This may be manifested by inflammation and foul odor.

"Oil of oregano outright destroys this disgusting fungus. The organism is defenseless against the oil's potent chemistry, since oregano oil contains solvents capable of disabling the cell membrane. Because of the chronicity [of the problem], it may take a relatively long period of treatment before the infection is eradicated. As long as improvement is noted keep using the oil. Even if it takes weeks or months before a resolution is noted, it is well worth the effort.

"Apply oil of oregano liberally to the affected regions of the feet, being sure to also treat regions between the toes. Repeat this application two or three times daily until the infection is cured. Always apply the oil to the feet after contact with public surfaces such as the floors of public showers, athletic clubs, and bathtubs/floors in hotels/motels.

"For toenail fungus apply the oil directly to the nail and nail bed in large amounts. Also, gently rub it between the toes. Take several drops of the oil in juice, milk, or water twice daily. Or fill a small gelatin capsule with the oil and take one or two daily with meals. Remember, toenail fungus is a chronic and difficult condition to treat. Don't expect results overnight." (For more information send a SASE to North American Herb & Spice, POB 4885, Buffalo Grove, IL 60089.

ATROPHIC VAGINITIS

Libyan Relief

A Delaware pediatrician, Halley S. (as in the comet), went to Libya on her own for a period of time to render badly needed medical service there free of charge to many young children. With menopause setting on, she soon developed vaginal inflammation with accompanying burning and itching.

One of the Bedouin women in an outlying village, upon learning of her dilemma, recommended that Halley use one of the following items to obtain relief: cold feungreek-seed tea, sesame-seed oil, cold camel milk, or cold goat's milk. She followed this advice and found that all of them worked about equally well once she had rubbed each of them around the inside of her vagina with her fingers.

Being a physician, she was amazed that such simple things could bring about such wonderful relief for a rather vexing problem following the transition to menopause.

AUTISM

World's Leading Authority

On April 12, 1992, I had a lengthy interview in San Diego, California with Dr. Bernard Rimland, who has a Ph.D. in experimental psychology. He wrote a definitive work entitled *Infantile Autism* (Appleton-

Century-Crofts, 1964), which has been widely recognized as a major contribution to psychology. He served as the primary technical adviser to *Rainman*, a film starring actor Dustin Hoffman in the role of an autistic adult.

Dr. Rimland is considered by many of his peers to be the world's leading authority on autism, a serious brain disorder. "It all began with my son Mark in 1956," he told me. "Mark was our first child. Gloria [the doctor's wife] and I were so proud of our newborn's extreme alertness. But that parental ecstasy we felt quickly flew out the window when we discovered what a violently upset little creature he had become. He would scream constantly, day and night, for hours on end for no apparent reason."

Dr. Rimland began scouring medical journals for anything he could find on autism. The leading theory, by since-deceased Dr. Bruno Bettelheim, blamed autism on problems with mother–infant interactions. But this theory struck Dr. Rimland as plain foolishness. "Gloria and I both wanted Mark very much, which ruled out that psychological nonsense of causation," he said. But with the publication of his book, Dr. Rimland replaced that old "standard hocum" with a more sound explanation attributing autism to a physical defect that impaired brain chemistry.

Vitamins as a Solution

Through much trial and error, Dr. Rimland eventually discovered that tryptophan (an essential amino acid) and vitamin B-6 were two of the best nutritional approaches to the problem. Later, when the former got a lot of bad press, he replaced it with magnesium and B-6, which have "proven to be real winners for solving autism," he stated with a great deal of confidence. His standard recommendations have been 250 mg. magnesium and 500 mg. vitamin B-6 on a daily basis for autistic children. While not totally curing the problem, "these nutrients definitely improve their lives a lot!"

Food Sensitivities

Dr. Rimland enjoyed calling attention to the work of the great Walter C. Alaverez, M.D. Alvarez worked at the famous Mayo Clinic in the 1920s and was the first to make the connection between food allergies and erratic brain behavior. But he was sharply disciplined by his supervisors for giving lectures on this subject and was threatened with dismissal. It was only through the intercession of one of the Mayo brothers themselves, who had a brain allergy, that saved Dr. Alvarez's job. That particular Dr. Mayo stopped eating wheat bread and cereal and drinking milk, and within a matter of days his former brain allergy had completely disappeared.

Later on, other courageous medical investigators such as William H. Philpott, M.D. *(Brain Allergies,* New Canaan, CT: Keats Publishing, 1987) expanded and refined the work initiated by Dr. Alvarez decades before. Besides grain gluten and milk proteins, doctors now specializing almost exclusively in autism know that food additives such as coloring and preservatives can also trigger mental disorders such as autism in children and even in adults. Folic acid, another important B vitamin, has come into prominent usage to alleviate such food sensitivities.

Frustrated Geniuses

Autistic adults can be incredible geniuses on one hand, but so intolerable in their behavior otherwise. I had a chance once in Lansing, Michigan, in the latter part of October 1996 to see one such person in action. His name was Kim Peek, who served as the inspiration for the Oscar-winning movie, *Rainman,* about an autistic savant reuniting with his brother. In a public demonstration of his incredible knowledge gleaned from some 8,000 books that he's read, he can freely recite for hours facts that absolutely draws gasps of amazement from bewildered spectators.

When I saw him in a school auditorium in company with his father, Fran, a student in the assembled crowd had just offered Kim his birth date. Almost instantly the kid was told the day of the week he was born, the day of the week of his next birthday, and the day he would turn 35. Another student queried Kim about Muhammad Ali and heard a rapid recitation of the years the boxer held the heavyweight crown. And just whom did Ali beat to win his first championship came a follow-up question. "Sonny Liston, TKO in 7," Kim hurriedly spat out. From another kid: "When was Michigan State University founded?" "1855," was the answer offered without hesitation. And when Mr. Peek asked the same kid if he would like to have his son rattle off all of the university presidents who served over the years and their respective lengths of tenure, the boy declined by shaking his head in disbelief.

As we left the auditorium later on, my Lansing host turned to me and remarked: "You know, John, it's really something to see someone who was considered retarded at one time but really is a genius at heart."

I nodded in understanding and added, "Yes, but a frustrated genius at that."

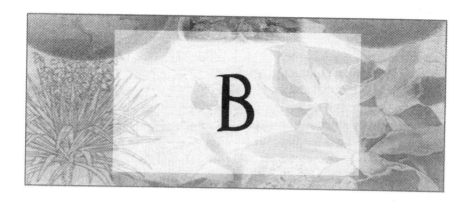

BACK PAIN (UPPER AND LOWER)

TV Funny Man Tim Allen's Approach

The year 1999 saw the final episode of one of television's most popular comedy sitcoms, *Home Improvement*. For eight seasons Tim Allen looked perfectly in character as Tim Taylor, the lovable Everyman. There he stood each week on the familiar *Tool Time* set (the fictional show within the show) wearing a clunky tool belt and hefting a no-nonsense power saw.

But behind the humor and goofy smile, there had been a lot of pain—back pain (both upper and lower), to be specific. Allen's solutions to finding relief for it include the following: yoga and tai-chi stretching exercises every day between takes; a daily one-hour Swedish massage with peppermint oil by a licensed masseuse; daily sips of *warm* peppermint tea; and sitting against a cushioned chair vibrator at home for 30-minute intervals, if necessary.

BACTERIAL VAGINOSIS

Changing "Ow" into "Ahhh"

Karina W. of New York City has worked for City Hall for seven years. She noticed a peculiar type of vaginal infection developing and reported the symptoms of this to her gynecologist. "There was a foul odor," she repeated for my benefit during a NewLife Expo at the Hotel New Yorker, where I was then speaking. "It made me smell as if I've just come from one of the local fish markets. There would sometimes be a gray or yellowish vaginal discharge. And sometimes I'd get a lot of itching down there, accompanied by low back pain, even pain when I urinated and irritation during intercourse with my husband, Jonnie."

She felt relieved upon being told by her doctor that this vaginal infection wasn't a sexually transmitted disease, but was caused by a common *Gardnerella* bacteria. Fortunately, her doctor was holistic-minded enough to suggest some natural solutions. "She told me to spray the area every day with a small solution of goldenseal-root fluid extract"—300 drops in two and a half tablespoons warm water. "I was also instructed to douche regularly with tepid hyssop tea"—steep two teaspoons cut, dried hyssop herb in two cups boiling water for 20 minutes; strain; and douche. "I also took two capsules each day of Kyolic Aged Garlic Extract," (see Product Appendix) she added. "The situation has pretty much remained under control with this treatment, but I sometimes take a vitamin C (3,500 mg.) if I feel the situation requires more nutritional assistance."

BAD BREATH

Back to Hackensack

A while ago I happened to visit Aylward's Natural Food in Hackensack, New Jersey, for a brief book signing. Prior to this I had just consumed a lunch dish loaded with garlic and onions, two of my favorite food spices. An elderly lady, discerning my smelly breath, dutifully reached into her purse and pulled out a crumpled box of Smith Bros. Cough Drops. She told me to take one and suck on it.

I momentarily hesitated, thinking to myself at the time, "But I don't have a cough or cold, just bad breath." However, to please her I removed one, politely thanked her, and slipped it into my mouth. Before she departed with an autographed copy of my *Natural Pet Cures* (Paramus, NJ: Prentice Hall, 1998), she leaned over and whispered, "I know you're skeptical right now on account of its being a cough drop. But trust me when I assure you that all of your bad breath will disappear in a few minutes. I call them my 'Altoid Substitutes.'" She then ambled off and before long, just as she had said, my breath smelled 100 percent better, albeit a little mediciny.

BAGS UNDER THE EYES

Used Teabags Are Good for Something After All

While seated in a large book section of Aylward's Health Food Center in Hackensack, New Jersey, one day in mid-January 1999, signing copies of one of my recent health titles for store customers patiently waiting in line, I had one of the clerks in the herbs section saunter over and casually flip through one of my books stacked on the floor beside me.

When the line had dissipated somewhat, she placed the volume down and complimented me on "a job well done." Then she inquired how I got all of the remedies mentioned therein. "Many of them are through my own practice and use of herbs over a lifetime," I replied. "Others come from ordinary people like yourself, who volunteer them freely. And a number of others come from numerous shamans and folk healers I've visited and worked with in more than 30 different countries."

She then said, "Well, I have one for your next book, Doc. It's a way to get rid of bags under the eyes, or where the eyes get kind of puffy." She said that instead of discarding used black- or green-tea bags, "I just squeeze out some of the excess liquid and place a couple of them over each of my closed eyelids while lying down. I place a small hand towel over them to retain the heat. I use them while still very warm and leave on until cool. Bags disappear, and those eyelids look good. A person may have to do this twice at one time if the puffiness is heavy. But I guarantee you it'll work *every* time."

BED SORES

An Anglo-Saxon Medical Text

Among the many priceless documents currently housed in the British Museum Library is an interesting collection of medico-magical recipes, charms, invocations and so forth, collectively known as *Lacnunga*. These survive in just one manuscript officially categorized by the uninspiring reference of MS. Harley 585. The document consists of 193 folios and contains several texts. The average size of each page is 7½ x 4½ inches. The number of lines per page varies between 13 and 24. The *Lacnunga* portion occupies only a part of the MS. Harley 585 volume, however.

MS. Harley 585 is believed by scholars to have been written sometime around A.D. 1000 by an unknown Anglo-Saxon leech, that is a folk healer who employed the use of leeches in his treatments, besides the usual herbal formulas, charms, incantations, and rituals. The author of MS. Harley 585 put together a collection of the favorite healing recipes which he and his brother leeches routinely used in their art. He first adopted the ancient and recognized plan of beginning with the head and working down to the feet.

While the first compiler of that portion of the manuscript designated as *Lacnunga a* was a monastery monk somewhat acquainted with the healing arts, the second compiler of *Lacnunga b* was not a monastery resident but of the common class. Evidence within the manuscript text indicates that this particular individual was heathen and not of the Christian faith, for there is a great deal of pagan magic interwoven with the many medical recipes given.

A later monk from a small monastery in the north of Great Britain somewhere and believed to have been of Irish descent contributed the material that forms *Lacnunga c.*

This composite volume, *Lacnunga a, b,* and *c,* was eventually rebound. During this process the page leaves were wrongly arranged and the contributions of the three previous compilers were thereby confused, though they still tended to adhere in groups. Finally, this rebound volume was copied shortly after the year 1000 by the scribe who produced the existing MS Harley 585. He also added some passages at the end that might be treated as a fourth stratum or as *Lacnunga d.*

A Cure for Bed Sores

Almost all the recipes contained in *Lacnunga* are interspersed with magical and religious elements. To preserve the flavor of the ancient document I have purposely retained them.

"For sores upon the body that come from lying in bed too long, take 1 part milk of any kind of animal upon the land, and mix it with 3 parts of good honey, and put 1 part holy water with them. Place these toward the altar and let a mass-priest sing four masses over them. Then apply upon each sore while repeating the names of Matthew, Mark, Luke, and John in unison."

Stripped to its bare essentials, the recipe would be as follows for modern application: Mix one teaspoon of milk with three teaspoons of honey and one teaspoon of pure water. Then apply to each sore with a clean object, such as a washed finger, tongue depressor, clean popsicle stick, knife, or the back of a wooden spoon. Do this twice daily. Cover lightly with some loose gauze to keep the material from sticking to bedding or underclothing.

Honey is extremely healing; the combination of milk and water tend to make the skin more supple. Ideally, *raw* milk and honey and distilled water should be used for the quickest results, but the other kinds are just as suitable, though healing may take longer.

BEDWETTING

Fig Water from West Africa

The Republic of Sierra Leone in West Africa is bordered by the Atlantic Ocean to the west, by Guinea in the north and east, and by Liberia to the south. Its Atlantic coastline consists of a belt of low-lying mangrove swamps, except for the mountainous Sierra Leone Peninsula on which the capital of Freetown is situated.

The country has an important mining industry that is largely controlled by large multinational corporations headquartered in Switzerland, Great Britain, and the United States. The chief minerals currently being extracted are diamonds, iron ore, gold, bauxite, and rutile; together they make up roughly 50 percent of this tiny nation's foreign-exchange earnings.

Diamonds are mainly found in East Sierra Leone, while iron is chiefly mined in the west-central part of the country. While generally a peaceful nation with a rather low crime rate, diamond smuggling has been its principal crime problem since the 1960s. Smugglers employ some rather ingenious methods to get them out of the country.

During a tour of West African nations many years ago, I happened to meet one such person, who showed me a few tricks of his trade. Being an enterprising fellow, he devised new ways to elude the authorities. One of the most clever of these was to secure the uncut diamonds in a goatskin leather pouch with a drawstring. As the bag was quite small in size, it wasn't too difficult for his wife to hide the bag *inside* their 14-year-old daughter's shoulder-length hair, which she carefully braided up on all sides and arranged into a rather nifty pile on top. This unusual hairdo actually made the girl look quite good, as a matter of fact.

Besides showing me a few good smuggling tricks, the father also gave me a simple remedy that the parents had used to curb bedwetting in some of their smaller children. Two or three figs would be boiled in two cups of milk for about ten minutes on low heat and then set aside to cool. Some of this syrupy liquid would be strained off and given to the children to drink about 30 minutes before their bedtime. After a week of this their bedwetting problems would usually cease for good.

BENIGN PROSTATIC HYPERPLASIA

Bathroom Explicitness

One of the most frequent compliments I keep hearing from many readers is the rich details I provide in my numerous health books. People seem to enjoy descriptiveness about others and the places they reside. Readers sometimes also prefer depth concerning particular remedies. For instance, in one of my more recent works, *Nature's Super Seven Medicines* (Paramus: Prentice Hall Direct, 1997), I provide little-known information about bees in general in the opening chapter devoted to "Gifts From the Hive." A number of readers have informed me just how fascinated they were by the data given about these little creatures.

The problem casually mentioned by a friend of mine and the solution offered by myself actually took place in such a facility some time ago when we both just happened to respond to "nature's call" at about the same time.

Suffice it to say, the rate of flow in my friend took almost five minutes, which led to our conversation on benign prostatic hyperplasia. A man of 47 may not urinate like a high-school boy, but he certainly shouldn't be forced to relieve himself with as much obvious strain as a 90-year-old might have to do.

A Total Program

My friend fell into the obvious trap that so many customers do these days when he asked the obvious question, "What supplement can I take to clear up this problem?" I gently chided him for thinking so narrowly upon the matter.

"There are several good supplements to choose from, but it really is a dietary approach you should be looking at for a permanent solution to your problem." On the supplement end, however, I recommended the Male Formula from ShapeRite, which tonifies the prostate rather nicely while at the same time building natural virility (see Product Appendix under ShapeRite).

I explained that in my long experience of folk healing, men who've had a high-meat, high-fat, high-sugar intake but with very little fruits, vegetables, or fiber tend to have a far greater incidence of enlarged prostate (as well as prostate cancer) than do those who regularly subsist on the latter. Other beneficial foods include tomatoes (in any form), nuts (especially hazelnuts or filberts and pecans), seeds (pumpkin seeds are wonderful for the zinc they contain), certain cereal fibers (especially cooked oatmeal and shredded wheat), fruits such as kiwi, mango, and papaya (isn't it interesting that South Sea islander men who eat these a lot have virtually no prostate problems to speak of?), root vegetables such as turnips, parsnips, carrots, and potatoes (baked, boiled, steamed, juiced, or raw), as well as dark leafy greens (parsley, endive, romaine lettuce, spinach).

He heeded my counsel and started a program consisting of many of the items mentioned in the foregoing paragraph. Within two months, he reported that he could relieve himself in one third the time and with far less pain and effort.

BLADDER INFECTION

The Pilgrims of Plymouth, Massachusetts

Besides the Founding Fathers (who gave us the Declaration of Independence and the U.S. Constitution), Betsy Ross (the seamstress who sewed up Old Glory), George Washington (who crossed the Delaware River in winter to rout out the British Army from Trenton, New Jersey, on Christmas night of 1776), and Abraham Lincoln (who freed the slaves with his Emancipation Proclamation act), the Pilgrims also figure heavily in early-American history.

The nucleus of the group came into being in the meetings of a number of Pilgrims at Scrooby, a village in Nottinghamshire, England. Opposed to the jurisdiction and the rites and discipline of the Church of England, the group had formed as a separatist church by 1606, with John Robinson eventually becoming their minister. The congregation was composed mainly of farmers and artisans, men of little education or position.

Although not actively persecuted, they were, nevertheless, subjected to ecclesiastical investigation and to the mockery, criticism, and disfavor of their neighbors. To avoid contamination of their strict beliefs and to escape the hated church from which they had separated, the sect decided to move to Holland, where other groups had found religious liberty. Life in Holland wasn't any easier, though, and the immigrants found the presence of radical religious groups there highly objectionable. Dutch influence also seemed to be altering their distinctive English ways. And the prospect of another war between the Netherlands and Spain loomed large on the horizon.

A small vessel, the *Speedwell*, was obtained to carry the Pilgrims to England in 1620, where that vessel joined the *Mayflower* for the long trip to the New World. The former ship proved unseaworthy and returned to port; however, many of the passengers and much of her cargo were crowded on the *Mayflower*, which set out alone. In December 1620 the *Mayflower* entered Plymouth harbor, where the settlers established dwellings. The name Pilgrim Fathers is given to those members who made the first crossing on that vessel.

Give Thanks for Ye Olde Cranberry

The winter of 1620 was incredibly hard on members of the Plymouth Colony. Food was in such short supply that to allay the impending starvation that faced everyone, Governor William Bradford ordered daily rations to be reduced by one half until the supply could be replenished.

The fall harvest of 1621 corrected this unhappy situation. Governor Bradford proclaimed a day of thanksgiving to the Almighty for their ample and bounteous supply. Four wild turkeys were caught and prepared for the sumptuous feast, to which members of the

Wampanoags tribe were invited. They brought with them wild cranberries, something the Pilgrims had never before encountered or tasted. And this is how the New England cranberry became associated with what has since become a national holiday celebrated on the fourth Thursday in November.

Add Some Lemon Power

Bladder infection (also know as cystitis or urinary tract infection) is usually caused by intestinal bacteria required for digestion. These bacteria, *Escherichia coli (E. coli)*, and others become incorporated into stool. Sometimes, though, they move from the anal area into the urethra, where they can work their way up into the bladder and cause infection. Other recurrent bladder infections, however, may involve other microorganisms, such as *Chlamydia trachomatis.*

Both sexes are subject to bladder infection, but women seem to be more prone to it than men are. A woman's urethral and anal openings are located closer together than are a man's, so it is much easier for anal bacteria to travel from the one to the other. And a woman's urethra is considerably shorter than a man's, which means that once the bacteria has been introduced into the urethra, they don't have far to travel to infect the female bladder.

Of all the natural things that have been proven to work best against this problem, cranberry juice (one-half cup twice daily) or cranberry powder (three capsules twice daily) are by far the best. True cranberry juice is best to use in spite of its obvious sourness. Some may even be available in your local health-food stores. Thawing out frozen cranberries and then juicing them in a Vita-Mix blender with a little water or a couple of ice cubes is the next-best thing to real juice. Commercial brands of cranberry juice aren't as effective because of the added sugar content to make them more palatable.

A favorite "cranberry cocktail" of mine calls for one tablespoon of lemon juice to be added to the thawed cranberry mixture here described. And Earth's Pharmacy makes a potent CranMax product with one 500 mg. capsule being equivalent to eight ounces of cranberry juice (see Product Appendix).

BLEEDING

A Terrible Tornado Experience

It is not very often that one gets to become a part of history while it is in the making. But such an opportunity came my way on Wednesday, August 11, 1999, shortly before 1:00 P.M. A freak tornado with wind speeds clocked at 137 miles per hour ripped a neat "surgical line" through downtown Salt Lake City and parts of the Capitol Hill and Avenues neighborhoods. This terrible twister narrowly missed my Anthropological Research Center by a mere city block!

My staff and I, on a high floor, heard the awful wind roar that sounded very much like a speeding train. We saw the blackened sky out of our office windows and witnessed big tree limbs being blown around into the air from the trees below with the greatest of ease. One person died, 89 were injured, and more than 300 homes, expensive high-rise apartments, and downtown hotels were damaged. The huge Delta Center where the Utah Jazz basketball team regularly plays sustained heavy damage.

The twister hit hard and fast before anyone could be warned. In a matter of minutes it tore apart buildings, shutting down power and scattering debris for miles in every direction. Tens of thousands of people's lives were disrupted by this unexpected natural holocaust. Insurance-claim adjusters estimated that this freak storm caused almost $200 million worth of destruction in less than four minutes!

Worst of all was the fact that a newly installed National Weather Service NEXRAD Doppler radar on Utah's Promontory Point could not be aimed low enough to detect this vicious tornado. This piece of sophisticated technical equipment is part of a highly advanced radar system and a much touted $4.5 billion Weather Service modernization overhaul. But since tornadoes aren't supposed to happen in Utah, the Weather Service computer software running this detection program couldn't recognize the radar "signature" for such an unlikely event.

Flying Glass and Bricks Injure Many

The massive wind power behind this F2 storm lifted roofs off buildings, blew out several thousand windows, hurled numerous bricks through the air, and uprooted giant oak and tall pine trees as if they were weeds. A great many people sustained serious cuts and bruises due to the flying glass and brick. Some consented to be treated by paramedics, but most decided to take care of their own problems.

A local off-duty police officer whom I've known for years happened to be near the center of this unfortunate action. At the time he was dressed very casually, wearing only a T-shirt, cut-off denim jeans, white socks, and a pair of loafers. He sustained cuts on both of his arms and legs from some of this whirling debris as he ran for shelter. Figuring he wasn't hurt that badly, the cop decided to walk over to my office, hoping I would be there.

I greeted him as he entered the premises. He apologized for his sorry state, but mentioned that he thought it was something I could help him with so paramedics could treat others with far more serious injuries. He patiently stood in front of our office washbasin as I cleaned away the dirt and bits of cut glass from the exposed parts of his limbs. I then disinfected everything with some apple-cider vinegar that we had on hand at the time.

Stopping the Bleeding

Several of my friend's wounds kept bleeding, however. So I fetched a bottle of cayenne pepper from the storage closet of another room and applied liberal helpings of the powder on these particular places. The cop was amazed at how quickly the bleeding stopped. "I knew you were good at writing about these things," he confessed, "but I didn't know something like this would work so fast!" He seemed pleased with the care and attention he was receiving.

We sat and chatted a while before he had to leave. He asked me what I owed him, and I replied, "Nothing . . . you owe me nothing." And then, as he got up from his chair, I had second thoughts about the matter and said, "Well, there is one favor I guess you could do for me. If you ever catch me exceeding the speed limit, I would appreciate it if you'd look the other way and not write me a ticket."

He laughed good-naturedly and half-promised to do this, but only "if you're not going more than ten miles over the speed limit." We shook hands and parted company with a unique experience that both of us could share with our grandchildren someday. That is the incredible healing power of cayenne pepper, and for *any* bleeding situations it works wonders that will truly amaze you.

For internal bleeding, just mix one-quarter teaspoon powdered red pepper in eight ounces of tomato or V-8 juice and drink. Bleeding should cease within minutes. CAUTION: For any kind of serious injury, always see a doctor before attempting self-treatment!

BLEEDING GUMS

Bog Cure

A brief history of the Pilgrims and their journey to Massachusetts was provided under Bladder Infection. The first wild cranberries they encountered were really no different from cultivated ones. They were found growing among sand dunes close to the roaring surf. Dunes are restless things that move like great slow waves. The wind blows away the sand above them until the surface is close to the water table. There the particles of sand are moist and cannot blow anymore, so a flat area of bare white sand develops.

Bogs are the promised land of the cranberry plant, which doesn't object in the least to salt sprayed ashore by the surf and demands little nourishment except light and an abundance of water. Gradually, the plant takes possession of the bare sand (the seeds are dropped by birds) and builds up to its dense mat of vines.

A natural cranberry bog among the dunes is (unlike a domesticated one on higher ground) impermanent and likely to be overwhelmed at any time by a slowly advancing wave of sand. Even if this does not happen, the vines have their domain to themselves for only a limited number of years. Few plants thrive as well in clean, damp beach sand, but little by little soil of a sort accumulates among the vines, and other plants take root in it. Sedges and marsh grasses grow into great bunches that crowd ever closer together. Bushes appear, then trees. Before long they shade out the low-creeping cranberry vines, which retreat to the edge of the deepening thicket.

If you have access to some of these wild or cultivated cranberries in their fresh state, crush a few of them and then rub the mixture across the gums with your forefinger after every brushing. This will halt the bleeding. Or else thaw a few frozen cranberries, mash them well with the back of a spoon, and do the same thing. Or empty the contents of a CranMax capsule from Earth's Pharmacy (see Product Appendix) and rub this over the gums. They all work in the same way.

BLISTERS

The Halcyon Days of Sail

When the War of 1812 ended speed at sea came into prominence. Until then most cargo ships were content to jog along in their own comfortable way. Speed was their last consideration, and merchants had been quite content to wait for their goods. Had they not been so patient, it's doubtful whether any difference would have been made. The only ships that attempted any speed were the ships engaged in what was known as the perishable cargo trade—fruit and slaves.

The exception to this rule had been the Americans, who had always built for speed for the purpose of evading the coast-guard cruisers that the Spaniards built in the vain hope of preserving their West Indian trade. During the war they continued to build for speed for privateering purposes; when peace was restored they saw the opportunity of using this quality in general trade. American ships made the fastest passage to the Oriental markets and profited accordingly.

American shipbuilders are generally credited with developing slim, fast schooners called Baltimore clippers because the Baltimore yards specialized in them. Clipper ships soon came into use as freighters, light naval cruisers, privateers, fishing vessels, smugglers, or slavers.

The Boston shipyards, in particular, started turning out even larger vessels equipped with more speed. These were the three-masted, ship-rigged clippers that came into service in time for the California gold rush of 1849. Ship after ship was crowded with those who preferred the sea passage round Cape Horn to a hazardous overland journey. Two years later (1851) gold was discovered in Australia. The demand for shipping rocketed to such heights that even British shipowners were willing to place orders with the Boston yards and forget that little Tea Party brouhaha that had erupted between their Parliament in London and the American colonists stateside.

"Working My Fingers to the Bone"

Sam Hall, a man in his forties, was one of many hundreds who made their living the old-fashioned way in those days—they literally "worked their fingers to the bone." At least that's what Sam said he did in his daily journal during his stint in one of these early New England shipyards.

He spoke of the many "painful blisters" his hands regularly sustained as shipyard owners worked their crews long hours and often seven days a week just to keep up with the increasing number of orders flooding in from abroad for these bigger and faster clippers. One of his entries, dated August 11, 1852, recounts how badly his hands hurt after a 13-hour shift in the shipyard. "I quit shaking hands today because the effort causes so much pain. I cannot even close my hand far enough to make a good fist. My wife is fearful that I may not be able to pick up a tool due to the many blisters covering both of my hands."

Then an interesting thing happened a few entries later. On August 13, he records: "This day my wife made me soak my hands in cranberry juice. Much of the pain went away. I was better able to grasp a writing implement and enter these few lines." On August 17 he happily writes: "Today most of my old blisters have gone. And the new ones do not seem to hurt me as much so long as I continue with my cranberry soak. Betsy's [probably his wife] insistence that I do so has rewarded me handsomely."

Based on this journal information, which I obtained from the Massachusetts Historical Society, I started recommending the cranberry treatment to others I met with similar blister problems. Farmers, carpenters, loggers, and weightlifters who tried the cranberry soak reported how quickly their blisters healed. It is certainly a remedy worth knowing about if you, like Sam Hull a century ago, "work your fingers to the bone" and blister doing so.

BLOOD CLOTS

The Pagan Way

Sondra N. is a bookkeeper by profession. But in her spare time she practices the Celtic brand of the religion known as Wicca. To be more blunt about the matter, she's a witch! Adherents of the Wiccan tradition really try hard to avoid this term because it has been twisted out of shape by the Christian world and charged with sensationalism. Wicca and other pagan creeds of ancient Egypt predate Christianity by at least 2,000 years. Generally speaking, these religions base their practice around the Goddess and the cycles of nature. As the 1999 "shield-bearer" for the Quicksilver community of pagans in her particular city and state (which she asked that I not identify), she organized all eight "sabbats" or pagan celebrations.

In our interesting dialogue, I found her to be neither fanatical nor funny, but very carefree in her style of delivery.

"Wicca is just a name for all the things I looked for in life," she began, "before finally finding them. And so it happened that I discovered all of them under the Wicca label. People just don't want to understand that all this Wicca business is about *reconnecting* yourself with nature, through the goddess of nature. There are quite a few deities to choose from if you're a pagan, male and female. I think it's good that people are permitted to identify with deities that represent both men and women. It gives a person more options. It's a more open way, and it's also highly individualistic. You can put a dozen Wiccans in one room and they'll never agree on everything.

"People I work with at my job love to kid me about going into the woods to dance naked under a full moon with the devil himself. But I tell them it's not about that at all. I remind them it's about *reconnecting* yourself with nature. And after I tell them that I never have, and never will, worship Satan, they feel a bit more relieved and find this statement reassuring."

Onions and Ginger

Sondra told me with a good-natured laugh in her voice: "If you intend using the herbal part of our discussion, then I want you to also include the other. Sorry, but you can't have the herbs without the witchcraft" (she followed this statement with another hearty laugh).

Becoming more serious at this point in our conversation, she told me about her mother, Dorothy, who lived just a few blocks from her house in the same community. Her mom had been to the doctor several times and was finally referred to the local hospital where further tests were ordered by the physicians on staff. The woman learned she had several large and very bad clots that could be life threatening at any time.

This strict pronouncement scared the living daylights out of Dorothy and she walked away from the hospital vowing to have nothing more to do with doctors. She came to her daughter for some much needed advice. "It just so happened that the day after Mom came to see me," Sondra said, "I went to the mountains with some other pagans for one of our sabbats. Here we were close enough to nature that our personal communions to her took on greater meaning. I was able in my own way to seek the counsel my mother required for her desperate situation."

What came to her as the natural remedies to use were onions and ginger. The instructions that followed (the specific method of communication was never mentioned) told her to have Dorothy finely cut enough raw onion and to grate just enough fresh ginger root to equal a tablespoonful each. These were then to be put into two cups of boiling water and simmered on low heat for seven minutes. After the mixture cooled and the liquid was strained off, Dorothy was to drink one-half cup three times a day. This daily ritual was to continue unabated for two months.

Everything was followed *"to the letter"* Sondra emphasized. She persuaded her mother to get some more medical tests done but in a different hospital with nicer doctors. When the test results came back everyone was astonished to find *no* further evidence of any existing blood clots. "That's the power of Wicca," Sondra claimed in a matter-of-fact way.

BLOOD POISONING

An Archaeologist's Remedy

A new breed of archaeologist was created as America expanded westward following the terrible Civil War that nearly broke this nation apart. The Bureau of American Ethnology, founded in 1879, pioneered a model of scientific archaeology and explored some of the continent's premier sites.

One of its stars was painter and photographer William H. Jackson (1843–1942), who lived to be almost 100 years of age. In 1875, he was the first to photograph, sketch, and measure the ruins of Chaco Canyon and its Pueblo Bonito Great House in New Mexico (part of the great Anasazi culture that flourished throughout the American Southwest from A.D. 900 to 1450).

Jackson also created precise models of these ancient dwellings. The models were carefully crafted by him, based on his own archaeological knowledge acquired through observation and considerable study. Through them the grandeur of the ancient Southwest was revealed, and a number of them may still be seen at different museums throughout the eastern United States.

When he was about 67 years old, Jackson developed a severe case of blood poisoning, most likely sustained by an accidental flesh wound caused by a rusty knife. His life seemed imperiled, and close colleagues attending him were beside themselves as to what could be done to rescue him. A Pueblo Indian shaman recommended using red-clover tea. Several pounds of clover blossoms were procured for this purpose and made into a strong tea.

Probably one cupful of red-clover blossoms were added to one pint of boiling water, stirred, then set aside, covered, and allowed to steep, then becoming sufficiently cool to drink. Jackson was given a cup of this tea four times a day for six days, after which he fully recovered from this awful ordeal. Since learning of this novel remedy myself some years ago, I have recommended it numerous times to others with similar problems and always with good effects. It goes to show how something as simple as red-clover flowers abate a potentially life-threatening situation.

Cure Given by Revelation

Among the numerous books in my huge personal library is a voluminous, four-volume set comprising 3,575 pages. It is entitled *Pioneer Women of Faith and Fortitude* (Salt Lake City: International Society of Daughters of Utah Pioneers, 1998; 4:2737). One of the many remarkable stories contained therein is about Harriett Orilla Austin Shaw. She was born in Cowlesville, Wyoming County, New York, on February 3, 1820, and died on January 20, 1896, in Ogden, Weber County, Utah. She and her husband and their family arrived in Salt Lake Valley sometime in the fall of 1848, settling in what was then called Great Salt Lake City.

"Orilla got blood poisoning in her arm and hand. She lay very ill for two weeks with her arm and hand so swollen and painful she could not move them. She got very little sleep. She was alone in the house one day when she heard a voice telling her to fry some onions and put them on her arm. When her husband came home she told him about hearing the voice. He followed the instructions, put the onions in a cloth sack and tied it around Orilla's arm. In one hour she was at ease and asleep. The swelling came down and she was completely well." (Used with permission.)

BODY ODOR

Going Straight to Your Head

If you're one of millions of people these days who goes around a great deal of the time with a cell phone pinned to your ear, then you'd better pause and read this page more carefully. In the early part of July 1999, I spoke by telephone with scientists at Bristol University in England who've been engaged in a rather startling experiment.

They have been testing model heads, complete with "liquid brains," to analyze the reaction of fake flesh and brain matter to the cell phone's high-frequency radio waves. One of them told me that the amount of harmful waves transmitted can differ between phone models by as much as a factor of 40. The heads, made from real skulls, saltwater, modeling clay, and antifreeze, have been monitored for the past two years with radiation-sensitive probes.

MRI images taken of these model heads were being compared with those of living patients. There clearly was evidence to show an alarming amount of damage being done to human brains by the high-frequency waves of cell phones. My informant suggested a higher risk of brain cancer and a much earlier risk of getting Alzheimer's disease in those who use such devices often.

Removing the Smell with Rubbing Alcohol

At some point in our interesting conversation, my informant and I engaged in a discussion on useful remedies for common health problems. He mentioned that he "was previously bothered with a common problem, which caused me much embarrassment"—this being the dreaded b.o. "It was the worst under my armpits and on my abdomen," he confessed.

His wife came to the rescue, however, with a solution she picked up from her grandmother. She bought a small bottle of rubbing alcohol and had her husband soak part of a clean washrag with it and then rub beneath his armpits and across his chest several times a day in the privacy of his university office. Surprisingly, the odor was eliminated in a jiffy. And all of this was accomplished without the benefit of a single commercial deodorant.

BODY PIERCING

Painful Piercing

In the last decade body piercing has become fashionable among many young people throughout the civilized world. Once a tribal custom relegated to the hinterlands of the African or Australian continents, body piercing is pretty standard fare in Europe and North America. Eyebrows, nose, lips, chin, and navel are common places for this to occur, as well as more unusual body parts that include the tongue, breast nipples, and a couple of other bizarre areas that I don't even dare mention in this text.

Even cartoonists are now getting around to satirizing this modern fad. The popular comic strip *Pirana Club* (formerly *Ernie*), drawn by Bo Grace and syndicated in hundreds of newspapers across the United States, poked a little fun at it in the strip that appeared in the comic section of the *Salt Lake Tribune*, Friday's edition for July 9, 1999. One of the regular characters, a pimply faced teenaged boy named Arnold, is seen arguing with his mother over the matter—she firmly resists the idea, and he is equally adamant about getting it done. The final panel shows him sitting at a table with his shirt off, while a body-piercing specialist (who himself is adorned with ten different rings across his naked upper torso) holds Arnold's left nipple down with a forefinger while raising his right fist in which is tightly clinched a wicked-looking ice pick. The boy warily looks at the instrument and inquires with obvious hesitation about his choice, "Is this going to hurt?" To which the other man casually replies, "Nah!"

Warding Off Infection

Body piercing is something I'm certainly very much opposed to. But there are many others who apparently feel differently and have submitted themselves to such bizarre mutilations. Ofttimes, though, the instruments used for piercing aren't always sterilized, and skin infections can result. Several young people who know of my reputation as a folk-healing expert and have encountered this problem for themselves during body-piercing episodes approached me for assistance.

I put together the following simple formula and gave them instructions as to how it could be used. In a *clean* small bowl or cup (preferably nonmetallic), mix together two tablespoons of apple-cider vinegar, one-half teaspoon of lemon or lime juice, and a pinch of sea salt. Using several cotton-tipped swabs held together, dip into this mixture and brush over the site(s) of skin infection.

It will definitely produce a mild burning sensation, but it's nothing to worry about. Be sure the area(s) in question are thoroughly washed with some of this solution. Repeat the application several times a day (three to four) for as long as needed.

The young people who followed these simple directions reported later that their skin infections had all cleared up. Unfortunately, none of them heeded my other advice to divest themselves of such silliness and become more responsible adults.

BOILS AND CARBUNCLES

Another Use for Pineapple

A boil and carbuncle are bacterial infections that begin deep in a hair follicle or an oil-producing gland and that gradually work their way up to the surface of the skin.

In the South Sea islands it is routine practice to lance such surface eruptions with a metal sewing needle or safety pin that has been previously sterilized by holding it over the open flame of a gas-stove burner, a cigarette lighter, a lit candle, or a match for about 45 seconds. Thick yellow pus will generally drain out after this procedure.

After this the skin surface is bathed with some freshly squeezed pineapple juice; sometimes a thin slice of *fresh* pineapple is even bound to the skin and kept in place for a while. Pineapple contains the wonderful enzyme bromelain, which reduces inflammation and expedites healing more rapidly. *Note:* It would be better if a medical professional incised such things rather than attempting to do it yourself.

BRAIN STRESS

Feed Your Head

During many years of innumerable free consultations with thousands of people, I've had more than my share of inquiries from those suffering from a variety of mental tensions that I've lumped into a single category and prefer calling "brain stress." A number of things can cause this: death of a loved one or favorite pet; loss of an old job or starting new employment somewhere else; marital discord; financial problems such as excess debt and not enough income; relocation to a new city or state; taking a school exam or driving test; behavioral problems with teenaged kids still at home; the prospect of undergoing surgery or visiting the dentist; and, of course, the much dreaded, universal feared IRS tax audit!

Well, there are ways to combat such "brain stress." Fatty-acid levels in the brain can be drastically altered by negative emotions and thoughts. That stress contributes to the destruction of long-chain fatty acids upon which the brain depends for much of its nourishment. Mental tension depletes essential fatty-acid levels by dumping them into the bloodstream from cell membranes in the brain; these eventually become oxidized and rancid. This may lead to free-radical injury if the body doesn't have enough antioxidants in the circulating blood plasma.

The obvious solution, therefore, seems to be to "feed your head" frequently with the one essential fatty acid upon which the brain depends so much, namely, omega-3. Ideal food sources for this include flaxseed oil (one tablespoon daily); dark, leafy, green vegetables or a good chlorophyll mix such as Kyo-Green (see Product Appendix under Wakunaga of America); canola and olive oils; fish (especially salmon, halibut, oysters, canned tuna, herring, sardines, mackerel, and trout); and eggs. Certain nut butters such as almond, cashew, and peanut, as well as whole nuts such as pecans, pistachios, and hazels, are also helpful. Brain stress can be easily corrected with these types of "smart foods."

BREAST CANCER

Frightening Stats

Investigative journalist Liane Chlorfene-Casten certainly didn't beat around the bush when she wanted to impress her readers of the seriousness of this disease in her aptly titled book, *Breast Cancer: Poisons, Profits and Prevention* (Monroe, ME: Common Courage Press, 1996). She titled her second chapter in the form of a question: "Are you the one in eight?" And then boldly marched forward with some frightening statistics that would alarm female readers.

"Breast cancer is now at epidemic proportions. *One in eight American women* has a lifetime risk of the disease. Each year, more than 44,000 women, or nearly one quarter of the 182,000 diagnosed, die from the disease. . . . Since 1960, more than 950,000 American women have died from breast cancer. To put this in perspective, only 617,000 Americans died in all the wars our country has fought in this century! And shockingly, almost half of these deaths have occurred in the last ten years, according to the 1994 Breast Cancer Health Project Fact Sheet, sponsored by the Massachusetts Department of Public Health."

A Plan of Action

If you are a woman and have been diagnosed with breast cancer, there are several options from which to choose: limited surgery and chemotherapy; radical surgery and chemotherapy; surgery plus chemo and radiation; chemo and radiation alone; *or* faith and prayer, a cancer-recovery eating plan, certain supplements and, if necessary, a VERY LIMITED "mix 'n' match" of the preceding three (surgery, chemo, radiation).

First and foremost is faith and prayer. There has *never* been a folk healer to my knowledge with whom I've worked in *any* culture worldwide who hasn't employed faith and prayer of *some kind* BEFORE, DURING, and AFTER natural treatments for different maladies. All those whom I interrogated and observed in more than 32 countries believed it was virtually impossible to successfully treat *any* disease without faith and prayer. Enough said for now on this issue!

The most basic plan for women with breast cancer to follow is this:

1. Reduce fat intake by a maximum of 25 percent of daily calories.
2. Increase daily fiber intake by no more than 40 percent.
3. Increase the daily intake of foods and supplements containing antiestrogens.

Let's look into the specifics of each of these general summaries to see what a woman *must do* in order to *permanently* defeat this disease ravaging her system.

First, replace *all* animal flesh with natural protein from a variety of plant sources. Soy makes one of the most ideal meat substitutes in this regard. A news report on the ABC Television *Good Morning, America* edition for Monday, July 12, 1999, mentioned how versatile soy can be in a number of different meal situations and how women with breast cancer should be eating more soy-based foods. Avocadoes and whole nuts and nut butters are excellent choices for protein needs. And though I did say to abstain from all *animal* flesh, this doesn't preclude the periodic consumption of certain fish, which should always be steamed, baked, or boiled but *never* fried or broiled. (I honestly believe that the iodine in seafood and assorted seaweeds such as kelp definitely help the female body in turning around a breast-cancer situation.)

Second, the intake of fiber should come mostly from cruciferous vegetables (cabbage, kale, kohlrabi, Brussels sprouts, cauliflower, mustard greens, watercress, spinach, broccoli, garlic, and onion), which are all very high in sulfur, a definite anticancer mineral. Additional fiber may come from squashes and pumpkin. Cooked (oatmeal, cracked wheat) or cold (Kellogg's Special K, All-Bran, Nabisco Shredded Wheat, Post Corn Flakes) cereals are equally valuable. Use soy, cashew, or goat's milk with them instead of regular cow's milk.

Finally, choose foods and supplements containing antiestrogens. Berries top my list in this regard: blackberries, blueberries, currants, grapes, and strawberries. Also include other fruits such as apricots, bananas, figs, cantaloupes, cherries, dates, oranges, pears, pineapple, and prunes. One must not forget the legumes either; I deliberately placed them here although they properly belong in the first "meatless" category as wonderful protein sources. Black beans, pinto beans, limas, and lentils are some of my favorites and can be made into delicious meals by cooking or baking them. Even something as simple as split-pea soup several times a week will provide the body with an amazing amount of antiestrogens to fight existing breast cancer.

In Japan, where breast cancer has always been historically very low in occurrence, women are prone to eating large amounts of algaes and seaweeds in the belief that such things will afford them protection against this disease. During the several trips I've made to Taiwan, I've noticed many women making and eating fish soup prepared with awonori; the whole fresh fronds impart a rich, nutlike taste to any food with which they are included. In some of the Japanese communities in Vancouver, British Columbia, and Puget Sound, Washington, the familiar red algae known as nori (or red laver with us) frequently graces many fish soups, fish wraps, and sea-vegetable tempuras. And during several tours of Japan, I always found the brown algae wakame being desalted and sun dried in prefectures stretching from south Ibaraki to north Miyagi Prefecture. Wakame is extremely popular with rice and bean-curd dishes. In Secul, South Korea, another type of brown algae, commonly called by its Japanese name of hijiki (nongmichae in Korean) imparts a lip-smacking nutlike flavor and crisp texture to whatever it is boiled, steamed, or simmered with.

On the American and European sides there is bladderwrack, dulse, and Irish moss, which are favorite ingredients in chowders, fish loaves, seaweed salads, hot lemonades and teas (believe it or not), shrimp cakes, puddings, and algae jellies. All of these variously described seaweeds (and many more) are rich in a number of trace elements that deactivate and help remove estrogenic compounds from the body that are definite breast-cancer inducers. No author that I know of who has written responsibly on this particular cancer has ever mentioned, let alone gone into depth on, so many seaweeds as I've done. I truly believe in them and am of the strong opinion that they could benefit women a lot if more were consumed in their diets, either to prevent getting breast cancer or in getting rid of the disease for good.

There are, of course, other supplements that have proven antiestrogenic activity to them that I like to recommend. Some of them come from Japan, such as Kyolic Garlic and Kyo-Green; others are medicinal mushrooms from the Orient such as maitake and reishi (various brands). Then there is Fat Complexer from ShapeRite for minimizing daily fat intake. A wonderful mineral blend called Concen-Trace is harvested from the Great Salt Lake and contains more than trace elements of known anticancer strength. And just about all the vitamins that anyone would ever need for a problem of this magnitude can be found in packet form in one handy box under the name of Total Care from Earth's Pharmacy. (Consult the Product Appendix for more information.)

A final favorite and an "absolute MUST" in *any* cancer-treatment program is red beets. This vegetable can be juiced or cooked. Pines International of Lawrence, Kansas, manufactures a very good Beet Root Juice Powder that has formed part of my "core program" intended for cancer therapy. There is something in the red pigment itself that works against breast cancer (and for that matter *all* other forms of cancer) in an unbelievable way. Use a Vita-Mix unit to shred and juice fresh beets after cutting them into small pieces first.

Let's Not Forget the Miscellaneous Either

Other activities that play a prominent role in any sensible cancer-recovery program would include drinking more water, moderately exercising (walking), meditating to put the mind at ease, and developing a HUMBLE determination to come off the victor in something not so easily conquered. Keeping the system clean and free of pollution always seems to be the first step in both cancer prevention as well as in treatment, irrespective of whatever form that pollution may appear in.

BREAST PAIN

What to Do Before You See a Doctor

Four of the most common sources of breast pain can be pregnancy and breast-feeding, premenstrual syndrome (PMS), lumpy (fibrocystic) breasts, and hormone-replacement therapy.

Many childbearing women are subject to sore breasts and tender nipples beginning from early pregnancy and concluding only when the child is weaned. Nipple problems can be greatly minimized if a woman will massage her nipples with the thumb and forefinger of each hand. Or she can vigorously rub them with a rough towel after bathing or showering. Nipples can also be massaged with pure lanolin and then exposed to fresh air and sunshine for a while to give additional relief.

Sore nipples may be gently rubbed with olive or flaxseed oil following each infant feeding. Used tea bags kept in their original water and then refrigerated until needed also help; these may be applied over tender nipples to relieve their soreness. The tannic acid in them toughens nipple skin. The best tea for this is a solution made by boiling acorns or oak bark, then cooling it down. Several cotton balls bunched together, soaked in such tea and then laid over the nipples really make the skin around them a lot tougher .

Nipples should never be washed with any kind of soap since it has a tendency to dry out the skin and promote cracking. Lactating breasts should always be cleansed with warm water. A good support bra with convenient flaps that can be left open should be worn.

During breast-feeding a mother's breasts may become painfully swollen. In the event such a thing happens, a breast pump should be used to remove the milk, or else the infant should be fed by hand. A hot washcloth put over the nipples will hasten milk flow. A nonnursing mom, however, needs to wait until all of her milk dries up for the painful swelling, tenderness, or hardness of the breasts to subside. Before this occurs, though, a woman might want to wear a tight bra and apply ice packs. To make an ice pack, a woman should wrap several ice cubes in a plastic bag. The bag should then be wrapped in a clean hand towel and apply over the congested breast for 30 minutes. The ice pack is removed for 20 minutes before reapplying. *Never* place an ice pack directly on the skin as this will result in frostbite damage.

If breast pain, soreness, or tenderness is due to PMS or fibrocystic breasts there are a number of self-help measures that a woman can safely employ to give her relief. Caffeine should be eliminated from the diet because it is a strong link to breast pain. This means NO coffee, tea, colas, soft drinks, coca, chocolate, herbal-energy formulas (containing kola nut), or over-the-counter medications with small amounts of caffeine in them. Fried and deep-fried foods should be curtailed. A woman should avoid smoking or inhaling secondhand smoke. Sugary foods should be severely limited. Moderate exercise gets rid of the excess fat that causes fibrocystic breasts. Alcohol and salt intake should be somewhat restricted as well.

Water-holding fruits and vegetables should form a necessary part of the diet of any woman who is troubled with breast pain. Such foods would include cantaloupe, watermelon, cucumber, cabbage, lettuce, spinach, watercress, grapes, and berries. Drinking herbal teas that are natural diuretics that help to eliminate excess fluids are also useful: chervil, chickweed, chicory, dandelion, juniper, pansy, parsley, peach leaf, sarsaparilla, and stinging nettle. An average of one to two tea-spoons of any one of these herbs steeped in a pint of hot water for 25 minutes makes a diuretic tea when cooled enough to drink.

Certain nutrients seem more beneficial at relieving breast pain than do others. Vitamin B-6 (100 mg.), vitamin C (500 mg.), vitamin E (400 IU), brewer's yeast (two capsules or tablets or one-quarter tea-spoon daily), and magnesium (600 mg.) are recommended on a daily basis for as long as breast pain lasts.

Aerobic Exercise

One of the things I've had some women tell me that has helped them relieve their breast pain is some form of aerobic exercise. This might include trampoline bouncing, horseback riding, rope jumping, stair climbing, swimming, or playing tennis or basketball. The constant up-and-down motions of the body (and the breasts) causes an inward re-lease of endorphins, which is the system's own natural pain-relieving substances.

Heat is yet another way to obtain comfort. A warm bath, heating pad, or hot-water bottle work nicely in the reduction of breast pain. The application of a few drops of eucalyptus or tea-tree oil or rubbing a little Mentholatum or Vicks salve on a sore breast and then covering it with a cotton cloth will engender a nice feeling of warmth in min-utes and will help to dispel pain.

Natural Alternatives to Hormone Therapy

There are certain herbs that are of especial value for those women seeking natural alternatives to hormone-replacement therapy. Alfalfa, black cohosh, clover, fenugreek, dong quai (dongguei), fennel, licorice root, and sage all manifest varying degrees of estrogenic activity in the female system. These herbs may be consumed in capsule or tablet form (two to three daily) or else maybe drunk as a warm beverage (one cup) away from a meal.

The ShapeRite company markets a nice Female Formula that assists hormone regulation inside a woman's body. It is recommended that one capsule of this product be taken morning, noon, and night with meals. (See Product Appendix for additional information.)

BREAST SWELLING

Exercising the Problem Away

If a woman discovers swelling in one or both of her breasts, she shouldn't draw the wrong conclusions and panic. Breast swelling may be due to birth-control pills or postmenopausal estrogen-replacement therapy. Also fibrous cysts, inflamed sweat glands, and other benign conditions can lead to breast swelling. Any significant swelling, however, should obviously be checked by a physician. If the swelling is a relatively harmless thing, it can be corrected by very simple stretching exercises.

Assume an easy standing position, with your feet parallel about 5 inches apart and the heels solidly anchored to the floor. Slowly raise the right arm to shoulder level in front of you; then raise the left one parallel to it. Bring one arm back behind your body as far as you can, then alternate with the other arm. Continue this procedure rhythmically. As one arm comes forward, the other one goes back as though you were resisting the wind or swimming in the air.

Keeping both heels well anchored to the floor, bring the arms down to the sides and position the head at a straight level. Now bring one arm forward to shoulder level; keep it extended in front of you. Then bring the other one parallel to it. Take a full breath. Exhale as you raise both arms overhead and bring the backs of the hands together, while at the same time shifting your full weight back over the balls of your feet.

Inhale as the arms flow wide apart and slowly outward to shoulder level. Exhale as they rise again and the hands meet back to back overhead. After repeating this a few times, you will start to experience a feeling of surprising rejuvenation, particularly in the upper torso of your body.

Stand in a relaxed position for a few minutes and gently shake various parts of your body in loose fashion. Gradually roll the head around the neck from left to right. This is to loosen any muscle tension that may be present.

Assume another standing position with the legs 10 or 12 inches apart. Raise the arms to an upward V position. Rise on the right toe and raise the entire right side of the torso. Carry the right arm over to the left side so that the palm of the right hand flows over to the palm of the left hand. The right arm returns to the open V position before the weight is shifted to the left toe. Do the same on the left side. Continue until the shifting is done with such ease and grace that the whole movement is a continuous flow from one side to the other.

These extensions from the tips of the toes to the tips of the fingers overhead are the longest of which the body is capable. Always remember to breathe when your arms are in the open V position and to exhale as they move from side to side. Do these few exercises every day for about ten minutes. You will be astonished at how effective they are in reducing not only breast swelling but also some breast pain, too.

A famous Russian ballerina shared some of these exercises with me many years ago when I visited her country with a number of other scientists. We were in Moscow at the time—the summer of 1979 it seems—and had watched her perform at the Kirov Theater. Afterwards, some of us had a chance to speak with a few of the ballerinas backstage. She spoke fairly good English. She told me about these exercises and even went to the trouble of demonstrating them for my benefit. Whenever she noticed a slight swelling in one or both breasts or experienced some minor breast pain she would do these exercises for a few minutes every day in her apartment or backstage at the theater.

BROKEN BONES

Emergency Treatment

A broken bone or skull fracture requires immediate medical attention. No physical movement of any kind should be allowed except by competent medical personnel. The affected area should be promptly immobilized as much as possible. Rolled-up newspapers, magazines, bath towels, and blankets as well as short, straight, and medium-thick pieces of sawed wood can all serve as temporary but adequate splinting materials.

In any injury such as this, the victim should remain calm and not become agitated. Consuming lukewarm water is one way of helping to achieve this. Diverting one's attention away from the injury to something else more pleasant keeps the mind from becoming panicky. Ice packs gently laid over the fracture or break will reduce swelling, inflammation, and pain.

X-rays will be necessary to determine the full extent of the injury. The fractured or broken bone may need to be set in traction by the attending physician. If the doctor wants to prescribe drugs to help control the pain, you can choose to decline them and instead opt for something more natural.

A Wonderful Tea for Pain Relief

Some years ago I was visiting with some friends in the eastern Canadian city of Sault Sainte-Marie in Ontario Province. Their rambunctious 13-year-old boy tripped outdoors on some stairs leading to their front door and broke his wrist. The parents and I worked together to make him more comfortable. I had them tape two wooden paint-stirring sticks on either side of the break, while I made a brew to help relieve the terrible pain the kid was feeling.

In one-and-a-half pints of boiling water I put two tablespoons wintergreen (Canada tea) leaves, one tablespoon diced celery stalk, one teaspoon skullcap plant, and three teaspoons valerian root. I stirred everything thoroughly, covered the pot with a lid, and reduced the gas flame to simmer for about four minutes. I then set it aside to steep until the tea became lukewarm. The boy was given a full six-ounce glass to drink. In less than five minutes he reported, with a happy smile on his face, that he no longer felt any pain.

He was then taken to a hospital emergency room some distance away, where the injury was properly set in a cast by doctors. They were astonished to find that he felt no pain and inquired of the parents what he had been given prior to being brought to them. The parents told the doctors about the herbal tea I had prepared, and one of them came over and quizzed me about it. I found this particular emergency-room doctor to be quite open-minded and I volunteered my formula, which he hastily scribbled down. Whatever became of that I never learned. But I know it worked well enough to relieve the boy's pain, and that's what counted the most.

Bone-Knitting Herbs

There are certain other medicinal herbs that have the unique property of hastening the healing of bone fractures and breaks. They are fenugreek seed, slippery-elm bark, comfrey root, boneset herb, and marshmallow root and leaves. Most of them are somewhat mucilaginous, meaning when cooked into a hot tea they demonstrate slick and slimy properties. They can be used together or paired separately with satisfying results. The tea is made exactly the same way as my pain-relieving formula.

Other plant foods that strengthen bone rebuilding include kale, watercress, endive, Romaine lettuce, and parsley. These dark, leafy, green vegetables are high in calcium, magnesium, potassium, phosphorus, and boron, all of which are bone-building minerals and necessary for injuries such as this. Trace Minerals Research of Roy, Utah (see Product Appendix) makes a Complete Calcium Hydrooxyapatite that includes all the above minerals and works wonders in situations such as this.

A Faith-Healing Episode

In my lifelong study of folk medicine, I have almost always found the element of faith present in whichever healers I've worked with or interviewed around the globe. I've also discovered similar dramatic episodes of faithhealing in action in the published autobiographies and family histories of different people.

One of the more remarkable true stories came from a book written by Irvin L. and Lexia D. Warnock entitled *Our Sixty Years Together: The Story of Our Lives* (Provo, UT: J. Grant Stevenson, 1973; p. 34). A son, D. Carl Warnock, Jr., related what happened to him as a young Mormon boy growing up in the south-central Utah community of Richfield many years ago.

"The time my arm was broken will always stand out as a truly faith promoting experience. . . . The Doctor cleaned up the wounds around the protruding bones as best he could and attempted to set the bones. Because of the problem involved, the Doctor thought it best to not completely set the arm and straighten it at that time. So, when we left the Doctor's office the bones were not in place. The Doctor said he'd let it heal as it was, then re-break it for a better set later on . . .

"Because of the pain in the arm and the accompanying restlessness I couldn't sleep that night. So, Dad was asked to use his priesthood to give me a blessing. Brother Sam Gurr was called to help with the administration. Athough it was not promised during the blessing, I felt assured that I would not have to have the arm re-broken.

"After I had gone upstairs to bed, Mother came to lie beside me on the bed because I was very restless and in much pain. Sometime, in the quiet of the night, I both heard and felt a movement take place in the bone of that arm. It was so real and so loud that I sat upright in bed. And I said, 'Mom did you hear that?' I was somewhat surprised when she said, 'Hear what?' I said, 'I heard the bones in my arm move, Mom. I know they moved.' Almost immediately I lay down and slept peacefully the rest of the night.

"When we visited the Doctor's office a few days later, the x-rays verified that the bones had moved and that, whereas they were not perfectly straight, they were near enough so that the re-breaking was not necessary." (See also "Fractures.")

BRONCHITIS

Something Yummy for the Tummy

Grasshoppers—naturally dried and salted like beer nuts—gave hunter-gatherers around Utah's Great Salt Lake a food source that surpassed even venison in terms of calories returned for hours invested.

The Utah State Historical Society, after finding bits and pieces of millions of grasshoppers scattered over once-inhabited levels of a cave alongside the Great Salt Lake, went hunting for an explanation. Prehistoric human feces revealed more grasshopper parts mixed with sand.

The mystery became clear when some archaeologists and this anthropologist noticed that dead grasshoppers were sometimes piled in neat rows with up to 100,000 hoppers per square meter (10.7 square feet) along the lake's eastern beach. They apparently had wound up in the salt water, died, and been washed up on the shore—sun dried, salted, and ready to eat.

The team I was with figured that Native Americans could have collected an average 273,000 grasshopper calories per hour at such bountiful times, while hunting large game provided just 25,000 calories per hour. Something yummy for the tummy, perhaps?

Bronchitis Broken

One of our small group at that time was a chronic smoker and suffered from serious bronchitis. You could hear his wheezing a mile away. The accumulated sputum in his bronchial tubes produced a dry hacking cough but refused to come up. Being made aware of my expertise with herbs, he came to me and inquired what he could do for his condition.

I suggested that he stop smoking or, at the very least, drastically reduce his nicotine intake. I devised a solution for him that was both easy and effective. It consisted of adding one teaspoonful of apple-cider vinegar and two drops of peppermint or tea-tree (melaleuca) oil to a cup of hot black coffee. After things were mixed up a bit, he was to slowly sip it. He was told to repeat the same procedure again in the evening.

He faithfully followed my instructions for about 11 days and reported large amounts of thick, yellow mucus coming up. His wheezing ceased, and he was able to breathe much better. He was somewhat amazed that such simple things could accomplish so much for relatively little cost.

As for those hordes of ready-to-eat grasshoppers . . . they're still floating in the briny waters of the Great Salt Lake or else resting in huge piles on its sandy beaches. Think of all that lovely protein going to waste!

BRUISES

An Eggs-Pert

Wally Hendricks knows a great deal about eggs. It is his job to convince Americans that they need to eat more of them. When we met at a recent food-industry convention in Las Vegas, he rattled off half a dozen egg facts. The color of the shell doesn't affect the quality, flavor, or nutritional value. The yolk color depends on the type of feed the hen consumes. Most recipes are based on "large" eggs, as are nutrition data (60 calories, 5 grams of fat, and 215 mgs. of cholesterol). Jumbo eggs are 25 percent larger; medium eggs, 15 percent smaller than large ones.

The yolk contains most of the nutrients, nearly half the protein, and all the fat and cholesterol. The white cordlike strands of egg whites that anchor the yolk in the center are called chalaze. Prominent, thick ones indicate high quality and freshness. It isn't necessary to wash eggs before storing or using them. They are routinely washed when commercially processed.

I congratulated Wally on being a true "eggs-pert" and knowing his subject well.

Bruising Made Easy

Wally is one of those people who bruises pretty easily. He showed me a couple of black-and-blue spots that he had casually sustained while at the convention. He asked what could be done for this problem.

I reminded him that he needed more calcium and vitamin K. To get more of these essential nutrients, I encouraged him to consume lots of dark, leafy greens, such as Swiss chard, collards, kale, spinach, mustard greens, and watercress. I advised him to invest in a Vita-Mix food processor and to juice some of these vegetables, too. I suggested he take at least 1,000 mgs. of timed-release vitamin C twice daily, along with citrus bioflavonoids such as rutin or hesperidin (60 mgs.).

He did this for a couple of weeks before calling me at my office one day to say how he didn't bruise so easily anymore and thanked me for my counsel.

BULIMIA

The "Binge-and-Purge" Syndrome

Much has been written about the final decline of ancient Rome. In the twilight years of its fading glory, Rome was a regular cesspool of debauchery and corruptions of every imagination.

One such extreme indulgence commonly took place during some of its frenzied pagan celebrations. As Edward Gibbon noted in his massive history, *The Decline and Fall of The Roman Empire* (London: 1807; 2:293), "on days of [such] general festivity, it was the custom of the ancients to adorn their doors with lamps and with branches of laurel and to crown their heads with a garland of flowers." The representations for all this signified "that the doors were under the protection of the household gods, that the laurel was sacred to the lover of Daphne, and that garlands of flowers, though frequently worn as a symbol either of joy or mourning, had been dedicated in their first origin to the service of superstition."

"The infectious breath of idolatry," as he aptly described it, filled the air everywhere. There was a strong sense of "riotous jubilation" in the Roman citizenry. Think Carnival days in Rio de Janeiro, Oktoberfest in Munich, or the much vaunted Mardi Gras week in New Orleans, and you begin to have a sense of sheer "crowd craziness" going on day and night.

In that long-ago era, bulimia was socially fashionable during festivals such as these. Numerous banquets could be found all over the city, and people went feasting from place to place as the night wore on. In many dwellings a special room called a vomitorium was set aside in which gluttonous Romans could go to deliberately disengorge whatever they ate and drank and then go back to the dinner tables for more helpings of food and beverage.

Today, though, the reason for such bizarre behavior, mostly among women, is an abnormal fear of becoming fat, an obsession with remaining (or becoming) thin, plus a fierce hunger for food. Continual vomiting can lead to dehydration, electrolyte imbalances, and serious malnutrition unless corrected.

An Italian Gastroenterologist's Guidelines

Dr. Lorenzo Paschetti is an Italian gastroenterologist who specializes in the treatment of bulimia. Ironically, most of his young female clientele between the ages of 15 and 30 come from Europe, the Middle East, and North America. In fact, he treats very few Italian girls with this problem. He has developed a sensible program that seems to be working for many of them.

He encourages his patients to eat many *small* meals every day. High on his list is snacking, which is done on a regular basis in between those other meals. He places heavy emphasis on leafy green salads with Roquefort cheese made of ewes' milk and ripened in damp caves. He believes that sliced apples and picked grapes accompanied with goat cheese and crackers makes tasty snacks. He encourages the consumption of root vegetables such as carrots, parsnips, radishes, turnips, and potatoes, eaten either raw or boiled or baked.

He gives unusual attention to the types of beverages his bulimic patients drink. He is a big fan of mineral water to help restore electrolyte imbalances. But he also reserves places for a little wine, a fair amount of grape juice, some herbal teas (chamomile and peppermint mostly), and, of course, spring water. The intake of mixed fluids such as these helps patients to overcome their food phobias, he believes.

He differs from his colleagues in Europe and North America in that he places little reliance upon supplements. But for those willing to spend the money, he recommends 500 mgs. of calcium citrate or microcrystalline hydroxyapatite and 300 mgs. of magnesium citrate or aspartate twice daily. Most bulimics are usually somewhat hypoglycemic, so 200 mcgs. of chromium each day is useful.

He's all for digestive enzymes, but feels a person does better by obtaining them from ripe fruits such as papaya, pineapple, guava, or mango. His approach to bulimia, while a little unorthodox for many doctors, does appear to have considerable merit because it has cured many women of their eating disorders *permanently!*

BUNIONS

Belly-Dancing Festival

Having been raised in a home where cultural appreciation was taught to my brother and me at an early age, I have become a strong supporter of the arts in my adulthood. I enjoy live theater, ballet, opera, concerts, sensible paintings, good books, deep poetry, fine libraries, and outstanding museums.

One of these arts, which is actually quite ancient from a historical perspective but may not be considered cultural by many people, is belly dancing. I dine at fine Near Eastern restaurants periodically where I can enjoy this particular art form, though some prudes may regard this as being bad due to the slightly immodest attire of the performers. But for this anthropologist it is certainly more than mere entertainment, and I take pleasure in the skill with which such dance maneuvers are so carefully executed.

The Middle East & International Dance Gala—indoors, with one stage—made its debut Friday and Saturday, August 13–14, 1999, at the Hellenic Memorial Building in downtown Salt Lake City. Included with this event was the Twentieth Annual Kismet Belly Dance Festival. Guest artists from around the world attended, including some from Egypt, Jordan, Lebanon, and Syria.

I spoke with festival organizer Yasamina Roque, who informed me that this belly dancing event is the largest and longest-running festival of its kind in North America. I watched with great fascination one evening as an Egyptian dancer named Delilah Aziz moved her way gracefully through a couple of numbers, the "Desert Orchid Dance" and the bawdier "Cairo Cabaret."

Belly-Dancer Bunions

As a specially invited guest, I had the opportunity to attend several workshops that featured Syrian-style belly dancing, veil techniques from Lebanon, and Jordanian percussion action. Delilah spoke pretty good English and shared with me a few of her health tips. She complained that the most frequent injury encountered in her profession was from bunions that invariably formed on the first joints of big toes. This was especially prominent in those who often chose to dance barefooted.

She told me what she did to treat such symptoms after each performance. First, she would reduce the redness and swelling with an ice pack kept at the base of the big toe for up to 20 minutes. After drying the area with a clean wash cloth, she would then anoint the afflicted area with a small mixture of fenugreek seed powder (one-eighth teaspoon) and olive oil (one teaspoon). This helped remove the pain and promote more rapid healing.

BURNS

An Effective Treatment from Vietnam

CAUTION: Burns are serious business and need immediate medical attention! Self-treatment of extreme burns should never be attempted without qualified medical assistance of some kind. While the following information is true and will work, it was used in a very rural setting where no regular medical help was available. Neither the author nor his publisher encourage the use of this remedy as long as regular medical care can be obtained.

Steve Forbush, a longtime resident of Cleveland, Ohio, and his Vietnamese wife, Sun, have several of my health books from Prentice Hall—*Anti-Aging Remedies, Nuts, Berries & Seeds, Miracle Healing Herbs,* and *Healing Juices.* He found my unlisted home phone number in the back of several of them and decided to give me a call on Thursday, June 24, 1999. He said, "I read every one of your books from cover to cover, and I want to thank you for the excellent work you've done helping others get well."

He has been a brakeman–conductor for the River Terminal Railroad that services LTV Steel Company for 26 years and likes his job a lot. Steve thought I might be able to use the following incredible remedy that his wife remembers being used many years ago by the local shaman in the small South Vietnamese village where she and her family then lived. Two boys between the ages of 10 and 12 were accidentally burned by some hot oil. Being far away from conventional medical facilities and in an extremely remote area, the only possible treatment available at the time was a particular folk remedy.

It consisted of soaking an unspecified number of banana skins in a ceramic vat filled with vinegar for several days and then straining the mixture into another ceramic container for storage. Both boys were treated with this solution every day for a few weeks. Their burns were washed and soaked with this banana-skin vinegar.

Sun testified that they experienced very little pain during the whole ordeal. And after they had fully recovered from their terrible accident, there was *no* evidence of any scarring. She has used this remedy a few times since coming to America for similar burns with very good effect.

BURSITIS

What Is It?

Located between our muscles and tendons or between muscles and bones are fluid-filled sacs called bursas. They secrete a lubricant to minimize friction occurring from frequent physical movements in the shoulders, elbows, wrists, hands, hips, knees, heels, and the base of the big toes.

When any of them become inflamed, bursitis results. Common symptoms include joint pain and swelling, restricted and painful physical motion, and pain that radiates into the neck, arms, or fingertips (due to shoulder bursitis). Sometimes these things may be accompanied by a slight fever if an infection is associated with the inflammation.

I had a touch of bursitis in the top of my left shoulder that left me in so much pain in January 1998 that I couldn't sleep properly, managed to shower only with the greatest of difficulty, and was barely able to finish typing the manuscript for my fifty-sixth book, *Natural Pet Cures*, which came out later that year. I was using some folk remedies as well as faith healing to overcome my torturous ordeal and was seeing some results occur, although rather slowly. Realizing, though, that I had several upcoming media and speaking events in New York City, I decided to end my pain more quickly and went to a local doctor who gave me several injections of corticosteroids. That alone produced such intense pain that I let forth a loud scream that nearly scared some elderly folks in the front waiting room half to death. But after that I was able to complete my trip relatively free of further agony.

Elbow Healed Naturally

Throughout 1999 I spent considerable time on our 400-acre family farm in the southern Utah wilderness performing many heavy chores that required a lot of physical labor. While the overall workout did me good, it also produced bursitis in my elbow. But this time I took capsules of fenugreek seed (two daily) and slippery-elm bark (2 daily) for a month as well as rubbing some consecrated olive oil that had been blessed by the priesthood on the site. This folk-medicine combination of herbal therapy and faith healing eventually proved to be just as effective as the corticosteroids, although not as quickly.

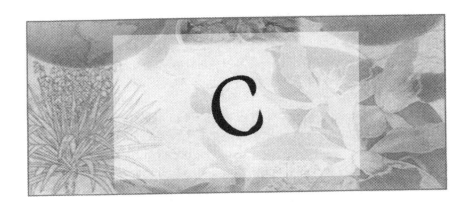

CAFFEINISM

Lock Up Juan Valdez!

For a number of years the National Coffee Association has been heavily promoting the robust flavor and stimulant virtues of Colombia coffee in the mythical advertising character of the simple peasant Juan Valdez and his favorite burro. Because of his humble charm and cleverly packaged message more Americans are drinking coffee than ever before. And the soft-drink world, in its quest for the next big hit, has turned to caffeine-spiked beverages. That can mean anything from colas blended with coffee to caffeinated orange juice. Even health food stores now carry energy-boosting supplements and drinks containing caffeine derived from kola or bissy-nut extracts.

Since smoking has fallen out of favor with many people these days, caffeine has supplanted nicotine as our nation's socially accepted drug of choice. Literally, Colombian java, Mountain Dew, and Pep! (an herbal energy booster) has replaced Joe Camel of previous cigarette fame. An ordinary 12-ounce serving of coffee yields 200 mg. of caffeine; the same size serving of Coca-Cola or Pepsi around 45 mg. The wide appeal of caffeine, according to an article in *The Wall Street Journal* for Tuesday, December 17, 1996 (p. B-4) is due to its "make-me-feel-good" aspect.

Mental Disorders

In 1996 the august American Psychiatric Association based in our nation's capital (an appropriate location, it would seem, considering all of the looney politicians based there), published an immense volume (886 pages) found in every shrink's office. Formally called the Diagnostic and Statistical Manual of Mental Disorders, it now goes by the catchy nickname DSM-IV.

On page 212, DSM-IV lists a rich menu of "Caffeine-Induced Disorders." Disorder #305.9 (every mental problem has its own serial number, something akin to what is found in an auto-parts catalog) is "Caffeine Intoxication." DSM-IV sets out in grim detail the "Diagnostic Criteria for #305.9 Caffeine Intoxication":

A. Recent consumption of caffeine, usually in excess of 250 mg. (e.g., more than 2–3 cups of brewed coffee).

B. Five or more of the following signs, developing during, or shortly after, caffeine use: (1) restlessness; (2) nervousness; (3) excitement; (4) insomnia; (5) flushed face; (6) diuresis (frequent urination); (7) gastrointestinal disturbance; (8) muscle twitching; (9) rambling flow of thought and speech; (10) tachycardia or cardiac arrhythmia; (11) periods of inexhaustibility; and (12) psychomotor agitation.

But the awful truth about this highly addictive substance doesn't end there; DSM-IV takes it to an even more severe level. Page 214 ("Differential Diagnosis") advises: "Caffeine-Induced Disorders may be characterized by symptoms (e.g., Panic Attacks) that resemble primary mental disorders (e.g., Panic Disorder versus Caffeine-Induced Anxiety Disorder, With Panic Attacks, With Onset During Intoxication)."

If you thought tobacco was addictive, just read on to find out what DSM-IV has to say about "Caffeine Withdrawal" (pages 708 and 709): "A characteristic withdrawal syndrome . . . Drowsiness, fatigue and mood changes from coffee withdrawal can mimic Amphetamine or Cocaine Withdrawal." Typical symptoms include "headache," "marked anxiety or depression," "nausea or vomiting," and "worsened cognitive performance (especially vigilance tasks)."

And whereas tobacco's ill effects are delayed for decades, the symptoms of caffeine intoxication are immediate: "during or shortly after caffeine use," DSM-IV says. Caffeine withdrawal symptoms "can begin within 12 hours of cessation of caffeine use, peak around 20–40 hours and last up to 1 week."

Based on this scientific information the Food and Drug Administration should be putting as much effort and funds into banning caf-

feine as the Drug Enforcement Agency has been in trying to ban cocaine and marijuana.

Alternative Solutions

Kicking the caffeine habit (or any other addiction for that matter) isn't
as difficult as it seems. Oh sure, there are going to be some ups and
downs along the way, but the process can be easier than realized if
strong will and a sense of determination are in place in the mind and
heart before the challenging journey begins.

First, there is a satisfying solution for coffee drinkers intent on
quitting caffeine: herbal coffee made from the roasted roots and grains
of dandelion, chicory, beet, barley, and rye. The search for this incredible blend is something of an adventure by itself and worth retelling
here. A colleague of mine, Dr. Peter Gail, a retired ethnobotanist who
taught for years at Rutgers, Princeton, and Cleveland State universi-
ties, became acquainted with some of my Prentice Hall health best-
sellers a while back and was impressed with my work.

On a trip to Wales one time, he discovered a peculiar beverage
product called Dandelion Coffee Compound by Symington and began
importing this to the United States and selling it to some of his friends,
family, and college students. In the meantime, on several trips to
Toronto, Canada, in an out-of-the-way health-food store I came across
another coffee alternative called Thuna Instant Dandelion Blend. I began recommending that to those who wished to quit the coffee habit
for good.

In the meantime my friend Dr. Gail began championing the lowly
dandelion in different ways. He wrote a book entitled *Dandelion Celebration: Guide to Unexpected Cuisine;* started the annual National Dandelion Cookoff in 1994; formed an organization, the Defenders of
Dandelion, with over a thousand members nationwide; and began
publishing an occasional newsletter for them and the media, *Dandelion
Doings.*

We eventually pooled our research talents and came up with a
unique beverage "Dandelion Java" that looks, tastes, and smells like
the real thing, but isn't. It comes in a one-pound container, and
slightly less than a teaspoon of the powdered blend will instantly dis-
solve in a cup of hot *or* cold water. A little cream and honey may be
added if desired, but it tastes just as good when taken plain. The ingre-

dients have been specifically designed to satisfy those receptor sites located within the brain that respond quickly to caffeine. Everyone who has gone on this beverage has not only quit drinking coffee but has also stopped smoking in many cases, not to mention quitting beer and hard liquor in other instances as well. (To order one pound of this Dandelion Java, contact the Anthropological Research Center, P.O. Box 11471, Salt Lake City, UT 84147.

Habitual coffee drinkers require three things to remain satisfied without coffee. The first is a need to satisfy the sense with a full-bodied flavor and roasted aroma accompanied by a deep, opaque color. The aforementioned Dandelion Java fills this role nicely. So does Postum (a roasted cereal grain-derived product) to some extent as well as herbal teas made from the roots of burdock, chicory, or dandelion or from roasted sunflower seeds; but as a rule these tend to be somewhat weaker in flavor and body. Dandelion Java, on the other hand, produces an ebony-black, full-bodied brew that has multiple flavor notes and an enticing aroma besides.

Second, ardent coffee drinkers are "hooked" on caffeine, and withdrawal can be tough under certain conditions. The familiar mid-morning migraine may become a common thing when the body starts missing its usual cups of coffee. To alleviate this somewhat, I've always suggested taking two to three capsules of white-willow bark at the onset of pain; it generally gives quick relief.

Exercise and water consumption is another way to combat caffeinism. Working up a good 15-minute sweat doing some simple aerobics and afterwards consuming eight fluid ounces of *cool* (but not cold) water will refresh and rejuvenate the body more than you can imagine.

Caffeinism produces not only anxiety and panic disorders (as cited in the DSM-IV report), but other symptoms as well, such as depression, irritability, nervousness, recurrent headaches, and heart palpitations. Many caffeine-craving individuals who have sought me out for different health advice usually are hypoglycemic and suffer from poor adrenal and/or thyroid function. I take them off *all* foods containing sugar (even fruit and fruit juices), stop their coffee and soft-drink consumptions, and encourage them to eat five to seven small meals regularly throughout the day or just enough to raise their energy levels again. I also require them to walk at least one mile every day. This simple regimen helps get rid of the "caffeine blues," rebuilds energy, and increases confidence.

Periodically I will suggest taking St. Johnswort (one to two capsules daily). A good deal of clinical research has already proven its value in getting rid of anxiety and depression. A suitable brand is sold by Earth's Pharmacy (see Product Appendix for details).

The Power of Prayer

In suggesting that prayer can be one of the most powerful tools in escaping addictions such as caffeine, I am not promoting any particular religious belief. Prayer is as universal and essential as rain or sunshine and to be found in *every* single culture and among numerous folk healers whom I've personally visited and investigated. It is *the* most potent spiritual discipline known to humankind. Each one of us is connected in some way with Providence. Because of this, when we pray we are doing so to something *and* someone. The glory of surrender to a will and presence greater than our own is a wonderful miracle in and of itself.

Sometimes I've encouraged believing souls to utter simple child-like prayers to Providence in the hope and faith that their addictions will be taken from them. In most cases this happens after some initial effort is put forth on the part of those praying.

Caffeine Can Control Asthma

A study published in the medical journal *Chest* (94(2):386–89, 1988) examined a randomly selected group of more than 72,000 coffee drinkers and nondrinkers; compared to the coffee abstainers, those who average one cup of java per day had 95 percent of the risk of having an asthma attack. But coffee drinkers who average two to three cups daily had less than 75 percent of the risk.

The explanation for this is fairly simple: one of caffeine's breakdown products in the body is theophylline, a substance widely prescribed for treating asthma. Air is delivered to and removed from the lung tissue by a network of bronchial tubes. These tubes spasm during an asthma attack, thus preventing the movement of life-sustaining air. Theophylline is a bronchodilator, which means it stops the spasm and reopens the bronchial tubes to restore normal breathing.

Once ingested, caffeine reaches its peak concentration in the bloodstream in about one hour. Its antiasthmatic effects continue to increase beyond that time, reaching a peak sometime between one and a half and four hours later, depending upon which measure of breathing capacity is used. The effect can last as long as six hours.

Just how potent is caffeine? In one double-blind study published in *Chest* (89(3):335–42, 1986), nine asthmatic patients drank brewed decaffeinated coffee to which varying amounts of caffeine had been added. Two hours later, the amount of caffeine normally found in a single cup of regular coffee (150 mg) had produced a 15 percent increase in the volume of air the patients were able to expire in one second. Caffeine's effect was judged to be 40 percent as potent as that of theophylline.

An asthmatic will definitely benefit from a few cups of *warm* black coffee (no cream or sugar) in the event he or she experiences an acute attack but has no regular asthma medication available to take care of the situation. I've occasionally used this remedy myself for lung congestion due to a cold or flu with terrific results.

CANCER

The Disease Defined

While cancer may seem to many of us as something of a modern epidemic, if the truth be known, it is really 5,500 years old. *An X-Ray Atlas of the Royal Mummies* [of Egypt] (Chicago: University of Chicago Press, 1980) mentioned tumors being found in some of the pharoahs of the Old and Middle Kingdoms. The Bible (II Kings 20:1–7) relates how Hezekiah, King of Judah (726–697 B.C.) was stricken with an unspecified malignant tumor and prepared to die but was healed of his affliction by the prophet Isaiah, who gave his servants a poultice of fresh figs to lay on the disease. *The Jewish Encyclopedia* (New York: Funk and Wagnalls Co., 1904; 6:381) suggested a number of mental and emotional issues that bothered Hezekiah and may very well have precipitated this disease—one of them being his lengthy unmarried status which was finally resolved when he took Isaiah's own daughter for a wife after recovering from his frightening ordeal. And Hippocrates (circa 400 B.C.), the eminent Greek physician, certainly knew about skin cancer, for he coined the term "carcinoma" for it, which comes from the Greek *karkinoma* meaning "crab"; this is how the cancer spreads, in crablike fashion, extending "claws" across cells, tissues, or skin.

Cancer is a disease that involves a number of different processes and steps. It occurs when healthy cells stop functioning and maturing properly. A mishap occurs inside these cells. But it goes even further than this: Cancer actually begins with a change (mutation) in the genetic blueprint of life itself, cellular DNA. This mistake is believed to happen when there is an irregular transfer of electrical energy to different cells. In other words, when the usual steady flow of body electricity to and between cells is interrupted for any reason, the cycle of cells is thrown out of whack. Their DNA becomes somewhat scrambled and as a result *mis*information and *ab*normal gene sequencing is passed on to other cells by this altered DNA.

The interruption in normal electrical current may come in the form of too little or too much flow to body cells. Inadequate flow may come as a result of mental and emotional disturbances in the mind and heart of an individual. Excessive amounts can be due to the presence of too many electrical devices such as cell phones, personal computers, hair dryers, radio headsets, microwave ovens, electrical blankets, photocopiers, video cassette players, color TVs, and similar high-tech gadgets.

Once DNA is negatively impacted with less or more of the electrical energy it needs, it's changed ever so slightly, which then makes cells become cancer prone. When the normal cycle of cell creation and death is interfered with, the newly mutated cancer cells begin multiplying uncontrollably, no longer operating as an integrated and harmonious part of the body.

Thus, in its simplest terms, cancer represents an accelerating process of inappropriate, uncontrolled cell growth—a chaotic process in the order of biology. Cancer cells, when examined under a microscope, are abnormally shaped, inconsistently formed, disorganized, and contain misshapen internal structures—the essence of biological disorder. Cancer, despite its horror for the unlucky person thus afflicted, is really a natural phenomenon: It represents the body's response to a continuous attack on its own balancing and regulatory mechanisms by numerous factors.

Some Factors Contributing to Cancer

Here is an abbreviated laundry list of some of the more important things involved in the cause of cancer. Some are natural such as sunlight, parasites, viruses, and oncogenes. Others, while also occurring naturally, can be substantially increased in the body and eventually make it sick; free radicals from fried, deep-fried, charbroiled, grilled, and refrigerated foods is the best example of this.

A surprising number of environmental factors take their toll on human health: electromagnetic radiation from all types of electrical devices; sick building syndrome; irradiated foods; pesticides and herbicides; industrial pollutions; chlorinated and fluoridated water; and air smog. Still others come as a result of things we do to ourselves: amalgam (mercury) dental fillings; X-rays and CAT scans; childhood/adult immunizations; hormone therapies; immune-suppressive drugs; poor diet or unwise food/beverage choices; excessive intake of sugary foods; immune-suppressive drugs; tobacco smoking; excessive alcohol consumption and caffeine drinking.

An astonishing number of cancers these days are due to social factors: loneliness, anxiety, depression, and guilt. All of these poison the system in slow but sure ways and invariably set the stage for the eventual appearance of some form of cancer. While stress in some form is always good (the human spirit loves being challenged), bad thoughts and negative moods can wreck the body more than many other things are capable of doing.

Finally, the failure of the body to adequately remove its own generated toxic wastes (urine and feces) plays a significant role in its own health and well-being. Harvard pathologist Guido Majno, M.D., discussed the ancient Egyptian take on this very thing years ago in his classic work, *The Healing Hand: Man and Wound in the Ancient World* (Cambridge: Harvard University Press, 1975; p. 129). The Egyptians "apparently took the anus as the center and stronghold of decay." "The most frightening aspect of the feces (as they saw it) was that they contained a very pernicious thing called *ukhedu*. Ukhedu lay there dormant, but might arise and settle elsewhere in the body. The word *ukhedu* cannot be [effectively] translated . . . [but can mean] rot [or] the rotten stuff par excellence. The ukhedu was either male or female, caused disease and pain, and could be killed. It could work its way into the vessels and travel around, setting up disease. In essence, what bacteria can do, it could do."

Hence, constipation was a thing to be greatly feared by these people. They did everything imaginable to keep the bowels working regularly. Normal evacuation meant greatly reduced risks of contracting cancer from traveling ukhedu.

The Curse of Chemotherapy

Despite occasional drawbacks and the customary tremendous ill side effects it causes, chemotherapy has proven to be extremely popular with the medical profession for nearly six decades. The National Cancer Institute estimates that about a quarter of a million patients receive cytotoxics nationwide on an annual basis.

About 40 different drugs are routinely used against cancer; these react with the genetic material of the cells to prevent further abnormal cell division. Once they used to be administered individually, but now it is more common to find them being given in various complex combinations, generally referred to as "chemo cocktails." These are known by their technical acronyms assembled from the generic or trade names of the drugs themselves. Hence many patients currently receive CHOP (a combination of cyclophosphamide, doxorubicin, vincristine, and prednisone), FAM (fluorouracil, doxorubicin, and mitomycin), or MOPP (mechlorethamine, vincristine, procarbazine, and prednisone).

According to An Alternative Medicine Definitive Guide to Cancer by W. John Diamond, M.D. and W. Lee Cowden, M.D. (Tiburon, CA: Future Medicine Publishing, Inc., 1997; p. 653) "the mainstream use of chemotherapy for cancer came directly out of Nazi war science and poison gas weapons research." It is a little known but significant historical fact that today's "chemo cocktails" were parented by poisonous substances originally used to kill millions of Jews in the Holocaust but later regained considerable respectability when used by modern medicine in the fight against cancer.

The final part of this great curse is never known to those who eventually die of cancer anyway in spite of the heroic measures employed by people of medical science who sometimes enjoy the ritual suffering connected with chemotherapy. That terrible unknown truth is recognized only by morticians and is this: A corpse previously exposed to long-term chemotherapy but *never* embalmed prior to burial simply *won't* deteriorate as nature intended it should. These various chemotherapy drugs sort of mummify or preserve the remains for long periods of time. I know this for a fact because I once worked in the funeral business for several years and was involved in the court-ordered disinterment of several corpses that hadn't been embalmed but were subjected to massive chemotherapy treatments on account of the cancers from which they finally succumbed. Additional evidence in support of this claim may be found in the enlightening article, "Judgment of the Bones" by socioanthropologist Loring Danforth, Ph.D., in *Science Digest* (September 1981, pp. 92–97) in which is mentioned this noteworthy observation: "Villagers in rural Greece are finding that the corpses of people who had undergone chemotherapy fail to decompose after five years."

The Fatality of Radiation

During one of my many trips to New York City in the past, I had a chance to visit with Robert C. Atkins, M.D., who has been practicing internal medicine and complementary medicine in the Big Apple since 1959. I asked for his opinion on radiation treatments. His response was that "generally they are futile." However, he occasionally uses a combination of radiation and hyperthermia (heat treatments delivered by ultrasound or microwave) to keep tumors from encroaching on vital parts of the body. He believes using a localized charge of electricity is much safer in destroying tumors than radiation would be. He agreed with my assessment that radiation nukes the body to such an extent that it can fry the immune system for good. And this is very unacceptable when attempting to help a recovering cancer patient regain his or her full strength.

Confessions of a Reluctant Cancer Therapist

Some years ago I wrote a book entitled *The Treatment of Cancer with Herbs* (Orem, UT: BiWorld Publishers, 1980). It was part of The Holistic Health Series in Medical Anthropology. It broke ground in several ways: (1) It was the first major work ever to deal with alternative approaches to this disease; and (2) it covered a broad number of unconventional cancer treatments then being used worldwide. It also earned the unhappy distinction of being one of the few books ever to have been put out of print by the combined efforts of the Food and Drug

Administration (because of the numerous cancer remedies mentioned therein) and the Federal Communications Commission (due to various radio–TV programs I was doing at the time based on material from the book). It subsequently went out of print and almost overnight became an instant health-book collector's item, selling for as much as $75 in some parts of the country.

I went on to write other health books and soon forgot about the government furor that this particular title had generated. But starting in 1993 our Anthropological Research Center here in Salt Lake City began receiving letters requesting copies of this book. They trickled in at first but within a year's time the demand had increased 400-fold. My staff and I were puzzled by this strange circumstance and wondered why so many requests were coming in for a book long since out of print. Of course, we started filling these orders but didn't fully solve the puzzle until there came with one inquiry in 1995 some photocopied pages from Richard Walters's *Options: The Alternative Cancer Therapy Book* (Garden City Park, NY: Avery Publishing Group, Inc., 1993). Finally, the mystery had been solved: Walters, a respected medical and science writer, had not only quoted from my book, but had also listed it as one of the best books ever published on the subject of cancer in general. (Today the book sells for $65; see Product Appendix under Anthropological Research Center for additional information.)

If Walters's book opened the door for public access to my out-of-print book, then John M. Fink's *Third Opinion* (Garden City Park: Avery Publishing Group, 1997) directory on alternative cancer treatments literally lifted the floodgates for many hundreds of people seeking further knowledge and enlightenment on this most controversial of subjects. I found myself in the uncomfortable position of having to inform each person who wrote or called me that I was not in the cancer treatment business by any means, nor was I even licensed as a medical doctor to help them. Still, I was willing to share whatever information I had free of charge as long as they understood the limitations and restrictions deliberately placed before them.

Consumer word-of-mouth publicity about my research eventually spread to parts of the medical and scientific communities that routinely deal with cancer from a more conventional basis. On Saturday, October 24, 1999 I was invited to present a paper on one aspect of this work at the fourteenth Annual International Symposium on Acupuncture and Electro-Therapeutics at Columbia University's

School of International Affairs in New York City. (The report was later published in *The International Journal of Acupuncture & Electro-Therapeutics Research* (Vol. 23, nos. 3–4, 1998; p. 300).

Then on Friday, March 19, 1999, I addressed an august body of doctors at the Canadian Health Association Conference then being held in Vancouver, British Columbia, on an expanded version of the New York presentation. Immediately after that I flew directly to Philadelphia where I was a keynote speaker at the Seventh Annual Advancement in Cancer Education Conference held at the Philadelphia College of Osteopathic Medicine. From there I went on to speak at a Health and Healing Seminar attended by many doctors and nurses near Atlantic City, which was sponsored by the Complementary Healthcare Consortium of South Jersey.

Several other important speaking engagements were filled by me later in the year before similar health and medical sciences symposiums held in other parts of the country. The significance to all of this is that since 1993 (the year Walters's book came out) a tide of concurrent events, for which I was not responsible, has reluctantly swept me along a course of action that I haven't been fully prepared to deal with. Cancer creates desperation and fear in those who have it and prompts them to reach out to anyone they think might offer them some help or even a little hope. And when certain things work and people begin seeing results, then they tell their friends, neighbors, families, and doctors about it. In time that individual and the work associated with him or her become rather popular. That is how I went from one fairly inconspicuous book on herbal cancer treatments to a "Core Program" (as I term it) with international flair and extremely broad appeal.

An International Cancer-Recovery Program

The following data are a concise condensation of my rather ambivalent work with cancer from several important sources: (1) My original book printed in 1980; (2) time spent with various folk healers in different countries; (3) a thorough search of computerized medical and scientific literature covering unconventional cancer treatments; (4) numerous testimonies from those who've had apparent success with some of my natural recommendations; and (5) actual results that I've personally witnessed with these ingredients.

The "Core Program" for cancer recovery that I've devised and refined several times over many years pretty much fits just about *any* kind of known cancer. It is astonishingly simple and easy to follow. As one gets into it, one will be amazed at just how practical and filled with common sense it is. There is a basic pattern to be followed and always needs to occur in this precise order: HEAD and HEART *first,* NERVES and LIVER *second,* STOMACH and COLON *third;* and THE BODY last of all.

I. Head/Heart

Back in the mid-1980s I became professionally associated with Laurence Badgley, M.D., author of *Healing Aids Naturally* (San Bruno, CA: Human Energy Press, 1987). He was one of the first and few doctors at that time willing and courageous enough to exclusively treat HIV-positive and fully matured AIDS cases. He had collected around him several health experts representing different healing modalities in a loosely knit organization called Natural Therapies Medical Group.

In the several years that I worked with him and his partners I learned a great deal about human compassion and the importance of always being nonjudgmental in regard to a medical pariah so controversial as AIDS then was. He would holds hands with his patients and even touch their external skin sores *without* the benefit of plastic gloves to show them that he wasn't afraid of them or their disease. And he *always* made a point of telling every afflicted male patient (99 percent of them were men) that their disease was not due to any personal sins or wrongdoings, but merely a biological happening of unfortunate consequence.

At first, I found this philosophy difficult to swallow, knowing that the good majority of them had contracted AIDS from sexual promiscuity among the same gender. So I put the question to Dr. Badgley one time as to his reasoning behind this approach. His answer caused me not only to marvel but made a great impact in my own life that has remained with me ever since.

"John," he told me, "my aim in telling them this is to *remove ALL feelings of guilt and fear.* For when the body is ravaged with something as vicious as this, *the mind and heart must be entirely emptied of anxiety and desperation* in order for our natural therapies to be of positive benefit for them. *Peace in the soul* helps to create the right kind of healing environment for the body."

II. Nerves/Liver

Sometimes a consideration of particular pieces of ancient folklore may be helpful in offering guidance toward the development of a more rational therapy from what may appear to be highly irrational sources. Some years ago the eminent German medical historian Jürgen Thorwald wrote a book entitled *Macht und Geheimnis der frühen Arzte* (Munich: Droemersche Verlagsanstalt, 1962; Section II, Ch. 3).

In the section covering Mesopotamian medicine, the author demonstrated that the ancient Summerians, Assyrians, and Babylonians all believed the gods sent demons to punish men and women for their sins by inflicting them with diseases of every sort. This same belief is still very much in vogue today among most folk healers with whom I've had the privilege of working. But educated people, for the most part, disbelieve this and regard it as mere nonsense.

Be that as it may, Thorwald pointed out that the internal pathway along which these presumed diabolical forces loved to travel was the human central-nervous system. Furthermore, these "demons took up their abode within the livers of men." Hence, a diligent and concerted effort was always made to root them out of these two places through exorcisms, prayers, and herbs such as garlic or onion.

In contemplating this quaint piece of irrational thinking from a biological perspective, it soon dawned on me that the nerves and livers of nearly all cancer patients were, to put it charitably, in great disarray. So I began an earnest search for things that would restore calm and order to both body systems. I came up with catnip, chamomile, and peppermint teas for the nerves and dandelion root and tomato juice for the liver.

The three herb teas may be consumed as a mixture (equal parts of each) or separately, but in liquid form. On the other hand, dandelion root (six capsules daily) should be taken with eight fluid ounces of tomato juice or low-sodium V-8 juice every morning upon arising or in the evening just before retiring to bed.

III. Stomach/Colon

A couple of years ago while in New York City I visited Argosy Bookstore, a long-established shop dealing in antiquarian books, and rummaged through a number of dusty old volumes in their basement. I found a rare copy of Elie Metchnikoff's *The Prolongation of Life* (New

York: The Knickerbocker Press, 1908) for which I paid a paltry sum of $25, a real bargain, indeed, considering its scarcity.

This Russian-born bacteriologist worked at the prestigious Pasteur Institute in Paris, France, for many years. Chapters four and five of this classic work are the most important sections of the whole book. He presented a compelling argument for the shortness of life which he blamed on "intestinal putrefaction" that arises from poor digestion and improper elimination. Eating food too quickly and not thoroughly chewing it before swallowing was one of those factors that promoted problem.

Metchnikoff insisted that lactic acid obtained from fermented foods such as live yogurt, cultured buttermilk, homemade apple cider, marinated foods (that have been exposed to apple-cider vinegar), sauerkraut, and rye bread was the best way to inhibit intestinal putrefaction. He noted that the friendly microorganisms found in the lower part of the gut were essential for the complete breakdown and absorption of food nutrients into the body. But this intestinal flora could be influenced by some of the foods we consumed and, therefore, vary in both content and quality.

He noted that bacteria in the gastrointestinal tract were essential for good digestion of food and the normal elimination of its waste materials. A unique probiotic discovered at the Pasteur Institute many decades later and now manufactured in Montreal, Canada, is based on Metchnikoff's research and nicely fills this need. One-half cup of refrigerated Bio-K+ before, during, or after a meal will guarantee better absorption and freedom from the usual constipation for those experiencing any kind of food-assimilation problems. (See Product Appendix under Bio-K+ for more details.)

In the course of his studies conducted with lactic acid, the good doctor discovered that those who were the most susceptible to cancer were the ones with very low intestinal flora counts. The best defense against infections such as cancer was to eat a variety of fermented foods that would keep this friendly bacteria level high at all times.

Metchnikoff wrote that fermented grains were also a good source of health-giving lactic acid. An important product from Germany called Kanne Enzyme Fermented Grain contains organically grown oats, rye, natural sourdough, and salt in a powdered form. This can be added to soups, sauces, juices, or mixed with plain water (two teaspoons in eight fluid ounces) and taken every morning before breakfast. A large jar sells for $49 and lasts about six weeks. (See Product Appendix under Anthropological Research Center for further information.)

The many cancer victims unfortunate enough to submit themselves to the barbarity of chemotherapy soon find that their digestion and elimination are thrown into utter chaos. They can't keep food down, much less eliminate satisfactorily. This is because potent chemotherapeutic drugs they're taking have destroyed nearly all of their friendly intestinal flora. They also are seriously deprived of the water-soluble B complex vitamins, which depend upon bacteria for their production.

Therefore, those fermented foods mentioned earlier and others as well, besides the several supplements listed here, will be helpful toward the restoration of normal stomach functions and bowel movements.

IV. The Body

Those features of the "Core Program" that have been outlined thus far consist of doing the following things for these parts of the body: (1) removing guilt, fear, anxiety, and desperation from the head and heart in order for peace to prevail in the soul; this creates the proper atmosphere for healing to take place; (2) the nerves may be soothed with herbal teas made from catnip, chamomile, and/or peppermint, while the liver is refreshed with dandelion root and tomato juice; (3) the gastrointestinal tract benefits from live foods that have first been fermented.

The cancer patient is now prepared to treat the entire body with a relatively small arsenal of useful things that should help to slow the progress of the disease, if not defeat it outright. These foods and nutrients will definitely reduce pain, improve appetite, give energy, promote better elimination, guarantee normal sleep, and generally create an overall feeling of wellness. As a result, the *quality* of life will get seriously upgraded, though the actual quantity of how much remains may still be in doubt due to a number of different variables (for example, age, gender, ethnicity, lifestyle, diet, geographic residency, spirituality level, sociability).

A few of the things mentioned in this section need to be taken every day, while others are varied enough in scope so as to be utilized interchangeably throughout any given week without much repetition. Here may be seen the full extent of the program's internationalism.

Hungary, Japan, Canada, Great Britain, India, Mexico, and China each contributed one or more items that will either reverse the disease to some degree or produce reasonable vigor and vitality or possibly do both.

HUNGARY—Beet root juice and the powdered concentrate were used extensively at the district hospital in Csorna (population less than 40,000), Györ-Sopron counties (situated in the extreme northwest part of the country) by Alexander Ferenczi, M.D., a doctor of internal medicine. From October 1950 to December 1959 he and his medical staff treated hundreds of different cases of cancer with very good results using mostly beet-root juice, grated red beets, or beet powder. This important research was translated from several articles published in leading Hungarian medical journals and reprinted in the Spring 1993 issue of *Folk Medicine Journal*. There was a notable regression in many tumors, which he attributed to the red pigment in the beets. He noted that too much (one glass) fresh beet juice could overwhelm the patient, so his staff administered a lesser quantity (one-half cup twice daily). I've recommended adding this amount to two cups of liquid chlorophyll. A powdered juice concentrate is available but due to its intensity only a level teaspoon should be mixed with two tablespoons of powdered chlorophyll in eight ounces of water and taken midday on a regular basis. (See Product Appendix under Pines International for further information.)

JAPAN—Wakunaga Pharmaceutical Co. of Hiroshima developed some years ago two products that have proven consistent in defeating cancer—a dry chlorophyll powdered-drink mix called Kyo-Green (includes cereal grasses, algaes, and seaweeds); and *liquid* Kyolic Garlic (aged garlic extract with vitamin B-12). (See Product Appendix under Wakunaga of America for further information.)

Also from the "Land of the Rising Sun" has come the world-famous Macrobiotic Diet. Originally pioneered by Yukikazu Sakurazawa, it was later introduced to the Western world by one of his most loyal disciples, Michio Kushi, who was born in Kokawa, Wakayama-Ken, in 1926. The macrobiotic philosophy behind cancer is this: Too much *yin* expansion or excessive *yo* contraction within the body creates a physiological imbalance that macrobiotics is intended to normalize again. These two forces or tendencies exist in all life forms and while clearly opposite of each other, still manage to work in harmony when everything is in balance. The Japanese classification of different cancer sites under one or both of these forces is interesting and worth reviewing here.

Yin Cancer	Yo Cancer	Yin & Yo Combined
Breast	Colon	Lung
Stomach	Prostate	Bladder
Mouth (minus tongue)	Rectum	Uterus
Esophagus	Ovary	Kidney
Leukemia	Bone	Spleen
Hodgkin's disease	Pancreas	Melanoma
Brain (outer regions)	Brain (inner regions)	Tongue
Skin		

To help offset the development of cancer or to correct an existing disease situation, it is vital to restore moderation and balance to the daily diet. To bring about such an equilibrium, one must consume certain amounts of those foods that can help achieve this: 50–60% whole-grains cereal (brown rice, wild rice, millet, whole wheat, oats, rye, corn, barley, buckwheat); 5 percent soups (two bowls daily seasoned with miso or tamari soy sauce but not too salty); 20–25 percent vegetables (green cabbage; kale; Swiss chard; watercress; Chinese cabbage; bok choy; dandelion greens/flowers; burdock root; carrots; daikon radish; turnips/turnip greens; onions; acorn, Hubbard, and butternut squash; red radish; cauliflower); 5–10 percent beans and sea vegetables (azuki beans, chickpeas, lentils, and seaweeds such as hiziki, kombu, wakame, nori, dulse, kelp, and Irish moss).

Supplementary foods are occasionally permitted several times a week. These include fresh- and saltwater fish (preferably steamed, boiled, or baked, a small amount of fruit (apple, peach, pear, kiwi, mango, papaya, raisins, grapes, lichi nuts), raw or roasted seeds (sunflower, sesame), and a few raw nuts or organic nut butters (almond, cashew, filbert or hazelnut, pecan, peanut, walnut). Suggested beverages would include roasted brown-rice tea, roasted barley tea, dandelion-chicory-burdock tea, Postum, and any cereal grain coffee substitute. If cooking oil is to be used at all in the preparation of food let it be high-quality sesame seed or extra-virgin olive oil. (I have added the latter oil, which isn't a part of the typical macrobiotic regimen.)

Meals should be taken in moderation and only to satisfy hunger. Careful chewing is important, and meal consumption should always be done in peaceful surroundings without any noise or agitation. Up to five small meals a day can be consumed. In lieu of other beverages water may be taken, but *never* icy cold, only lukewarm.

CANADA—In the 1920s, a Canadian registered nurse named Rene Caisse introduced a nontoxic herbal tea for treating cancer. The tea was originally named Lasagen by the Ojibway, a Native American tribe in Ontario, Canada, and the Great Lakes region. Caisse obtained the formula for this natural herbal combination from a breast cancer patient who had been healed by an Ojibway shaman; she renamed it Essiac (which is her name spelled backward) and used it to treat over ten thousand cases of cancer until her death in 1978 at age 90. According to Richard Walters' book *Options* (cited earlier in this section), Nurse Caisse was invited to the Brusch Medical Center in Massachusetts at age 70 to treat terminal cancer patients under the close supervision of 18 doctors. At the end of these initial tests clinical doctors produced a document testifying that "on patients suffering from pathologically proven cancer, Essiac reduces pain and causes a recession in the growth; patients have gained weight and shown an improvement in their general health." Furthermore, "remarkably beneficial results were obtained even on those cases at the 'end of the road' where it proved to prolong life and the quality of that life. . . . The doctors do not say that Essiac is a cure, but they do say it is of definite benefit."

Essiac's principal herbal components include burdock root, Indian-rhubarb root, sheep-sorrel leaves, and slippery-elm bark. It is still made in western Canada today by a Hungarian pharmacist but is very difficult to find here in the States. It goes by the name of Essex Botanical and sells for $75 a quart. (See under Anthropological Research Center for ordering instructions.)

GREAT BRITAIN—Red clover tea has been used by a number of homeopathic doctors for a number of decades to successfully treat existing malignancies. Red clover works in a much different way from the way other anticancer herbs do. Instead of aiming to destroy tumors, red clover sets out to limit their blood supply by attempting to shrink them and prevent further growth. Certain potent compounds in red-clover blossoms stop new vessels from forming around a tumor and break up the existing network of abnormal capillaries that feeds the cancerous mass. Boil one quart of water in a stainless-steel or enamel pot. Turn off the heat and add four tablespoons of cut and dried clover flowers. Stir and add one teaspoon of cut and dried oat-straw. Cover with lid and steep for 30 minutes. Strain and drink one eight-fluid-ounce glass three times daily between meals.

INDIA—Turmeric root is the main ingredient in curry powder. I devoted an entire chapter to it in my book, *Nature's Super 7 Medicines* (Paramus, NJ: Prentice Hall Direct, 1997; pp. 201–216). It is one of the top four herbs for the liver (the other three include the roots of dandelion and goldenseal and milk-thistle-seed extract). Take three turmeric capsules daily—two in the morning with breakfast and one in the evening with dinner. (See Product Appendix under Anthropological Research Center for more data.)

MEXICO—For many years Charlotte Gerson has carried on the work of her deceased German-born physician father Max Gerson, M.D., at the Gerson Clinic in the backwater border town of Tijuana. While the clinic employs a number of different healing modalities in its sometimes rather bizarre approach to cancer, one of the central themes that has a lot of common sense to it is the food-therapy program. Dr. Gerson believed that a lifetime consumption of cooked, canned, frozen, and packaged *dead* foods could initiate cancer, while a raw or lightly cooked foods diet could reintroduce *life and vitality* into the system, thereby driving the cancer out. Besides the organic foods utilized, the *forms* in which they're prepared is just as interesting: fresh juices, homemade soups, and garden salads are the mainstays. (Having a Vita-Mix machine on hand is quite helpful in preparing each of these things. See under Vita-Mix in the Product Appendix.)

Space doesn't permit listing favorite recipes given to cancer patients at the Tijuana clinic. (Recipe booklets may be ordered by calling the Gerson Institute in Bonita, California: 619.472.7450.) However, by mentioning some of the primary foods involved, it is hoped that readers can use their own clever imaginations to create for themselves or loved ones delicious meals that will fight cancer while rebuilding sick bodies. Such foods include carrots, apples, green peppers, red cabbage, escarole, Swiss chard, parsley, chives, celery, spinach, watercress, onion, scallion, radish, endive, romaine lettuce, broccoli, cauliflower, artichoke, tomatoes, potatoes, beets, dill weed, corn, string beans, lima beans, squash, eggplant, raisins, sweet potato, apricots, zucchini, rice, flaxseed oil, and apple-cider vinegar.

CHINA/JAPAN—Thanks to the recent media hype given medicinal mushrooms, people are only now beginning to become more familiar with what I term "the fungus amongus." Most of the research concerning medicinal fungi originates in Asia. While the Chinese use a great deal more of this natural substance than the Japanese do, it is the latter culture that has been primarily responsible for doing most of the scientific research on it.

There are more than 20,000 species of mushrooms, of which 2,000 are edible. At least 300 of the edibles are presumed to have medically active constituents; 50 alone are widely employed in the medical systems of mainland China, Taiwan, Hong Kong, Singapore, Malaysia, and Indonesia.

Their major health advantage is believed to be their high polysaccharide or sugar polymer content. These complex carbohydrates stimulate the immune system to help combat bacterial and viral infections. All mushrooms contain some amounts of these polysaccharides. But only a handful have proven themselves clinically capable of retarding cancer and other diseases.

These include reishi *(Ganoderma lucidum)*, turkey tail *(Trametes versicolor)*, shiitake *(Lentinula edodes)*, and maitake *(Grifola frondusa)*.

Mushroom nutrition can be especially valuable for those who are immune-compromised or who are just starting to recover from chemotherapy and radiation treatments. In fact, mycological therapy is very popular in the Orient among doctors specializing in cancer. They frequently prescribe one or several of these medical fungi to their patients to help reduce the terrible suffering associated with conventional chemo drugs and radiation as well as to promote physical improvement.

Some of these mushrooms can be found in most health food stores. Recommended intake is two to four capsules/tablets/pill daily with meals.

Only Clucks Eat Chicken

One final observation needs to be made with regard to the prevention and treatment of cancer. It concerns the consumption of animal protein. The current belief for many holds that eating red meat can be very bad for you if you've already been diagnosed with cancer. Medical science has already declared in the appropriately published literature that charbroiling or broiling red meat can definitely increase the risk of cancer.

So the trend has been to consume more chicken and leave red meat alone for the most part. The assumption here is that fowl is somehow healthier for the body and less risky. *But nothing could be further from the truth!* The late doctor–biologist Virginia Livingston, M.D., pointed out in her mind-awakening book *Cancer: A New Breakthrough* (San Diego, CA: 1972; pp. 107–32) that a new but hidden cancer-causing microorganism she classified as *Cryptocides* could be found lurking in most poultry and nearly all eggs. Since much of the American population are heavy chicken and egg consumers, she felt that better than half of all diagnosed cancer cases could be attributed in some way to *Cryptocides* infection.

My own research into this matter came from a cultural perspective as a medical anthropologist. In conjunction with several Seventh-Day Adventist physicians and a few other non-SDA doctors who had worked for many years in providing medical treatments for the Navajo and Havasupai Indians in northern Arizona, I conducted thorough research of numerous medical records representing thousands of patients to find out just how many cancer cases there really were over a 30-year period. For all of our efforts, we could come up with only about half a dozen at most.

Tracking down the relatives of the deceased proved to be a little trickier and more time-consuming than I had imagined. But hard work, determination, and lots of patience finally paid off in a big way. Those few (and I do mean FEW) who had passed away from some kind of cancer had all eaten chicken and eggs at different periods in their lives. But the great majority of tribal members from both Indian nations have managed to resist the temptation for such delicacies as long as they stay on their respective reservations. (The same can't be said, however, for those who wander away into the white person's world and begin eating that kind of food, especially the finger-licking fried chicken that everyone seems to rave about.) Navajos and Havasupai deliberately avoid poultry (including turkey) for religious rather than health reasons, believe it or not. In their peculiar belief systems, such feathered fowl are thought to inhabit the underworld and carry in them evil apparitions during their short mortal existences. Since they're considered so unclean, neither tribe will dine on them, which is curiously commendable in one way. But the rest of their diets leaves a lot to be desired: both Indian nations have atrocious eating habits and junk food cravings that promote obesity, diabetes, heart disease, hypertension, and alcoholism big-time! Still, *cancer is virtually absent among them* because they refuse to touch eggs or chickens. (For a complete report on Dr. Livingston's and my own research regarding the cancer–chicken connection, contact the Anthropological Research Center, POB 11471, Salt Lake City, UT 84147.)

Thank God I Have Cancer!

Many years ago a California woman named Edie Hunsaker wrote a small book with the startling title *Thank God I Have Cancer!* Like so many others I was intrigued enough with the heading alone to investigate the text. Her entire premise for the highly unusual position she took of being grateful to God for letting her get this disease (she eventually recovered) was that it taught her meekness and humility, increased her faith in God, and gave her greater compassion for others. "When death finally stared me in the face, I was able to truly start living *right* and beginning my life all over again!" she wrote. This is the attitude that everyone should be taking when faced with a health crisis of similar magnitude. It's good for the soul they say, and you come out of the ordeal a much better person in the end.

CARDIAC ARREST

Yellow-Bellied Sapsuckers Are for Real

A friend of mine, Maynard Rasmussen, is a professional birder—that is someone who is in the business of watching and studying birds for a hobby. Maynard's wife gave me a call some time ago and asked that I come over to visit them and make some recommendations for dealing with a case of cardiac arrest that he had just recently encountered.

Maynard chose to talk about birds, particularly one of his favorite kind, before I had a chance to counsel him and his wife on herbal therapy appropriate for his health crisis.

"Sapsuckers have been the butt of jokes for too long," he began. "But, as a matter of fact, they are very real and belong to the woodpecker family. They get their odd name because they *do* consume sap from trees as part of their diet. Their strong, straight, chisel-like bills are uniquely adapted for drilling into trees, and a greatly elongated tongue permits entrance into nooks and crevices and excavated borings.

"Most woodpecker tongues end in barded tips with sticky secretions to help extract prey. But sapsucker tongue tips are brushy for soaking and lapping up tree sap." I grunted a slight "humph" sound through my nose in surprise to this distinct variation. Maynard concluded by observing that the male and female William's sapsuckers have the brightest of yellow sapsucker bellies and, therefore, qualify for the official name given them.

Cayenne and Ginger Always Work

His wife then suggested that he be still and listen to what I had to say. I told them that cayenne pepper and ginger root were always the two best herbs to use in situations such as this, once the patient has sufficiently recuperated in intensive care and is ready to be discharged. Maynard began taking one capsule of each herb in the morning before breakfast and again at midday for the next six months.

I also added to the protocol raw garlic and onion on a fairly regular basis, at least three times a week by itself or with food of some kind. I strongly recommended that he curtail eating fried and deep-fried food and encouraged his wife to start preparing meals that were steamed, baked, or broiled. I advised some raw foods, but because too many raw vegetables gave him gas, I had to limit this to just a few things such as carrots, parsley, and celery.

There was no further recurrence of those symptoms typical for an absence of mechanical cardiac activity in older men: unconsciousness, lack of pulse in the larger arteries, breathing gasps, and skin pallor. After six months he went for another checkup and it showed much improved cholesterol/triglyceride readings and a reduction in his formerly elevated blood pressure.

CARPAL TUNNEL SYNDROME

Black Forest Spa Remedy

The Schwarzwald, the Black Forest, is a mountain range in southwest Germany, extending 90 miles between the Rhine and Neckar rivers. The range is covered by dark pine forests and cut by deep valleys and small lakes. The Danube and Neckar rivers rise there. Lumbering and woodworking are important economic activities. Orchards and cattle are found in the valleys; grains are grown in the highlands.

The Black Forest is famous for its clock and toy industries (cuckoo clocks, music boxes). It is a year-round resort area, known for its winter sports and mineral springs. Baden-Baden and Freiburg are the chief cities there.

Idyllic Baden-Baden has been a summer residence of aristocratic Europeans for 150 years. The Brenner's Park Hotel offers the ultimate in pampering and health treatments in the luxurious environment of a grand hotel. When I was there some years ago I found the swimming pool to have been modeled in the Roman style in celebration of Julius Caesar, who it is said once came here for some badly needed R&R following the fierce Gallic Wars (58 B.C.–51 B.C.) in which ancient Gaul (modern France) was finally conquered by him.

A massage therapist I met at this fine hotel by the name of Helga Ulrich demonstrated her own technique for treating *and* curing carpal tunnel syndrome. She had never heard of the vitamin B-6 therapy commonly used in America for this, but assured me that her method worked much better and didn't cost anything.

Applying a little extra-virgin olive oil to the front and back sides of my left wrist and hand she then began slowly massaging in a gentle, circular motion with her right thumb and index finger the flexor tendons and the median nerve located within the carpal tunnel itself. Helga gripped the fatty part of my hand with her index finger while at the same time slightly pushing on the backside of my hand with the bent tip of her thumb. After a couple of pushes with her thumb, she would then grasp this part of my hand with the left side of her index finger and bottom part of the thumb in a slight grip, while at the same time sliding her left thumb over the back part of my left hand located between my thumb and index finger.

She kept up this procedure for several minutes before switching to the other hand. She insisted that by doing this simple massage for three minutes at least five times a day, those suffering from carpal-tunnel syndrome would experience a reduction in tingling and burning sensations. I started applying this technique to myself after long periods of typing and discovered just how wonderfully well the peripheral-nerve compression due to repetitive wrist actions was relieved. And while vitamin B-6 (four tablets daily) certainly helps, too, this particular treatment is free and easy to do any time you feel like it.

CATARACTS

What the Germans Know that We Don't

During my visit to different European health spas some years ago, I had a chance to stay at the Schlosshotel Bühlerhohe located slightly over half a mile above Baden-Baden. I found this splendid turn-of-the-century hotel to be like some great baronial palace tucked away in its own park. The view from almost any window made my trip worthwhile: I could see in the distance pale mountains rising gently over thick forests, lush river valleys, and lively little villages.

There was an intimacy about the place that I found very appealing. The facility had only 90 guest rooms, including 20 suites and junior suites. The spa was even more appealing, accommodating only a dozen guests at a time, so that individual attention was virtually guaranteed.

My body was treated to some of the best natural therapies to be found anywhere on earth: aromatherapy, fango pack, herbal wrap, loofah scrub, lymph drainage, Kneipp shower, thalassotherapy, and thermal baths.

Oskar Schmelz was one of the instructors who took the time to answer some of my probing questions about folk treatments in the region. He told me of a "wonderful treatment we have in the area for getting rid of cataracts in their *early* stages," with emphasis on the word "early." He explained that mineral-water consumption and daily bathing of the eyes with the same kind of water was the "echtes Geheimnis" or real secret for the prevention or reduction of *early-formed* cataracts.

He explained how the rich minerals in such water helped to remove the thin milky-white film that gradually causes the eye lens to grow more opaque with the passing of years.

CELIAC DISEASE

Something Good from Budapest Besides Goulash

My tour of European spas included some in what was still then considered to be "Iron Curtain" countries. But with the fall of Communism all of that has since changed. Hungary is rich in medicinal thermal springs that have been an integral part of the culture since Roman times. Budapest, the beautiful capital, has several famous baths where people still gather. The most splendid baths, I soon learned, are located on Margaret Island, which is gracefully wedged between Buda and Pest in the Danube River.

I met an old gypsy lady there by the name of Margarit Slyza. She told me of a cure that her people sometimes used for cases of celiac disease, which was fairly uncommon in that part of the country at the time. She told me that just one item was used, it being the famous spice paprika that gave color and flavor to the typical Hungarian *gulyás*—a beef stew made with assorted vegetables.

She said that those who were troubled with the gluten in wheat products should season their grain foods liberally with paprika, as well as to take it orally every day. I had never heard of such a thing before and frankly doubted that it would work. But after timidly suggesting it to a few individuals here in America who suffered from celiac disease and getting back glowing reports from them on just how well it worked, I no longer was reluctant to suggest it for this problem. The usual dosage is three capsules daily when consuming anything with gluten in it.

CEREBRAL PALSY

A Treatment That Works

Cerebral palsy is a nonprogressive disorder of movement or posture that is a result of a central-nervous abnormality that occurred prenatally, perinatally, or during the first years of life. The disease is lifelong, although changes occur as the patient matures.

In looking over my extensive notes made while on Margaret Island near Budapest, I noticed some things that had been jotted down from a visit I had with a medical doctor named Bela Lazar. He worked at one of the medicinal thermal springs and told me how various cases of cerebral palsy had been *improved* or *remedied*, but *not* necessarily cured. He said that a combination of therapies was involved in bringing about better motor nerve and muscle skills and deep-tendon reflexes.

Thermal-spring soaking, sauna treatment, underwater jet massage, carbon gas bath, Swedish massage, mud packs, and solarium therapy were incorporated into a daily or biweekly regimen that showed noticeable improvement, especially in young children up to five years of age who suffered from this muscle-nerve disease. Muscle spasticity was reduced by as much as 40 percent, while incidents of epilepsy usually cleared up. Behavioral problems and mental retardation often attributed to this disorder also experienced apparent reductions.

However, no more specific information was furnished by the doctor during our short interview that might have provided for a more detailed program of treatment for interested readers. Dr. Lazar stated that many of these spa treatments provided "electrical excitement" (or stimulation) to dysfunctioning muscles and nerves.

CHAPPED HANDS AND LIPS

Isle of Capri Beauty Secret

Situated in Anacapri, the most exclusive and unspoiled part of Capri, a famous Italian island resort, is the luxurious Europa Palace Hotel. Housed adjacent to the hotel in an ultra modern building is the Capri Beauty Farms. Here Francesca Molini shared with me one of her world-famous beauty secrets.

For chapped hands and lips she mixes *equal* parts of extra-virgin olive oil and lanolin together, then has her customers rub it between their sore hands and upon their lips. The dry soreness is promptly relieved.

CHARLEY HORSE

Remember the Seaweeds

My body was purified and my spirit elevated within an atmosphere of total relaxation and wonderful healing during my stay at the Capri Beauty Farm in Anacapri, Italy's charming island where the wealthy and carefree come to vacation and get themselves rejuvenated. Although women tend to outnumber male customers about 9 to 1, there was an adequate number of gentlemen present so I didn't feel like the only man around.

An Italian–German physiotherapist by the name of Max showed me what they use at this lovely facility for treating Charley horse or severe muscle cramps in some of their patients. A combination of yoga stretching, water massage, and, most important, seaweed consumption helped to clear up this excruciatingly painful discomfort.

The most common seaweeds were bladderwrack, laminaria, dulse, and kelp. These were always cooked or steamed and served with lunch or dinner. But I later discovered that some of them could be used in powdered form, either in loose bulk (one tablespoon added to water, juice, or soup) or taken by capsules (four per day). Max explained that their rich mineral content, particularly the iodine–calcium–magnesium connection, enabled the body to rebuild its mineral reserves and thereby counteract any further development of such painful cramping later on.

CHEST PAIN

Mullein Tea

An old folk remedy my grandmother used a long time ago for chest pains was a warm glass of mullein tea. She would boil a pint of water and then add two large tablespoons of dried mullein herb and flowers, after which she would stir the contents, cover with a lid, and simmer for one minute before setting aside to let steep for 20 minutes. She would strain the lukewarm tea into an eight-ounce glass and give this to the person to drink. It would *always* make the pains disappear and the chest feel a lot better.

CHICKENPOX

Cures from Northwestern Africa

The nations of Northwestern Africa have contributed much to our own understanding of ethnobotanical medicine in general. Morocco,

Algeria, Tunisia, Libya, Western Sahara, Mauritania, Senegal, Gambia, Guinea Bissau, Guinea, Sierra Leone, Liberia, Mali, Niger, Chad, Cote D'Ivoire, Ghana, Burkina Faso, Togo, Benin, Nigeria, Camaroon, and the Central African Republic are those countries that comprise this particular region of the continent.

In past years I've visited many of them when they were known by other names—that is, the Ivory Coast (Cote D'Ivorie) and Upper Volta (Burkina Faso). It is a fascinating part of the world where many different kinds of food spices and medicinal herbs may still be purchased for a mere pittance in any number of open-air marketplaces. Their rich and pungent aromas intrigue the mind while stimulating one's gustatory sense. It is an aromatherapy adventure definitely worth pursuing and experiencing if one has the time, patience, and finances to do so.

Children or adults suffering from chickenpox are given several very effectual remedies that hasten the recovery process. A soup or tea is made from chopped chicken livers and chicken bones to which are then added tiny pinches of both cayenne and black peppers. When the liquid cools down, the patient is given some to eat or drink by the resident witch doctor. This always helps to break the fever accompanying such a childhood ailment.

Now, the more interesting part to this twofold treatment comes with the external applications used for relieving the itching. These vary and may include the *warm* urine of cows, camels, donkeys, or even humans, as well as the more conventional milky latex from milkweed stalk or dandelion stem. Oh, and did I forget to mention the rubbing of saliva on skin sores? Another more practical solution is the use of gel from the aloe-vera plant. But, strange as some of these may seem to be, they all work quite well in relieving skin itch and helping to dry up weeping sores.

CHLAMYDIA

Most Common STD

Chlamydia is the most common sexually transmitted disease (STD) in America today. Roughly four million new cases are discovered each year and nearly 20 percent of American adolescents have had it at some time or another in their lives.

An estimated 12 percent of men and 73 percent of women have no symptoms at all in the early stages of the infection. But as it progresses, both genders suffer inflammation, itching, difficulty urinating, and pain during sexual intercourse. All too frequently *Chlamydia* occurs as part of a combined infection with gonorrhea or another venereal disease. Once the other infection is treated, a previously hidden chlamydial problem may show up.

This is the leading cause of infertility in women today. About 50,000 American women have become infertile because of it. If a woman with chlamydial infection does become pregnant, the disease can cause problems for her newborn.

Herbal Antibiotics

Conventional treatment usually consists of drugs of the tetracycline class—Achromycin, Doryx, Monodox, Vibramycin, Vibra-Tabs, and others. For those unable to tolerate drugs of this class, erythromycin is used. Some doctors even prescribe a much more expensive antibiotic called Zithromax. While all these drugs are effective in controlling this infection, they have a huge downside to them: They wreak havoc on the body's beneficial bacteria. What this means is that an overgrowth of *Candida* may manifest itself in the form of vaginitis or oral thrush and that a variety of gastrointestinal problems result—that is, indigestion, flatulence, diarrhea, constipation.

Over the years I've developed my own botanical treatment program for tenacious STDs of this sort. My regimen includes three spices, two medicinal herbs, and enzymes in the following suggested dosages (I've listed some commercial brands beside each of them that readers can learn more about in the Product Appendix):

BOTANICAL THERAPY FOR SEXUALLY TRANSMITTED DISEASES

Herbs	Daily Dosages	Brands
Echinacea	2 capsules	Earth's Pharmacy
Garlic	2 capsules	Kyolic-EPA
Goldenseal	2 capsules	Earth's Pharmacy
Oregano	1 capsule	Oregamax
Turmeric	1/8 tsp. in juice	Schilling
Enzymes	3 capsules	ShapeRite

Other Treatments

Other nonsupplement recommendations that can greatly alleviate this problem and prevent further recurrence later on include the following:

- Practice monogamous sex; multiple partners are very dangerous!
- Strive to control excessive sexual desires.
- Wear loose cotton underwear that permits air circulation.
- Avoid wearing pantyhose or tight, hip-hugging jeans or pants.
- Take 30 mg. of zinc along with 2 mg. of copper each day for two months.
- Take 1,500 mg. of nonacidic Ester C twice daily for three months.
- Take 1 tbsp. of cod-liver oil every other day.
- Take 1 tsp. Red Wheat Germ Oil daily (see Product Appendix under Anthropological Research Center).
- Consume 1 cup of Bio-K+ in the morning and again in the evening. (See Product Appendix.)
- Inflamed tissues can be easily treated with tea tree or melaleuca oil.
- Eat a high-fiber, low-fat, and low-sugar diet.
- Drink a minimum of six big glasses of water daily.

CHOKING

Recognizing the Choking Victim

Prior to the Heimlich maneuver choking was the sixth-leading cause of accidental death in the overall population and the leading cause of accidental death in the home for children under one year of age. But even with worldwide knowledge of this life-saving technique, between 3,000 to 4,000 people still die every year in America due to upper-airway obstructions, according to the *University of California at Berkeley Wellness Letter.* That's still far too many deaths when something as simple and effective as Dr. Heimlich's maneuver could be applied to save them.

Foreign-body obstruction of the airway usually occurs while the victim is eating. This is what happened to the famous American trombonist and bandleader Tommy Dorsey and Cass Elliott, of the recording group The Mamas and The Papas—both died while choking on food during meals. However, others such as Ronald Reagan (when he was governor of California) and actress Elizabeth Taylor have had their lives saved with the Heimlich maneuver when they accidentally choked on a small piece of food (for Reagan it was a peanut and for Taylor a grape).

If the victim is a child, however, choking may also occur during play, when a small toy or object such as a marble is being mouthed and suddenly slips back into the airway. Within four minutes of the onset of the attack, the victim will be dead or will suffer permanent brain damage. Thus, the rescuer must make the diagnosis immediately.

There are three signs that indicate complete obstruction of the airway: first, an inability to speak or breathe; second, pallor followed by a bluish skin color; and third, loss of consciousness and collapse. As soon as the rescuer notices the first of these signs, that individual should immediately perform the renowned maneuver developed years ago by Dr. Heimlich.

The History Behind the Maneuver

I have known Henry J. Heimlich and his wife, Jane, since 1982. Our first meeting was through a mutual friend at Alta Ski Resort in the mountains east of Salt Lake City. During subsequent trips of his to the Beehive State later on during the ski season, I became better acquainted with them and we've remained friends ever since. In one of these later visits, I asked Hank how he came by way of his maneuver. The following is a synopsis of what he related then.

"As a chest surgeon, I knew that there are twelve hundred to seventeen hundred cubic centimeters of air in the chest, plus another five hundred or so if the person has inhaled. So I took an endotracheal tube, closed off the upper end, and put it down the throat of an anesthetized dog. When I compressed the air in the dog's chest, the tube moved out of the airway. It wasn't immediately apparent where I should push. I tried pressing on the chest, but got getter results by pushing up under the diaphragm.

"Then I had to figure out how this maneuver could be devised in such a way that people could do it very quickly and it would work. There are several positions from which you can push on the diaphragm, but it became clear that the best way would be to stand behind the victim, wrap your arms around him, and squeeze upward. That became the maneuver. I also came up with a method that works when the victim is lying unconscious on the floor. You simply press on the diaphragm with the heal of your hand."

Now that Hank had the concept right, he had to figure out a way to try it out. "I wasn't about to tie a string to a piece of meat and put it down someone's throat to find out if it worked or not," I recall him saying with a chuckle. "So I went ahead and published the study in a journal, *Emergency Medicine*, and asked the editors to bring it to the attention of certain people in the press.

"A week later I was sent a front-page story from the *Seattle Times* about a restaurateur who had read about the maneuver. One day his neighbor came running out of the house, screaming that his wife was having a heart attack. The restaurateur ran over, saw the woman unconscious, with her face literally in her mashed potatoes and gravy, and performed the maneuver right there at the dinner table. A piece of chicken popped out of her mouth and she survived. After that, the maneuver spread like wildfire and the rest, as they say, is history."

I asked Hank to estimate about how many lives his maneuver may have saved. He thought a moment before replying. "We have documented around thirty-six hundred so far, but we know there are at least six thousand from what we hear" (up to 1984, that is).

Saving Lives Different Ways

I am indebted to Hank for the following information, which he kindly provided me with years ago. The basic maneuver can be performed upon a victim who is situated in different positions, including a technique for saving yourself, if necessary.

VICTIM STANDING

When the victim is standing the rescuer positions himself behind the victim and encircles the victim's waist with his arms. With one hand, he makes a fist and then places its knob against the victim's abdomen, slightly above the navel and well below the lower tip of the breast plate. The rescuer then grasps the fist with his free hand and presses into the victim's abdomen with a quick upward thrust. It may be necessary to repeat the thrust as many as six times to clear the airway. Each new thrust should be a separate and distinct movement. Resumption of breathing, return to normal color, and restoration of consciousness indicate that the airway has been cleared of the offending obstacle.

Once the airway has been cleared, the bolus of food or other obstructing object should be found and identified.

VICTIM SEATED

The technique for the sitting and standing victim is almost identical. When the victim is seated, the rescuer stands or kneels behind the chair, encircles the victim's waist with her arms, positions her hands, and delivers the thrust just as she would if the victim were standing. The only difference is that now the back of the chair is interposed between the rescuer and the victim. The chair back provides a firm support for the victim's back and seems to enhance the effect of the subdiaphragmatic thrust.

If the victim is sitting in a dining booth, an airplane seat, or a chair that is too large for the rescuer to reach around, the rescue can still be performed while the victim remains seated. He is simply turned sideways in the seat so that the rescuer can get behind him and then perform the maneuver upon him that way.

VICTIM SUPINE

There are only two situations in which the supine position is indicated: first, when the victim has already fallen unconscious to the floor; second, when the rescuer is too small to reach around the victim or too weak to deliver an adequate thrust. When the victim is already lying unconscious on the floor, vital time can be wasted trying to pull her to a standing position. And when the rescuer is too small or too weak, the maneuver can't be performed effectively unless the victim is supine.

If the victim is unconscious and lying facedown on the floor, the rescuer should roll the victim onto his back, with his face up. Facing the victim, the rescuer kneels astride the victim's hips and positions her hands against the victim's abdomen slightly above the navel and just below the rib cage; the right hand is pressed flat against the skin (unless the rescuer is left-handed) while the left hand is placed directly over the other hand. She then presses into the abdomen, toward the diaphragm, with a quick upward thrust.

The same procedure can be used with a conscious victim if the rescuer is small or weak. While kneeling astride the supine victim, the weak or small rescuer can use his own body weight to achieve sufficient force for the necessary thrust. Using this position, children have saved their parents and petite wives their big, husky husbands.

It is vital, though, that the victim's head be facing up and aligned to the midline as much as possible, although it does not need to be held rigidly in position. The head is not deliberately turned to the side to prevent aspiration should the victim vomit because turning the head twists the throat, blocking the expulsion of the obstructing foreign object. If vomiting does occur during the rescue (and the incidence of vomiting is quite small), the victim's head is quickly turned to the side and his mouth cleaned out.

The only time that the head position is not crucial is when the maneuver is performed on a drowning victim. Water can pass through the airway even if the throat is contorted.

SAVING YOURSELF

Both of the self-save techniques are simple adaptations of the basic subdiaphragmatic thrust. In the first variation, the victim simply performs the standard Heimlich maneuver on himself. He places his hands in the same position as he would if he were saving someone else. (The knob of his fist should be directly against his own abdomen, slightly above the navel and well below the rib cage.) He then presses upward, toward the diaphragm, with a quick motion to clear the airway.

The victim can also attempt to save himself using a firm edge instead of his hands. He positions himself over the edge of a horizontal object such as a chair or couch back or table edge and presses his abdomen against the edge with a quick movement.

The Maneuver on Animals

The Heimlich maneuver can be used efficiently on dogs and cats to help save them from choking to death on wrongly swallowed objects. The following two stories illustrate how true this is.

In late December 1987, Randall P. Sinclair, then 62 years of age, told me the following tale by telephone. He said he was walking along a downtown Toronto, Ontario, sidewalk with his five-year-old German-shepherd companion, Duke, when the dog suddenly commenced coughing. "I could tell poor Duke was choking on something, but I didn't know what to do," Mr. Sinclair said. He had been blinded in an industrial accident four years before this episode occurred.

"I yelled for assistance, and that's when this kind young man came to my dog's rescue." Randall was referring to then 15-year-old David Dockerty, who happened to be standing on the opposite side of the street when the cry for help came.

The teenager rushed over and picked the guide dog up in his arms and squeezed real hard a couple of times until a chunk of hamburger and bun came flying out of his mouth.

"I guess someone had thrown a half-eaten burger onto the ground, and Duke ate it," Randall related. "But he couldn't swallow it, and it became stuck in his throat somewhere. I offered the young man $20 Canadian for his good deed, but he refused to take my money and said he was only glad to be able to help someone in need like this."

In late February 1994, Clearfield, Utah, resident Sandy Otteson found her kitten choking on a cigarette butt and nearly dead. Sandy dialed 911 but the confused dispatcher turned her over to an animal-control director. As a certified emergency-medical technician, this female county employee knew how to perform the Heimlich maneuver on a baby. But on a kitten? Well, that seemed an entirely different matter at first.

The woman decided, however, to calmly instruct Ms. Otteson to hold the cat so its head was pointing directly toward the ground. Then she told the cat's owner, who was crying hysterically at the time, to squeeze the cat's diaphragm "like you're trying to squeeze something out of a bottle."

It worked. The cigarette butt popped out like a champagne-bottle cork and the kitten was able to breathe normally again. The recent divorcee calmed down after this and couldn't thank her adviser enough. "That kitten is all she has in the world. It's more than a cat. It's her whole family," the animal-control director told me later in an interview.

CHRONIC-FATIGUE SYNDROME

A New Name for the Same Old Malady

Recently I received a new health title to review in *Folk Medicine Journal* (a publication I've edited several years). Entitled *The Downhill Syndrome* (Garden City Park, NY: Avery Publishing Group, 1997), it essentially was a renaming of an old problem, chronic-fatigue syndrome. The book was more diagnostic than remedial, which may have accounted for its rather slow sales.

The authors, Drs. Pavel Yutsis and Morton Walker, attributed this widespread problem to a type of herpes virus (Epstein-Barr virus or EBV), which in more aggressive phases can mimic flulike symptoms. The primary one, though, "is fatigue" but not the type "most people recognize as tiredness." They differentiated between normal fatigue and this: "The primary symptom of the Downhill Syndrome fatigue is an inveterate depletion of energy, draining of strength, and total wearing out of a person to the point of absolute disability."

Health Advice from an Old Rockhound

In my own many consultations with those suffering from chronic fatigue syndrome (CFS), I have always emphasized one particular group of nutrients over anything else and that is *minerals*. While it is true that vitamins, amino acids, enzymes, certain herbs, good food, and adequate rest also play major roles in correcting this condition, it is minerals that are the real key to successfully coping with it. Strangely, just about all of the popular health literature that has been written about CFS virtually ignores or pretty much downplays their significance. For instance, the authors of the book just cited give a measly five lines to minerals and then ignore them in the rest of their text.

Sometime in the summer of 1961 when I was 15 years old, my father, Jacob, took my brother, Joseph, and me from our home in Provo to the small farming community of Lehi in the northern part of Utah County. It was on a Sunday after church and we spent several hours visiting with an elderly gentleman named John Hutchings. At that time this locally born naturalist was in his seventy-second year of life (he died at age 88).

He showed us through several outbuildings on his property that housed a massive collection of Indian artifacts, several hundred antique guns, and just about everything imaginable to represent everyday pioneer living: pine furniture, intricate glassware, butter churns, flat-irons, boot-pullers, fluters, mechanics' tools, razor strops, hoop dresses, quilts, spinning wheels, treadle sewing machines, and the like.

As a youth Mr. Hutchings had studied and practiced mounting birds and animals of various sizes until these skills have become finely honed. He showed us lifelike mountings of nearly 50 Utah County birds, which included perchers, swimmers, divers, waders, seed eaters, carrion eaters, birds of prey, gnat catchers, flycatchers, quail and grouse, woodpeckers, goat suckers, and tiny hummingbirds. As part of this wonderful avian collection, he had more than 400 sets of mostly local bird eggs, with each clutch carefully mounted in a glass-covered container.

My father and he soon became engaged in a short conversation on health-related matters. My father, who then owned and operated an antiquarian bookstore in Provo (Cottage Book Shop), inquired of the older gentleman what he did to have so much energy and stamina at his age. Mr. Hutchings informed him that his "secret" for having so much vitality lay in the fact that he took minerals on a constant basis. He claimed that minerals and eating three regular meals a day consisting of good, solid food (mostly tuber vegetables and whole grains, some dried fruit, and a little meat) was all that was needed to give an individual the kind of vigor and vitality he or she was looking for.

The man wasn't into taking vitamins or using herbs (except for serious ailments) or going to a health-food store (which in those days were few and far between and sometimes hard to locate). He has spent much of his life outdoors, working some 30 years for the U.S. Postal Service, first as a horse-and-buggy-driving rural carrier and then later as a walking mailman. He spent nearly all of his available free time on numerous adventurous exploring expeditions in the surrounding mountains, foothills, and receded lake beds looking for more items to add to his ever-growing collection. He claimed that walking and hiking, breathing good air, eating the right kind of food, and having a strong faith in God was all that anyone needed to "grow in style while retaining your youthful vigor" (as he aptly put it).

Minerals Are Everything

I remember Mr. Hutchings had a passion for minerals. Besides consuming mineral-rich foods and adding some powdered minerals to his cereal, juice, stews, or soups occasionally for guaranteeing himself extra vitality, he also collected minerals in a B-I-G way! He showed us one of the most impressive gem and mineral collections I have ever seen in my life. It consisted of precious and semi-precious gems, gold, silver, and platinum specimens, rare pearls, and numerous crystals of every intriguing shape and size imaginable. It was from Mr. Hutchings that I learned as a boy the real meaning of the adage, "a diamond in the rough." I remember him placing into the palm of my hand what appeared to be a rather unimpressive looking pebble of no particular distinction. He watched as I turned it around with my fingers before making the wisecrack about how nice it would be to send skipping across the surface of a pond several times. He chuckled and said that if I ever did such a thing, it would be the most expensive stone ever thrown to satisfy such boyish antics. But the real surprise came when he told me I was holding a diamond worth half a million dollars! I about dropped it in astonishment and meekly handed it back, feeling a little foolish for my careless remark.

The gentleman consoled me by saying that my reaction had been typical for most of those who had seen this particular stone before. He said that the untrained eye would never know the true worth and beauty that lay beneath its plain, uncut, and unpolished surface. He then related a little piece of history that I found fascinating. He said that history's largest diamond, the Cullinan, 3,106 carats before cutting, was so unimpressive in the rough that King Edward VII of England haughtily remarked, as he held it up to the light for closer inspection, "I should have kicked it aside as a lump of glass if I had seen it in the road."

Mr. Hutchings stated that the world's best diamond cutters were in the Netherlands and that they were a small and select aristocracy of expert lapidarists. It was their job to skillfully cut, grind, and polish the many facets of such stones, to which with their precision they were able to allow their stones to take full advantage of light's effects passing through them. He finished his brief lecture to me by saying that those who've suffered the most in life ofttimes make the best gems because, like the stones, they've been skillfully worked by the Almighty to the point where their best virtues show.

I have been recommending ionic minerals from the Great Salt Lake as well as mineral-rich foods for years for those suffering from CFS, with many good results. Minerals, indeed, are the centerpiece of energy production and vitality maintenance just as John Hutchings said they were almost four decades ago. I typically advise CFS sufferers to add 15 drops of liquid ConcenTrace to a glass of tomato or carrot juice or mixed greens twice daily for that extra boost they need. (See Product Appendix under Trace Minerals Research for more data.) I also encourage them to eat more baked or steamed root vegetables (with the skin left intact, where most of the minerals are), squashes and pumpkins, whole grains, nuts and seeds, and various edible sea-weeds such as kelp (which can be used as a food seasoning in place of salt and pepper). Then, too, there is a wide array of seafoods ranging from fish to shrimp that will supply additional trace minerals not al-ways obtained from food sources raised on the land.

CIRRHOSIS OF THE LIVER

A Naturalist's Simple Approach

During 1966–1968 I worked in several Salt Lake area restaurants as a line cook and apprentice chef. One time I drove down to Lehi, Utah, and visited again with naturalist John Hutchings, who was by then an octogenarian. The city had helped to raise the necessary funds for a museum named in his honor. I knew of an older morning line cook at work who suffered from cirrhosis of the liver due to a bad drinking problem and inquired of Mr. Hutchings what might be good for this fellow to use.

He told me of an old pioneer remedy given to him by a Greek im-migrant many years ago when he worked in the mines as a young man. It consisted of making a tea from equal parts of fenugreek seeds, crushed olive pits, and the roots of burdock, yellow dock, and dande-lion. One-half teaspoon of each of these was simmered in one quart of boiling water for 15 minutes and then covered, set aside, and allowed to steep another 15 minutes, after which the liquid was strained and taken five times a day.

I thanked my host for this information and passed it on to the fry cook, who decided to give it a try for three months. He said it helped his liver a lot and even made him eventually quit his drinking habit.

COCKROACH INFESTATION

Catnip for the Roach Motel

Cockroaches as a whole are extremely cold; fossil evidence indicates their extreme abundance during the Carboniferous period, approximately 350 million years ago. These ancient cockroaches were able to fly and were undoubtedly the first flying animals. Today's roaches are worldwide in distribution and invade food supplies as well as emitting foul-smelling glandular secretions. Their shape enables them to use tiny cracks as hiding places. They are definitely creatures of the night and are believed to be carriers of a number of contagious human diseases.

A team of entomologists at Iowa State University in Ames now believe they have stumbled upon the best roach repellent of all, because it's natural, safe to use, and works effectively. Chris J. Peterson and Joel R. Coats tested the reaction of German cockroaches to two forms of nepetalactone, the herbal compound in catnip that drives cats up the wall with ecstasy. The researchers gave insects a choice of walking on either a piece of paper treated with nepelactone or untreated paper. For driving away roaches, one form of this catnip compound was 100 times as effective as deet, a toxic chemical ingredient found in commercial insect repellents. They are currently testing catnip's effect on mosquitoes in the hopes it might do the same thing.

They recommend keeping *fresh* catnip around the house in places where roach motels are likely to be found. But they warn of a possible side effect: too much of it might draw unwanted attention from all the neighborhood cats.

COLD HANDS AND FEET

Keeping Warm in Cold Weather

John Hutchings (1889–1977) was one of those remarkable individuals who was a self-made man in everything he did and in what he accomplished in his long and illustrious career as a famous Utah naturalist. It was he who discovered Timpanogos Cave in American Fork Canyon many years ago despite what park rangers say to the contrary.

Mr. Hutchings related to me that early one winter he ascended the rocky ledges of the flank of Mount Timpanogos in search of Indian relics. In doing so, he came up to a natural opening in the rock face. With the aid of a lantern he ventured inside and found the interior to be breathtakingly beautiful.

He said that groundwater trickling through limestone hidden deep inside the mountain had dissolved the cave's three-chamber system over many millenniums and decorated them with fantastic mineral deposits. He found the underground passageways and various rooms to be floored with colored stalagmites and the dripping ceilings studded with uncounted crystal stalactite formations.

Emerging sometime later, he felt numbness set into his hands and feet. To correct this he made a small fire and brewed up a pot of Postum (a noncaffeinated cereal-grain beverage) and added a pinch of cayenne pepper to it. After slowly sipping two cups of this warm brew, he felt life and circulation returning to his cold extremities. After this he climbed back down without suffering any further stiffness.

COLD SORES

Try This Zinc Sandwich

Cold sores (also known as fever blisters) are an external manifestation of the herpes simplex virus (HSV-1). It causes chickenpox and shingles. Once the herpes virus enters the body, it can remain dormant within the central nervous system for a long period of time. It can then be reactivated by fever, physical or emotional stress, excessive exposure to sunlight, and some foods or drugs. Herpes outbreaks can recur for life, but they generally taper off after age 50.

Naturalist John Hutchings of Lehi, Utah, was in his eighty-fifth year of life when burglars broke into the municipal museum which housed his priceless collection of gems and minerals, jade, ivory, Chinese vases, soapstone carvings, antique guns, prized fossils (including some dinosaur footprints), numerous stuffed birds and animals, and even relics from King Arthur's Round Table. They stole a number of valuable objects after gaining entry by forcing a lock on the west entrance, cutting a chain, and then disabling the alarm.

It made the entire community sick at heart, but especially so for the collector himself. Just the thought of knowing that thieves had plundered and made away with some of his lifetime treasures was more than his aged system could bear. He soon came down with a bad case of cold sores and was unable to do much about them.

One of his children had been to one of my first health lectures in the Provo City Public Library and contacted me in regard to the man's unhappy predicament. I felt it an honor to be able to return something of service to a gentleman who had shared so much with me in past visits made to his place beginning when I was a teenager.

I recommended crushing a zinc tablet and then mixing it with a little vitamin E oil to make a suitable paste that could then be applied to the fever blisters. Since some of them were inside his mouth, I advised that this simple paste be applied over a small piece of soft white bread and peanut butter. Half a slice of the bread would have a thin layer of creamy peanut butter smeared over it. Then a small piece about an inch square was to have the vitamin-mineral paste spread on top of the peanut butter and inserted into the mouth with the fingers and firmly affixed to each cold sore site; the purpose of the peanut butter obviously was to help hold the paste in place.

This was done for about a week's time after which the elderly gentleman's cold sores completely cleared up and disappeared for good. I had also recommended to one of his children that he often be given warm chamomile or peppermint tea to drink in order to calm his nerves, which was done per my instructions. About a month later the burglars were captured and arrested in nearby Salt Lake City, but unfortunately most of the stolen items were never recovered.

COLIC

A Frontier Remedy

All babies are naturally prone to cry—that's their way of self-expression. But when otherwise healthy babies cry incessantly, usually after a feeding, they more often than not tend to have colic. Gas produces colic and abdominal pain, which occurs in an estimated 25 percent of all babies.

When this happens, mothers should cease giving cow's milk or formula to their infants; instead they should opt for soy or goat's milk, always given warm and never cold. Warm catnip or peppermint tea may be bottle-fed to anguished infants with astonishingly great success noticed within a matter of minutes. Babies should be burped and persuaded to rest on their stomachs for a short time with a small folded towel placed underneath them. Stay in the room with the baby while he or she is on the stomach, and then lay the baby on his or her back to sleep.

COLITIS

Similar to IBS

Simply put, colitis is inflammation of the colon. In reality, though, it can indicate one of two diseases: Crohn's disease (regional enteritis) or ulcerative colitis. Symptoms typically occur episodically in "attacks" and include pain in the lower abdomen and diarrhea, which may be bloody. Other symptoms may include fatigue and anxiety during such spells.

In its early phases colitis is difficult to distinguish from irritable bowel syndrome (IBS). But there are a few major differences. Colitis tends to flare up, then subside, whereas IBS tends to be a recurring problem. In colitis, the abdominal pain tends to be more severe and more localized on the left side (the descending colon). In colitis, the other chief symptom is diarrhea, whereas in IBS, often both diarrhea and constipation may occur. And IBS often causes increased belching and bloating, which rarely happen in colitis cases.

Same Basic Self-Care Program for Both

Dietary readjustments are mandatory: Stay away from high-fat foods such as butter, hot dogs, sausage, bacon, pizza, and ALL fast foods. Eat low-fat, high-fiber foods instead: salmon, no-butter popcorn, fresh fruit, carrot and celery sticks, radishes, cherry tomatoes, cooked beans, baked apples, cooked oatmeal, oat bran bread and cookies, tossed green salads, and so forth. Also remember to drink more water and *always* start every day with breakfast built around whole-grain or bran breads, muffins, and cereals, fresh fruits, and yogurt.

If diarrhea persists, drink some boiled rice water to stop it. If there is excessive gas, drink some warm peppermint tea or take two ginger-root capsules to alleviate it. When the urge comes to defecate, do so without any delays. If constipation is a problem, drink prune or carrot juice, eat one-half cup Bio-K+, or take some Fibre System Plus from ShapeRite (see Product Appendix).

COLON CANCER

Science Proves Garlic Works

On Thursday, August 12, 1999, I attended the last graduating class of the twentieth century from Brigham Young University in Provo, Utah with a friend. Graduates from almost every state and 51 countries received bachelor's, master's, and doctoral degrees. There were a great many black gowns and colored tassels gathered in the Marriott Center for these commencement exercises.

The class of 1999 happens to be the largest graduating class since the inception of Brigham Young Academy. It also has—for the first time in 50 years—more women than men graduating.

One of the graduates whom I had a chance to meet from this one hundred twenty-first class proved to be anything but ordinary. David Frantz began his master's work on the effects of garlic on colon cancer in 1995. Shortly after he began his research, his wife, Deborah, was diagnosed with scleroderma. Frantz studied the rare illness from a professor's textbook and learned that it is generally a fatal one that immobilizes its victim's limbs and organs. The disease progressed rapidly in his wife and she died in 1998.

This experience left Frantz determined to return to the lab and do what his wife had wanted him to do: finish graduate school. His determination paid off last spring when he presented a paper at the annual meeting of the Federation of American Scientists for Experimental Biology. Frantz discovered that garlic stops colon cancer during a phase of the cancer's growth cycle.

Frantz said that based on his initial research he wouldn't hesitate recommending raw garlic often to anyone with a background history of family colon cancer or those who may be at higher risk than the general populace. While he never said anything about garlic supplements, I suggest supplementing the diet with Kyolic aged garlic extract from Japan. (Also see "*Cancer.*")

COLOR BLINDNESS

The Delightful Dandelion

Everyone knows dandelions. They dot fields, lawns, and meadows with their bright-yellow flowers and downy-white seed heads. There is hardly a more versatile and practical plant to come by than this one. Ironically, though, many gardeners, landscape specialists, and extreme lawn lovers consider this to be one of the most cursed and despised of any herbal weed around. And yet as the loveable infant comic strip character Marvin (drawn by Tom Armstrong) once observed while crawling on the front lawn of his parents' home: "Dandelions are nature's way of giving dignity to weeds!"

Sometime in July 1992, while lecturing in the state of Maine, I happened to have had the good fortune of meeting Adrian Wells of Wilton. He told me he had a unique problem: He couldn't keep the grass out of his dandelions. Or, put another way, Wells grew edible dandelions as a cash crop; but he just couldn't get them to grow where he wanted them to. Oh sure, the pesky perennials prospered on his lawn—exactly where he *didn't* want them. But they weren't flourishing in his three-acre dandelion field, where they helped him earn part of his then cool $100,000 annual revenue. "The trouble is," he lamented, "too much is known about how to kill them but not enough on how to grow them."

He related to me that a local herbalist used the *fresh* yellow blossoms that he regularly supplied her with in a type of green vegetable drink for people suffering from color blindness as well as night blindness. Her primary vegetable juice bases were tomato or carrot. She would blend three tablespoons of cut dandelion flowers to every eight ounces of juice. People reported being able to distinguish colors a lot better after 30 days on this regimen.

COMA

An Indian Powwow

In July 1994, on a hot Sunday afternoon, I stood with Max Bear Paw and Jolene Little Deer on the shore of Flathead Lake at Elmo, Montana, and listened to the sound of bells and jingles ringing to the heartbeat of distant drums. This cacophony of sounds reverberated against the expanse of an incredibly blue sky and majestic mountains. We were all here for a Red Earth Celebration: there was a field full of cars, campers, tents, and teepees around us. And off to one side were a circular arena with a metal roof where competitors were dancing, some shedlike buildings where people played gambling games with sticks and small hand drums, and a cluster of plywood buildings and trailers where one could buy coffee, jewelry, Indian tacos, beads, elk teeth, or snuff-can lids for dancers' regalia.

"We go to powwows to experience the kind of peace and joy we can't find in the white man's world," Mary Bad Wolf explained to me later in the day. The phrase *pau wau* once meant medicine man or spiritual leader to Algonquin tribes. But Europeans who viewed these medicine dances believed the word referred to the entire event. What those Europeans saw, however, didn't resemble what goes on today. The tradition of Indian dancing is ancient, but today's powwows developed only in the last century. Powwows are gatherings—often held on weekends—in which Native Americans of many different tribes come, usually from great distances, to dance, sing, gamble, and visit friends and family.

The focus is dance—a series of open social dances called intertribals mixed with competition in several dance categories. The categories, such as Men's Fancy and Women's Jingle Dress, are based on traditional dances that were once part of spiritual ceremonies, preparation for war, healing rituals, or celebrations of triumph. Today's powwows are more of a salute to ancestral rituals. They're definitely not shows or features of entertainment. These celebrations may at first appear to be somewhat loud, rambunctious, and a bit disorganized to a non-Indian outsider. But for someone such as myself who by professional training is an anthropologist and has followed such events for many years over the entire Western Hemisphere, they are fraught with considerable meaning and purpose.

Toma's Coma Remedy

Toma Medicine-in-the-Wind is a Crow medicine woman. We had a chance to exchange some information regarding the use of certain common herbs that are popular in this part of the country. Toma related an interesting case in which she was called to assist in 1992. A 32-year-old white woman had been in a car wreck and sustained some serious head injuries, which had left her in a coma. The attending doctors had attempted to bring her out of it but were unsuccessful. The woman's husband, however, hearing of Toma's skills, requested her presence through an intermediary who happened to know both parties pretty well.

Because of the husband's strong persuasiveness, doctors reluctantly gave their consent for Toma to treat this woman in her room at the hospital. The medicine woman mixed together some peeled, crushed garlic cloves, a pinch of cayenne pepper, some finely ground fresh yerba santa leaves, and a few crushed pine needles with a little wintergreen oil and bear grease (Vaseline can be substituted for the latter). After mixing these together in a ceramic bowl using a wooden spoon, she obtained a smooth paste.

The compound was strongly aromatic, and its odor filled the entire room. She mentioned that sometimes she has added a little Mentholatum ointment or Vicks Vaporub for greater smell intensity. She then proceeded to rub some amounts of this mixture on the comatose patient's forehead, throat, inside the arm bends, on both wrists, inside the palms of the hands, and upon the soles of the feet. After this, the patient was turned on her side and the remainder of this strongly scented mixture was liberally applied from her neck to the base of her spine through the open hospital gown she was wearing at the time.

"All it took was 15 minutes for the medicine to work," Toma stated. "The white woman began making stirring motions which eventually brought her to a full wakeful state." Toma indicated that the husband was extremely pleased with what had just happened and offered to pay her several hundred dollars cash on the spot for her services, which she refused to take. She told him that accepting such a token of payment would offend the Great Spirit. The doctors were totally baffled by what she had accomplished, but obviously elated and happy for their patient and her husband.

COMMON COLD

American Indian Dances

In mid-summer of 1994 I attended an authentic powwow held at Flathead Lake near Elmo, Montana. Several hundred people representing numerous tribes were in attendance. I watched a number of Native American dances with awe and fascination.

These dances were intricate and varied. Women in fringed buckskin dresses danced slowly—the Women's Traditional Buckskin Dance, as it is appropriately called. Men wearing fur-and-feather headdresses and bustles later danced a story of an animal hunt or of ancestral scouting before a great battle—the Men's Traditional. I found the Men's Grass Dance to be sinuous and smooth; it looked to me like wind blowing across a prairie of men dressed in flowing streamers of yarn. In the Jingle Dress Dance—an Ojibwa dance originally used in healing—the women wore dresses adorned with hundreds of jingles made from the lids of snuff cans. In the flamboyant Fancy Dance men wearing double bustles, ribbons, and bright streamers of yarn danced wildly as color swirled around them, making each seem as if he were on fire.

Toma's Better Brew to Kill That Cold

I met a number of interesting people at this event. One of them was a female Indian shaman named Toma Medicine-in-the-Wind. We shared botanical information for a few maladies. She asked me what white folks did when they got a cold. I told her some of the herbal and vitamin–mineral supplements that are popular in health-food stores these days. She asked me how much they cost and I gave her an approximate figure for two leading brands.

She was astonished that people would dare to pay so much for what she called "dead medicine." She shook her head in disappointment and then wondered aloud just *who* was doing the scalping to whom with these inflated prices. She said that the Indians she knew almost *never* paid for such medicines when they came down with a cold. Instead they turned to reliable remedies handed down from their ancestors.

One of her favorite remedies called for adding two tablespoons each of chickweed herb and mullein leaves to a quart of boiling water. After stirred, the pot was covered with a lid and set aside to steep for 30 minutes. The brew was consumed *warm*, one cup at a time every three hours. The patient would rest for the entire day and by the following day all symptoms would be gone.

COMPULSIONS

Bitter to the End

A remedy periodically used among some western American Indian tribes to help allay compulsions for gambling, hard liquor, or loose women calls for a strong tea to be made out of pine needles (four tablespoons) and some pine sap (one-half teaspoon). Both ingredients are added to one quart of boiling water, covered with a lid, and allowed to simmer five to ten minutes on low heat before being set aside to steep another 40 minutes. This intensely bitter brew is strained and slowly sipped one-half cup at a time two to three times daily on an empty stomach. The compulsion usually goes away when the full bitterness of the tea sets in.

"COMPUTER-SCREEN" EYES

A Grandmaster's Solution

A "first-ever" experience for Salt Lake City occurred during a three-week period stretching from August 23 to September 10, 1999, when the U.S. Chess Championships opened at the downtown Holiday Inn. Sixteen men and ten women participated in an invitation-only competition. I attended the event as a spectator one afternoon for several hours.

The gallery numbers were in the dozens, not in the thousands. And nobody in the sparse crowd yelled out, "We're Number 1" or "You suck." None of the players talked trash or mugged in front of TV cameras. In fact, they didn't do much of anything except sit, scratch, yawn, stretch, belch, occasionally pass wind, and periodically get up and walk about for a little exercise.

By now, you've probably got the idea that chess isn't a contact sport and is played with a great deal of dignity by men and women who respect one another's skills. But I wasn't fooled. The level of intensity and concentration here rivaled anything that The Masters (golf), Wimbledon (tennis), the World Series (baseball), or the Super Bowl (football) were capable of generating. And the mind games were at an entirely different level altogether.

I spoke with one grandmaster—there were 15 of them in attendance, which is half the total number in America alone (there are 450 worldwide)—who commented, "You won't find anything more rigorous. It can be quite physical, too. I've seen players drop weight during these championships. Once you get locked into a battle of the minds, it's an incredible thing to experience and see."

This particular gentleman told me that he enjoyed playing chess by computer via the Internet and the World Wide Web with grandmasters in other countries. "Often I will be in front of a computer screen for hours on end," he admitted, "and my eyes will start to hurt and sting quite a bit." So what does he do in such instances? "I brew myself a cup of chamomile tea by taking *two* teabags and letting them soak in a cup of hot water for about ten minutes. I remove and discard the bags and then get some clean cotton balls, soak them in a little of the tea, and gently squeeze them into my eyes, while my head is tilted back. I make sure the tea is *lukewarm* so as not to damage my eyes. I repeat the process several times on each eyeball. It is so soothing and relieves the symptoms of my 'computer screen' eyes very quickly. I do this at least twice a day when I'm using the computer a lot."

For those unacquainted with the intricate game of chess, a grandmaster is the highest title to be awarded by the World Chess Federation to top winners. Chess originally was played in ancient Egypt several thousand years ago by the pharoahs and other members of the royal class.

CONCUSSION

A Russian Chess Champion's Remedy

Not too long ago (late August to early September 1999) the U.S. Chess Championships were held at the Holiday Inn in downtown Salt Lake City. A little over two dozen men (16) and women (10) participated in this invitation-only tournament. I went for part of one day to watch them in action; the experience required a great deal of patience and absolute quiet and was something akin to watching a snail race.

I met 52-year-old Grandmaster Boris Gulko, who has won national championships in both the United States and Russia. He spoke pretty good English. I steered a portion of our brief conversation toward folk remedies. He related this to me. He said that an aunt of his sustained a serious concussion in Moscow a few years ago from a bad fall. Doctors were concerned she might not fully recover from its effects—headache, dizziness, blurred vision, and mental confusion.

One of his *babushkas* (Russian grandmothers) was skilled in the healing arts. She made a porridge for the aunt by cooking equal parts (one-half cup) of fenugreek seed and oatmeal in hot water. She also gave the woman the same items in powdered form (a teaspoon of each three times daily) mixed with a little jam and spread on some dark rye bread to eat. Within four days his aunt had totally recovered from the symptoms of her concussion and was pronounced well by her doctors after that.

CONGESTIVE HEART FAILURE

A Polish Approach

Some of my best sources of health information generally have come from large gatherings where many people assemble for various purposes. That is why I make an effort to attend such events, especially those with an international flavor to them. One such happening occurred at a local chain hotel in downtown Salt Lake City the latter part of the summer of 1999. It was the U.S. Chess Championships, a first ever for this city.

I spoke with one Polish strategist who said it was his aim "to get into my opponent's head and try to discover his tactical and psychological weaknesses, so I know where I can attack him." He then opened up a laptop computer and showed me a database of several of his expected opponents that included their histories and playing tendencies. "Nobody just walks into this room and starts playing," he mused.

We watched several players in action that day. It was a grueling process, to be sure. Divided into two divisions, the men played a round-robin, with the top two players from each division advancing to the semifinals and championship (each four-game matches). The women played nine rounds to determine their champion. Though under a time limit, it wasn't unusual for games to last four, five, or even six hours.

"It gets to be pretty intense sometimes," my Polish informant suggested. He had just come from Las Vegas, where the world championships concluded with Russian grandmaster Alexander Khalifman clinching the title with a draw against fellow countryman Vladimir Akopian. "Some of the players paced like crazy down there [in Vegas]. Others just stayed quiet. But everybody has his own style. It's a wide range."

When he inquired what I did for a living, the conversation turned toward alternative health matters. Upon discovering that I was a doctor of folk medicine, he volunteered the following information about his own physical health. He said that he had suffered in the past from symptoms of congestive heart failure; his included extreme fatigue and weakness, rapid heartbeat, shortness of breath, swelling in his ankles and feet, rapid weight gain, swollen neck veins, and restlessness. He stated that his poor health affected his game and frequently kept him from winning as he had used to do.

An old woman in the city of Gadansk whom he consulted for advice, told him to brew a tea made of the cockleburs and leaves of the burdock plant. He did this on a daily basis for six months. He boiled one quart of water and added one-half cup of *fresh* cockleburs and one and a half cups cut leaves. He simmered the brew on low heat for approximately five minutes and then steeped it, and covered it with a lid for another 30 minutes after this.

My informant drank one cup of this tea every three hours or five times daily between meals or on an empty stomach. He also started walking more often and completed a 45-minute stroll every morning and evening. Half a year later the fluid retention had disappeared and he had more vigor and vitality than before. His mental clarity significantly improved, as did his chess-playing skills.

CONJUNCTIVITIS

Something from My Childhood Days

In 1954–55 my father, brother, and I lived in Salem, Utah. (At that time my mother, Jennie, lived separate from the rest of the family on account of her mental illness and the fact that children made her exceedingly nervous.) I attended Mr. Thomas's third-grade class in a historic-looking, turn-of-the-century three-storied brick schoolhouse complete with a wooden bell tower and bell.

One day in class my eyes started itching, and so I rubbed them with my unwashed fingers. The next morning upon awakening at home, I discovered that I couldn't open my eyelids. They were glued shut with a yellowish sticky material. My father became aware of my situation and got some boric-acid powder from the cupboard and mixed it with a little warm water.

With this simple solution in hand, he washed off both of my eyelids and around the corners of my eyes with some tufts of clean cotton soaked in the liquid. He did this morning and evening for a number of days until the condition had completely disappeared. I was never bothered with it again after that.

CONSTIPATION

Food Laxatives

I'm very much a fan of food therapy and believe that foods are ofttimes just as good as, if not better than, nutritional supplements for different health problems. While herbs such as cascara sagrada, buckthorn, and senna are proven potent laxatives, they also can be habit-forming and can be injurious to pregnant women and the elderly.

But certain foods can certainly move the bowels efficiently: a bowl of prunes, a small glass of prune juice, orange juice, or carrot juice, a bowl of cooked oatmeal, one medium banana, one ripe avocado, one medium-sized raw carrot, one celery stalk, an apple, or a bag of unbuttered popcorn.

CONTACT-LENS PROBLEMS

Nutrients Fight Infection

Those who wear contact lenses sometimes experience problems with eye infection due to dirty or improperly cleaned lenses. Vitamins A and C are very good for fighting infection and should be taken if such a problem occurs. Generally 25,000 I.U. of vitamin A and 1,500 mg. of vitamin C taken orally every day should help to clear up this condition.

Problems of redness and itching may be due to badly fitting lenses or wearing contacts for too long. Such problems result from either injury to the extremely sensitive layer of cells that cover the eyeball or irritation of the conjunctiva, the thin membranes that line the inner surface of the eyelid and cover a portion of the eyeball itself.

To avoid such things from happening, be sure to clean your contacts frequently with a solution made especially for them. Don't use saliva for wetting. That's a bad idea since it contains bacteria that might bring on infection. And also think twice before using homemade saline solutions. They contain no preservatives and have been associated with eye infection. (Also see under *Conjunctivitis* for additional information.)

COUGH

A Short History of Watches

Watches evolved from portable clocks sometime in the late 1500s. The first ones were suspended from belts or worn around the neck, and later they were carried in pockets. The mass production of pocket watches in America began in the 1860s. By then watches on bracelets had already appeared, but they were mostly worn by women. They didn't become popular for men, who believed they were too decorative. But with the advent of World War I that attitude changed, as soldiers soon discovered just how difficult it was to reach inside their bulky coats to check the time.

Today watches pour off the assembly lines in unbelievable numbers: more than half a billion a year, with some 300,000 sold daily in the U.S. alone. Some tend to believe that more timepieces have been built than all other machines combined.

The Great Swiss Tea That'll Cure Your Cough Like Clockwork

Franck Gerhard worked for many years as a Swiss watchmaker in the city of Basel until he relocated his family to New York City, where he now works part-time as a watch repairman. The preceding history of the watch was his small contribution to this book as well as a remedy for a nagging cough.

"I recommend several warm herbal teas depending, of course, on what type of cough you have," he began. "If a mucus condition exists within the lungs and you wish to expel it, then sipping some warm tea made from mullein leaves or pine buds or thyme herb is very good. On the other hand, if you wish to suppress that same cough and have nothing to expectorate, than a warm tea made from fennel seed and aniseed is ideal. You should remember to simmer the seeds a few minutes before steeping afterwards.

"If a more soothing tea is desired to heal the delicate mucous membranes lining the throat and lungs, a combination (equal parts) of mullein leaves and yarrow herb makes a wonderful remedy for this." Any of these herbs may be obtained from your local health food store or a major mail-order herb supplier such as Indiana Botanic Gardens in Hammond, Indiana or Frontier Herbs in Norway, Iowa.

CRABS

Getting Rid of Pubic Lice

Crabs is a nickname for body lice found in the pubic area. Sometimes, though, the eyelashes, trunk hair, and armpit hair may become infested. To get rid of them apply a shampoo or lotion (A-200 Pyrinate) liberally from waist to knees to guarantee adequate coverage. Or add one tablespoon of tea-tree oil or melaleuca oil to one pint of warm water. Mix thoroughly and then sponge the body well with the solution. Or bathe with a soap or shampoo containing melalueca. The lice die quickly after contact with either of these medications, but it may require a week for the itching to subside. New bedding may also be needed to prevent their recurrence.

CRACKED HEEL

Rose Vinegar

Some years ago I bought a copy of *Cést la nature qui à raison* (Paris: Opera Mundi, 1972) by the renowned French herbalist Maurice Mességué. His inspired use of ordinary plants and herbs helped thousands of ordinary men and women achieve good health again. Among these were a small number of celebrities that included popes (John XXIII), presidents (Herriot of France), poets (Jean Cocteau), prime ministers (Churchill of England), kings (Farouk of Egypt), artists (Maurice Utrillo), and statesmen (Konrad Adenauer of Germany).

He spoke affectionately of his Grandmother Sophie in his book and how she used rose vinegar to treat numerous skin afflictions including cracked heel, rough elbow, pimples, and warts. To make her rose vinegar he advised macerating ten handfuls of dried petals and then soaking them in seven pints of red-wine vinegar in plenty of sunlight for up to three weeks before straining and bottling.

This rose vinegar makes a wonderful skin lotion and should be rubbed on those areas needing specific attention morning and evening for several months. After doing this each time it may be a good idea to rub the cracked or toughened skin with a little virgin olive oil to help soften things a bit. Also taking a high-potency B-complex (two tablets daily) helps nourish the skin nutritionally from within.

CROHN'S DISEASE

Kampo Medicine

The folk medicine of Japan is known as kampo; it originated in China about 12 centuries ago. While traditional Chinese medicine (TCM) has always had an elegant theoretical system, Kampo medicine is a greatly simplified approach to both diagnosis and treatment as compared to that found in the TCM. The idea behind it is quite simple: Combinations of herbs can correct combinations of imbalances within the body, thereby relieving the combination of symptoms that a person may be experiencing.

Today kampo is the officially government-sanctioned alternative medicine in Japan and is now beginning to find some favor in North America as well. Most of those who currently practice kampo in Japan are physicians who've been trained in Western medicine. Patients obviously benefit from this since they are getting the best of two worlds, orthodox and holistic medicine combined. Keisetsu Otsuka, M.D., recorded his own personal experiences with kampo in the book *Thirty Years of Kampo: Selected Case Studies of an Herbal Doctor.* In this important healing manual he recorded 374 case studies in which kampo was applied to medical conditions as defined by Western medicine. First published in 1959 in Japanese, the book was later translated into both Chinese and English.

Dr. Otsuka had great success with the herb hakka (peppermint). Warm peppermint tea consumed during or after a meal helped to relieve the cramping, intestinal inflammation, and diarrhea accompanying both Crohn's disease and irritable bowel syndrome (IBS). Or he would prescribe peppermint oil (eight drops in six ounces of warm water), which would pretty much accomplish the same things. More often than not multiple herbs rather than single herbs are used to treat both disorders due to their complexities. In this case, dandelion root is paramount to the successful treatment of either disorder, since kampo theory teaches that both digestive diseases result from an "overcontrolling liver." Dandelion root can be drunk as a tea or taken as capsules (two to three daily with food).

Those suffering from either disorder should avoid alcohol, wheat, cold or raw foods, greasy foods, coffee, carbonated beverages, chocolate, butter, margarine, ice cream, and citrus juices. Moderate fiber intake is recommended. High protein (fish and poultry) and vegetables (carrots, turnips, rutabagas, squash, cabbage, and broccoli) should be eaten frequently.

CROUP

A Common-Sense Approach

A pediatrician from the Czech Republic passed this information along to me a while back at an alternative medical convention we both were speaking at in New York City. Vaslov Havilicek, M.D., explained to me what he always tells parents who come to him with a child who is suffering respiratory problems at night.

First, he instructs them to calm down and not become panicky. Second, the croupy child's throat needs to be exposed to hot-water vapors. To do this the child should be taken into the bathroom by one of the parents. The door is closed and a towel pushed up against the bottom edge. All of the hot-water taps should then be turned on full blast and allowed to run for up to ten minutes. The parent holds the child in a comforting position and reassures him or her that everything will be okay if the child is upset or worried. The child's breathing will return to normal the more he or she breathes in the warm, misty air. Sitting in a steamy bathroom is quicker, much safer, and a lot easier than exposing a child to steam from a tea kettle, which can be very dangerous in that the child and parent might both get scalded.

Dr. Havilicek added that if warm mist fails to help the child to sufficiently recuperate, then a window should be opened so the child can breathe cool night air. Croup improves in the daytime but returns at night.

CROW'S FEET AROUND EYES

A Vinegar Trick from Hungary

My father's mother, Barbara Liebhardt Heinerman, emigrated to America from Temesvar, Hungary (now Timisoara, Rumania) with her husband Jacob Heinerman in 1906. She was an eighth-generation folk healer. One of her best-kept secrets for looking so young even in her late eighties and nineties was to rub the skin near the corners of both eyes with some wine vinegar or apple-cider vinegar morning and evening. She would soak a washcloth with this solution for that purpose. She was careful never to get any in her eyes. Being very astringent, vinegar helps to tighten skin, thereby removing most age lines.

CUTS

Ranchero Remedy

In the center of Spain is the huge *Meseta Central* that extends from the Cantabrian Mountains in the north to the Sierra Morena chain in the south and from the Portuguese border in the west to the low ranges that separate the plateau from the Mediterranean coast in the east. This vast central plateau contains some fertile valleys in which cattle and sheep are raised.

Pedro Almeira has worked as a ranchero (ranch hand) on one particular ranch for almost 30 years. A ranchero's life isn't easy, as I learned from him some time ago. He was visiting America for the first time in 1996 and stayed with his Basque sister in Idaho while here. It was through her that we met. He informed me that because a ranchero spent much of his time outdoors on horseback far away from regular medical services, it became necessary to improvise and do much of one's own doctoring.

Whenever any ranchero suffered cuts of any kind in the line of his work, he would first disinfect it with beer, wine, or some kind of hard liquor. After this a pinch of powdered red pepper would be placed on the cut and then left alone to heal of its own accord. He said this remedy always worked.

CYSTIC FIBROSIS

General Measures

This is the most common lethal genetic disease affecting mostly white infants, children, and young adults. In 1998 there were more than 35,000 known cases of cystic fibrosis.

Peppermint tea daily is required for respiratory functioning. No dairy products, sugary foods, or white-flour products should be allowed in the diet. An enzyme supplement is required every day to help food digest better. Room air should be sprayed with strong eucalyptus-tea solution. Oxygen therapy may be needed from time to time. A complete mineral formula such as ConcenTrace is highly advisable in juice or water (ten drops three times daily).

My own success in helping others with this problem has been largely confined to diet. The right kind of food is the best therapy for the successful management of this disease. Foods should always be more alkaline than acidic. This means fresh leafy greens and tuber vegetables take precedence over greasy foods and most fruits (some exceptions) every time. Protein sources such as whey, colostrum, nuts, seeds, and beans are especially valuable here. Fats can come from plant oils such as olive, sesame, or safflower as well as from avocado and certain nut butters.

No consumer health books that I know of have ever dealt with this problem. It would be safe to say that 99 percent of them ignore the matter altogether. This may be due to the seriousness of the problem itself or simply to a fundamental lack of knowledge concerning it. Even though I've generalized with most of the data given here, it is sufficient for an individual to apply in order to see good results and expect better-than-average management of an autosomal recessive disorder.

CYSTITIS
(See "BLADDER INFECTION")

CYSTS

Different Types

Cysts are fluid-filled sacs. Epidermal cysts are simple painless bumps under the skin that slide with the skin when you pull it. But they can become painful and tender if an injury breaks the cyst wall.

An ovarian cyst forms in the ovary, is quite common, and is usually noncancerous. It can vary in size and may occur at different sites within the ovary.

Cysts may develop within the tissues of the kidneys singly or in groups. They are usually spherical, thin-walled sacs filled with fluid.

Medical science is still baffled by cysts. How they originate and can then disappear just as mysteriously remains unexplained.

Diet Is a Factor

As I've observed numerous cyst cases over the years, I've come to the conclusion that poor diet is the leading cause of cysts. I've recommended a diet principally filled with water-holding fruits and vegetables: all melons, cucumbers, certain leafy greens (lettuce, watercress, parsley, spinach), pulpy fruits (kiwi, pears, peaches, grapes), berries, pumpkin, and squashes. I believe that they have a remarkable "rinsing effect" inside the body and can clean up "dirty" blood and polluted tissue nicely.

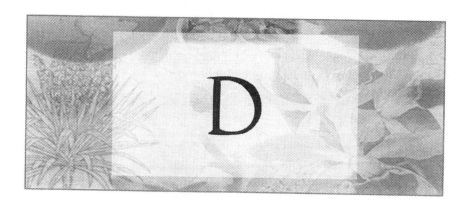

DANDRUFF

Meet the Future Techno-Cop

Lonny James is a police officer in a midsized community somewhere in the Intermountain West. Recently I had a chance to ride along with him one night in his patrol car while he was on shift. I was amazed by the technology currently at his disposal. We started out at 10:17 P.M. At 11:31 P.M. we tracked down a burglary suspect in a well-to-do neighborhood (the homeowners were then vacationing in the French Riviera). As usual the suspect gave a fictitious John Doe. But all Lonny did was fingerprint the guy and then transmit those prints from his squad car via computer to a national database for identification. Within 72 seconds (because I timed it) word came back that the man had several outstanding arrest warrants and also gave his real name. He was arrested on the spot and hauled off to jail.

The particular police department Lonny works for just bought 55 laptop computers with a federal technology grant of $340,000 that officers now use in their cars . Lonny used his laptop computer to scan in a digital picture of a suspected Peeping Tom whom he detained at 1:14 A.M. and had taken a photo of with his new digital camera. Several other officers some blocks away received it through their own computer e-mail and then showed the likeness to several witnesses who testified that this was the man who had been snooping around their homes an hour earlier. He was arrested and taken to jail by another officer who arrived on the scene for this purpose.

The latest piece of equipment, which Lonny had received just a day prior to our ride-along, was a digital video camera that allows him to digitally videotape the scene of an accident or crime and then send it back to police headquarters through his e-mail.

Dandruff Gone

During the course of our busy night shift together, I asked my police host if he knew of any folk remedies. His immediate reply was in the affirmative. "Yah, I got one for you," he said while at the same time running one of his hands through his thick blond hair. "I used to have dandruff real bad until my mother-in-law told me to rinse my hair with distilled vinegar every time I finished shampooing my hair. She told me to leave the vinegar in for five minutes while I washed the rest of my body and then to rinse it out with warm water. I did this for several weeks per her instructions and my dandruff disappeared for good. Now I need to do it only a couple of times a week to keep it from coming back."

DEEP-VEIN THROMBOSIS

Kanab Lassoes Western Legends

Our family has a 400-acre ranch in the wilderness of Southern Utah, about 65 miles north of Kanab. I made a trip there September 1–4, 1999. On Friday, September 3, I drove to Kanab to attend the first annual Eastern Legends Round-Up set amid the splendid red-rock country close by the Arizona border.

There was an inauguration of Kanab's "Little Hollywood Walk of Fame," honoring those who left their mark on Kanab filmmaking. At 9:30 A.M. producer Howard W. Koch was honored in the Century 21 parking lot. He was in attendance and I had a chance to briefly chat with him afterwards. Koch brought 11 productions to Kane County. His Kanab Westerns included *The Yellow Tomahawk* (1954) with Rory Calhoun, *Fort Yuma* (1955) with Peter Graves, and *Fort Bowie* (1958) with Ken Johnson.

One of his most famous numbers, however, to hit Kanab was *Sergeants 3*, directed by John Sturgis (*The Magnificent Seven*) and starring "the infamous Rat Pack"—Frank Sinatra, Dean Martin, Sammy

Davis, Jr., Peter Lawford, and Joey Bishop. "Oh, that was quite a bunch to be working with," he exclaimed with some reverence in his voice.

An Indian Remedy

I asked Koch if by chance he knew of any folk remedy that might have passed his way during those years of exciting filmmaking. He didn't have to think very long to give me a response. He recalled that a close relative of Peter Lawford's was suffering from deep-vein thrombosis at the time that *Sergeants 3* was being filmed in Kane County.

One evening after the day's shooting had been done, Lawford was in one of the town bars downing a few beers with one of the locals. Somehow mention of his relative's malady became known in the course of barroom conversation. A half-breed Indian by the name of Jasper Mule Deer sashayed over to the bar and told Lawford he couldn't help but overhear that part of their conversation. He said he had a remedy that might help Lawford's particular family member.

Lawford was wise enough to stop and listen respectfully to what the other man told him. Jasper instructed the actor to have the afflicted person take one-half teaspoon each of red powder and finely grated ginger root and one teaspoon of finely grated white onion in tomato juice every day for two-and-a-half months—and to be sure to take it with food because of the remedy's intense flavor and taste. He promised that would effect a cure. When Lawford inquired as to how much he owed the man, Jasper waved his hand and said the information was being given free and then walked back to his table and sat down where he resumed his drinking with some other Indians.

Koch said Lawford told him about this peculiar situation next morning on the set and didn't quite know what to make of it. Koch's advice was to have his sick relative give it a try and see if it worked. Lawford passed the information along and sometime later informed Koch that his relative's deep-vein thrombosis had disappeared for good.

Koch's take on all of this was simply, "You never know what you'll find or pick up in a bar!"

DELIRIUM

Red-Rock Country Medicine

On Friday, September 3, 1999, I went to Kanab, the seat of Kane County in southern Utah, to attend part of the first ever Western Legends Round-Up. Dozens of Westerns have galloped through the red rocks around this town, including John Ford's 1939 classic *Stagecoach* (which was also shot in Ford's favorite location, Monument Valley), *Union Pacific* (1939), *Brigham Young, Frontiersman* (1940), Clint Eastwood's *The Outlaw Josie Wales* (1976), and the 1993 big-screen remake of *Maverick*.

Non-Westerns filmed in the region include the Revolutionary War drama *Drums Along the Mohawk* (1939), the biblical epic *The Greatest Story Ever Told* (1965), the science-fiction classic *Planet of the Apes* (1968), and John Travolta's 1995 action flick *Broken Arrow*.

One of the local cowboy poets and I chewed the rag a while after his poetry reading in the Old Barn Playhouse located behind Parry's Lodge. Jones (as he wanted to be called) said that a couple of years ago he and some of his cowboy poet buddies got roaring drunk one night. One of their number became mentally affected by the hard liquor he drank and started hallucinating really badly and showing nerve-muscle disturbances, too.

"None of the rest of us were in too good a shape ourselves to really help out," he stated. "We thought maybe if our friend took 'some more hair of the dog that had bit him' [drink more alcohol] that that might do the trick. But the bartender advised against doing it. Instead, he gave our sick buddy a mug of hot water and honey and told him to sit down and slowly sip it. He did this, and it took about ten minutes before he finished the whole thing. Imagine our surprise when his delirium mellowed out some 30 minutes later."

"That's some mighty fine red-rock country medicine, don't you think?" he asked. And I nodded in agreement that it was.

DEMENTIA

Putting Your Money Where Your Heart Is

Turn on any financial talk show and you'll probably be deluged with advice about how to make more money. You'll learn which kind of retirement plan is best for you, and you'll hear arguments about the pros and cons of no-load mutual funds. Undoubtedly this can be helpful information, but it doesn't seem to go far enough.

Given the central, powerful role of money and business—in both our society and our personal lives—it is astonishing that so little attention is given to money's social, ethical, and spiritual dimensions. Even the most caring commentators seem oblivious to the enormous impact that our financial decisions exert on communities, the earth, and our individual peace of mind. Our money carries our voice to the world, a fact we often ignore.

Entering the picture at this point is an unusual Wall Street stockbroker. His name is Reginald Stuart, and he is an import from the London Stock Exchange of seven years ago. We recently met in New York City where I happened to be filming a one-minute television commercial for the Rubicon tin bracelet made and sold in Vancouver, British Columbia (see Product Appendix under Rubicon).

He acquainted me with something called Natural investing in which people seek to integrate their money and their values. Natural investing avoids some of the contentiousness that arises from the term "socially responsible," which can make others feel they are being labeled irresponsible. Natural investing simply encourages investors to identify their ethical values and to consider them when making financial decisions.

For most people, this approach does, indeed, feel quite natural. For example, a 1996 survey of mutual-fund investors found that 83 percent want their financial adviser to understand their concern for social and environmental issues before making an investment recommendation. Reginald claimed that data furnished to him by an organization called the Social Investment Forum indicated that well over one trillion dollars of today's investments—one tenth of all investment dollars— rely on some sort of ethical criteria. Nearly every mainstream investment option, he noted, now has a values-based equivalent.

I mentioned it was reassuring to hear something like this, because I had naturally assumed that most investors were just a bunch of cold-hearted and money-grabbing capitalists.

Something for His Grandma's Dementia

Mr. Stuart then turned the tide of conversation my way by telling me something of his grandmother's dementia, which he said had been getting progressively worse in the last year. He made it clear, though, that it wasn't Alzheimer's disease.

I informed him that his grandmother needed to increase her consumption of fresh vegetables and *some* fresh fruits. I also suggested five small meals per day instead of the conventional three big ones. I recommended a high-potency B-complex vitamin supplement (two tablets) daily, as well as an additional 500 micrograms of vitamin B-12 twice a day.

I recommended some good sources of essential fatty acids and those nutrients that augment them. I told him to have her caretaker give the woman one teaspoon each of evening primrose oil and flaxseed oil per day and to accompany these with 400 mg. of L-carnitine for breakfast, 750 mg. of choline for lunch, and 600 mg. of lecithin for dinner. I encouraged him to have her given 600 mg. of gotu kola and 200 mg. of ginkgo biloba daily and to make sure she ate plenty of cooked fish.

Almost five months later he called my home to tell me that my recommendations had helped her regain much of her memory and her old personality back. He said he appreciated what I had done for her and promised me some free "hot-stock tips" if I ever needed them.

DENTAL CAVITIES

Kangaroo Company

Wally Bradford lives "Down Under" in the Australian Outback. His business, to put it delicately, is kangaroo hunting. "It's not for the squeamish, matey," he told me some years ago as we lay on the beach in Bali, Indonesia, after a short ocean swim. Numerous Aussies clamor to this attractive vacation spot much as Americans do to Hawaii or some of the Caribbean Islands.

"I track 'em down, lasso the buggers, and haul 'em back to me place. There the gang and I skin 'em live," he said with a deliciously mischief smile, "before we sell 'em to fancy restaurants." Noticing I didn't so much as flinch a bit during these gory details, he praised my courage by saying, "You got good, solid backbone in you, mate!" I gave him a nonchalant glance and drawled, "Why should it bother me seeing as how I once was in the funeral business."

To which he roared a good laugh and retorted, "You got me there, mate. That's a good one, for sure!"

Some time later he told me of an old Outback remedy learned from the Aborigines. "If one of your teeth is bad and start's hurting like the devil," he said, "just cut yourself a small plug of chewing tobacco, wet it with a little of your own spit, and then jam it next to that tooth and leave it there. In a good and proper time it will take away the pain."

DEPRESSION

Crash Course for Feeling Happy

These condensed recommendations work and have a 15-year track record of proven success. Omit sugary foods from the diet. Get as much sunlight as possible. Eat more fish and fiber-rich foods. Consume organ meats such as heart, liver, kidney, and brain more often. Walk at least 15 minutes twice a day. Visit or call friends and relatives. Become involved in meaningful projects in your own neighborhood. Watch old comedies that can make you laugh since laughter is one of the most powerful antidepressant medicines known. Learn to relax by listening to classical music that is uplifting to the spirit and ennobling to the soul. Eat five to six small meals regularly every three hours or so. Have your doctor prescribe lithium if necessary.

DERMATITIS, DIABETES, DIAPER RASH

One Plant Does It All

The Maya Indians occupy an area comprising the Yucatan peninsula and much of the present state of Chiapas, Mexico; much of Guatemala; and parts of El Salvador and extreme western Honduras. Speaking a group of closely related languages, the population of Maya land today is roughly four million.

Maya prehistory is divided into the Formative (1500 B.C.–A.D. 300), Classic (A.D. 300–900) and Postclassic (A.D. 900–1500) periods. Most of the elaborate carvings, relief and full-round, and the paintings, murals, and ceramic that are the hallmarks of Classic Maya art come from various civic centers. These were once quite numerous and included such present historic sites as Copan in Honduras, El Mirador; Tikal, and Uaxactún in the northcentral Petén region of Guatemala; and Palenque, Piedra Negras, and Uxmal in Mexico.

I have visited most of these places on one or more occasions and have marveled at their breathtaking beauty. Truly, the ancient Maya had architectural design and building skills far beyond our comprehension. At the same time I have availed myself of interviewing natives residing in each of these regions who are descendants from these ancient craftspeople. My main interest has always been in their local materia medica, of course.

One of the most common herbs still in use after many centuries is *xabila* (also spelled *zabila*). This is the aloe vera plant. The clear gel secreted from the plant's succulent leaves is applied to dermatitis to help relieve the itching and promote healing of the skin. A watery liquid is made of the gel and consumed daily to help in the management of diabetes; various brands of liquid aloe vera can be purchased from health-food stores or through networking companies for the same purpose—one-half cup is taken in the morning with breakfast and the same amount again at night with dinner. Mothers periodically rub some of the raw plant gel on their babies' behinds to help clear up diaper rash. There are a few good companies in the United States who market a nearly pure aloe gel that can achieve the same results, but consumers need to do a little investigating for themselves and read product labels carefully before choosing a brand they feel comfortable with. If an aloe product seems to have too many chemical ingredients in it, then chances are its aloe content is rather sparse. Opt for another brand with few ingredients and where aloe is listed first on the label.

DIARRHEA

Boiled Rice Water Never Fails

Any number of herb books (including some of my own) will give you quite a variety of herbs from which to choose to stop diarrhea. Most of them are effective to varying degrees for this problem. However, some aren't always readily available and those that are may be a bit expensive.

Well, I like to keep things as simple and affordable as possible. During numerous visits to the Orient in more than two decades, I've discovered one easy "foolproof" remedy for getting rid of diarrhea in a hurry. Why, even a small child can make it. It is boiled rice water that has been cooled down before being drunk.

Follow the directions on the box or sack in which the polished white rice comes. Always be sure to *triple* the amount of water indicated. So, for instance, if the instructions call for one-and-a-half cups of white rice to be cooked in five cups of water, then be sure to add 15 cups instead. Cover the pot with a lid, turn the heat up high, and boil the contents for about 15 to 20 minutes. Strain the water, and refrigerate the rice for a later meal. When the rice water has sufficiently cooled, drink two cups. Usually the diarrhea will cease within 30 to 45 minutes. If need be, drink another two cups three hours later.

DIFFICULT URINATION, DIVERTICULAR DISEASE, DIZZINESS, DOUBLE VISION, DRUG ABUSE BY THE ELDERLY, DRUG ADDICTION, DRUG AND ALCOHOL WITHDRAWAL, DRY SKIN, DYSLEXIA

Introducing New Orleans's Two Cultures

New Orleans is Louisiana's largest city and one of the busiest and most efficient international ports in all North America. The picturesque *Vieux Carré* or French quarter of the old city, located north of broad Canal Street, is a major tourist attraction. In the heart of the Vieux Carré is Jackson Square; fronting upon the square are the Cabildo (1795), St. Louis Cathedral (1794), and other eighteenth- and nineteenth-century structures.

Several world-famous restaurants, specializing in shrimp, oysters, and fish from nearby waters, uphold the New Orleans tradition of good living. And the annual Mardi Gras is undoubtedly the best-known festival in America. Also adding to the local color are the many parks, museums (including a voodoo museum and the New Orleans Museum of Art, both of which I went to), and gardens.

The Cajun and Creole cultures that dominate much of this city are quite distinct. The former are descendants of French Canadians whom the British, in the eighteenth century, drove from Nova Scotia and adjacent areas. They eventually settled in the fertile bayou lands of southern Louisiana. Today the Cajuns form small, compact, self-contained communities and speak their own patois. This is a curious admixture of archaic French forms with idioms taken from their English, Spanish, German, Indian, and black neighbors. They generally prefer keeping to themselves as a rule, but can be sociable and hospitable when called upon to do so.

Louisiana creoles, on the other hand, can be one of several things: French-speaking white descendants of early French and Spanish settlers; mulattos speaking a form of French and Spanish; or simply people of color who have adopted a European way of life.

The cuisines of each culture are similarly diverse and distinctive. Cajun cuisine is generally characterized by the use of wild game, seafoods, wild vegetation, and herbs. From their association with the Indians, the Cajuns learned techniques to best utilize the local products from the swamps, bayous, lakes, rivers, and woods. Truly remarkable are the variations that have resulted from similar ingredients carefully combined in the black iron pots of the Cajuns. Jambalaya, grillades, stews, fricasees, soups, gumbos, sauce piquantes, and a host of stuffed-vegetable dishes are all characteristic of the new Cajun "one-pot meals."

Creole cuisine is noted for its rich array of courses indicating its close ties to European aristocracy. Creole cuisine is indebted to many unique people and diverse cultures who were willing to contribute and share their cooking styles, ingredients, and talents. Obviously then, this particular cuisine represents the history of sharing in southern Louisiana. The subtle influences of classical and regional French, Spanish, German, and Italian cooking are readily apparent in Creole cuisine. The terminologies, precepts, sauces, and major dishes carried over, some with more evolution than others, and provided a solid foundation for Creole cooking to evolve. For instance, bouillabaisse is a soup originally from the Provence region of France and plays an integral part in the creation of gumbo in Creole food. The Spanish endowed Creole food with paella, which was the forefather of Louisiana's jambalaya. Paella is the internationally famous Spanish rice dish made with vegetables, meats, and sausages. The Germans helped establish the boucherie and fine sausage making in South Louisiana when they came in 1690. The same things also applied with the Italians, Haitians, and Native Indians.

Food Is Your Best Medicine

Of all the American cities I've visited over the last two decades, none stands out so prominently or has created as many rich experiences as New Orleans. I suppose it's the great diversity of culture, cuisine, *and* folk medicine that has been so appealing to my scientific, culinary, and doctoring instincts. Some years ago a prominent American physician by the name of Henry G. Bieler, M.D., wrote a book entitled *Food Is Your Best Medicine* (New York: Random House, 1966). In it he maintained that with the proper foods any number of diseases could be cured. He held the view that the right kind of food was far better for you than any number of vitamin, mineral, or herbal supplements.

To a large extent this same philosophy prevails within the Cajun and Creole cultures. While it is true that they have their tinctures and tonics for this and that ailment, it is also equally valid to say that they have a number of simple food dishes that are regularly prescribed by local folk healers from both cultures. As I have so often worked with these people over the years, I became aware of this fact—that certain specially prepared "one-pot" meals were prescribed more often for various illnesses than were alternative things such as nutritional supplements.

I found that while different folk healers have their own food preferences, when I did an inventory of these items from my notes later on I was pleasantly astonished to find how similar many of them were. Also the methods of preparation were essentially the same: Prepare the food as a liquid stew in a large heavy pot in about an hour.

An Explanation of the Ingredients

Since there was so much commonality among a number of different "food remedies" that had been collected over an extended period of time from both Cajun and Creole folk healers, I decided to combine them all into one basic stew for the multitude of problems mentioned at the beginning of this section. I was struck with awe at the number of sulfur-bearing and beta-carotene-rich vegetables that were repeatedly utilized by various individuals, although sometimes in slightly different preparation ways.

Equally astounding was the all-too-frequent use of crawdads or crayfish, which are exceptionally high in iodine, an important nutrient for the thyroid and other "master" glands of the body. Crawdads are ugly little buggers, but quite tasty. The big ones in Louisiana have golf-ball-sized bodies and Popeye forearms. These little lobster-looking crustaceans can rip at a piece of meat in no time with their sharp little claws.

Gathering them is hunter-gathering at its most basic, fun and social. Several of my Cajun and Creole informants took me out to nearby bayous at night to show me how it was done. With lanterns, some buckets, waders, and a cooler full of ice, we set to work to catch them. Lines were thrown out a few feet from shore with a chicken drumstick tied around the knuckle bone. We waited a few minutes for the chicken to disappear from sight in the light (that meant the crawdads had covered it) and then began scooping the whole mess up with a long-handled dip net. We caught dozens and dozens, several pounds at a time. I and one other person had the task of ripping off tails and claws, then stashing them in the open cooler while discarding the bodies. (Oh, did I forget to mention the local custom of sucking the heads?)

The tails must be mixed immediately with lots of slushy cold water to keep them fresh. Sometimes they're tossed into boiling water right after being caught, which keeps them better. A few minutes of boiling turns these "mudbugs" a brilliant red.

I believe that the combination of minerals in the vegetables accompanying these iodine-rich crayfish promotes better urination, relieves diverticular distress, helps overcome dizziness and double vision, greatly reduces the physical craving for prescription pharmaceuticals in the elderly and illicit drugs in young-to-middle-aged people, helps cut back the painful symptoms associated with the withdrawal from drugs or alcohol, definitely gives the skin better texture, and certainly enhances the cognitive skills of poor readers.

It is unfortunate these days that many folks are tied too closely to pills, capsules, and tablets from the drugstore or health-food store instead of assorted food options by which to get well. Does this particular recipe work for the ten conditions previously listed? Absolutely! Of course, since individual metabolisms are different, each person may experience varying degrees of success with this single meal. But *some* improvement in ALL of these ten categories *will* be evident with the fairly consistent consumption of this particular stew; it is recommended that a bowl be consumed once a day minimum of three times per week for six weeks straight.

A Fantastic Food Remedy

Well, here is the recipe as promised. It takes approximately one hour to fix and yields half a dozen servings. I am indebted to my friend Chef John D. Folse, CEC, AAC, of Lafitte's Landing Restaurant in Donaldsonville, Louisiana, for his assistance in combining a number of different recipes into one simple stew. He is considered a great authority on Cajun and Creole cuisine and culture.

Medicinal Crawdad Stew

2 lbs. cleaned crawdad tails   1/4 cup tomato sauce
2 cups chopped onions   3 quarts spring or filtered water
1 cup chopped celery   1 cup chopped green onions
1 cup chopped bell pepper   1 cup chopped parsley
2 tbsps. diced garlic   1 tsp. granulated kelp to taste

In a large stainless-steel or enamel stockpot, heat one quart of the water at medium-heat level. Then add the onions, celery, bell pepper, and garlic and cook just long enough for them to appear wilted, which takes less than five minutes. Next add the crawdad tails and cook until the meat is pink and slightly curled. This should take another five minutes. After this, stir in the tomato sauce and slowly add the rest of the water. Be sure to stir constantly until all of it is incorporated. Bring to a low boil, reduce to simmer, and cook 20 minutes, stirring constantly with a wooden spoon. Now add the green onions and parsley and season to taste with some granulated seaweed kelp.

When done, it can be consumed as a watery stew. Or some of it can be mixed with a little cooked wild rice and eaten that way. Some

New Orleans folk healers have insisted that their patients strain the liquid out and just drink that. But I'm inclined to think that eating the vegetables and crawdad provides additional fiber and nutrients to the body that it may not be getting otherwise from the broth alone. For those who like their stews a little zestier, this dish can be tweaked with a few dashes of Louisiana Gold Pepper Sauce, which is worth about two fire-alarm bells once it gets settled in your system.

Cajun and Creole chefs who prepare similar dishes prefer to add roux in the beginning to give it thickness. Roux is simply a little heated butter and flour constantly stirred on the bottom of a large pot with a wire whip until the desired color is achieved. But I don't think that is very good for a person's health. None of the folk healers whom I interviewed for this section ever used it and always administered their particular stews in a watery form.

It is no exaggeration on my part to say that those who've taken the time to try this medicinal stew for themselves or their loved ones have always testified as to wonderful healing properties and to the many satisfying benefits that have come from it for various health situations.

EARACHE, EAR INFECTION, EAR PAIN, EARWAX BUILDUP

The K.I.S.S. Principle at Work

Just about everyone has heard at some time in his or her life the meaning to the acronym K.I.S.S., which signifies (in a slightly altered form) "Keep It Simple, Silly!" And that's basically what most folk healers around the world manage to do. They utilize only a *few* things but manage to accomplish a lot with what they use. In other words, out of just a couple of items can great things be achieved many times.

Nothing Smaller than Your Elbow

The otolaryngologists that I know have always specified to their patients that nothing smaller than an elbow should ever be inserted into the ear. Although the advice is probably good considering the delicate state of the ear, such ear–nose–throat specialists are usually being facetious when giving such absurd counsel.

It is important for readers to understand that any serious ear disorder should be checked out by a doctor at once. This isn't to say that some forms of self-treatment may not be warranted. But at least a person should find out first from a specialist the type of problem and its seriousness before anything else is attempted. Certainly making casual inquiry as to the appropriateness of a particular folk remedy wouldn't be out of line either. If the doctor is open-minded, he or she will work with you; if just the opposite, then lectured warning will follow demonstrating the other's obvious bias toward folk remedies as a whole.

Using Common Sense for Getting Relief

When attempting self-treatment for any of the these conditions, always remember the following rules: (1) Make sure whatever is being put into the ear canal is pure; (2) Liquid material works best and requires just a *few drops* to work effectively; (3) The liquid matter should be lukewarm and never cold; (4) The head should be tilted at an angle in order for the liquid to remain in the ear canal for several minutes without running out; if both ears require liquid in them, do one at a time, and then insert a little tuft of clean cotton to keep it in while the head is upright.

The three herbs I've enjoyed working with the most for ear disorders (including wax buildup) are garlic clove, mullein leaves, and a tiny amount of tea-tree oil or melaleuca (to fight infection). To make an ear oil at home, pour two-thirds cup of olive oil in a clean glass pint jar. Peel and finely chop one garlic clove. Cut one-half *fresh* mullein leaf (identified by its tall stalk and soft, furry leaves) into very tiny pieces. Add both of these to the olive oil, seal with a screw-on metal lid and set in the sunlight for ten days. The sunlight will extract the medicinal virtues from both plants into the oil.

After this, strain out the oil, first through a fine-mesh wire sieve and then again through a clean muslin or cotton cloth into another small container, preferably made of dark glass. Add four to five drops of tea-tree oil and shake the contents thoroughly. Cap and store in a cool, dry, dark place away from heat or light. When needed, use a glass dropper and squeeze out just enough for the ear problem. *No more than* five drops should ever be used for a young child's ear and no more than eight for an adult's ear.

To get the oil lukewarm, heat a small amount of it in a clean metal tablespoon over a burning candle or lit cigarette lighter for one-and-a-half minutes, or until it is comfortable when dropped on the back of the hand. The oil can be put into the dropper from the spoon if the dropper is held on an angle while the rubber end is being gently squeezed.

Don't hesitate to confer with your doctor on a procedure such as this if you feel any uncertainty about what you are doing. While this remedy is quite effective and safe enough to use, YOU need to feel confident enough *in yourself* and in the remedy to use it with wisdom and discretion.

Street Minstrel and Remedy Man

There is a colorful fixture on the streets of a major Texas city whom I met a while back, and who has been in the habit of playing the keyboard in the busy downtown area for a number of years. I watched from a distance as some passersby stopped long enough occasionally to throw a few dollars into his open hat sitting on its brim on the sidewalk in front of him. This middle-aged African-American gentleman intrigued me enough to prompt an acquaintance with him following several minutes of distant observation.

I found out that his given Christian name is Samuel Johnson Williams, but he prefers going by the name of Sam or just plain S.W. He left a bad marriage in Arkansas 27 years ago. "My ole lady did me wrong and the younguns all sided with her," he quipped. "So's I got myself outta that fix in a hurry and came back to my hometown of Dallas here. I did a bit of traveling around after that on the bus, going to places like Albuquerque, Phoenix, and Las Vegas. But I eventually found my way back here where I've been ever since."

S.W. bought a used keyboard from a Goodwill thrift store and taught himself how to play by reading the instruction booklet that came with the instrument. I noticed that S.W.'s voice was somewhat gravely in places, making him sound like a hoarse Ray Charles. But like any true blues singer, he had a knack for belting out the tunes as if he meant it. He sang for my benefit "Let the Good Times Roll" and did it with such conviction and flair that it commanded my entire attention. (And I am *not* a fan of jazz by any stretch of the imagination!)

I've never known anyone who was able to milk the vibrato and let slip some of the most beautiful musical phrasing the blues has ever seen as this guy could. That is the power and magic of the old gent's gift: He has taken an old musical form, adapted it to his own style and infused the same with his lively personality—at once classic and visionary. To my way of thinking the man possessed that quality that has always been so interesting in blues singers: He appeared to have lived what he sang.

S.W.'s not the kind of fellow who sings on the street for spare change. This transient minstrel was a good performer the last time I heard him. He sang "Nobody's Blues But Mine" right before a funked-up "You Are My Sunshine" and never missed a step of emotional transformation. "I ache, break, and shake every song I sing," he laughed good-naturedly. Watching him do his stuff that fine autumn day in the heart of the Dallas business district was like watching Billie Holiday or Bessie Smith (real blues artists), only *live*.

I managed to catch him long enough between his musical numbers when he was "resting to catch my breath" to inquire about some of his personal history. Upon learning that my business was writing alternative health (which I had to explain the meaning of) books, he cracked a wide ivory grin and said, "Well, youse come to the right place, young man. I am both a blues singer *and* a remedy man to boot." He then proceeded to share with me some of the medical folklore that "my mom and grammaw used years ago to treat the complaints of many folks with."

At that time I was working on the E section of this book and decided to ask questions pertaining to certain problems needing to be covered here. S.W. was very accommodating and without hesitation volunteered the folk medical advice I sought. Sometimes I would have to pause and define something for him such as encephalitis or endometriosis. But at other moments, he would redefine a problem in his own particular lingo. This was quite evident when I threw out "erection problems"—his prompt response was, "Why don't you jest say 'gettin' your nature up'; that's how we use to call it where I come from."

Some African-American Folk Remedies

I came unprepared to interview this watershed of useful health information and so had to scrounge around in a garbage bin in an alley
close by to find enough suitable paper to write on. S.W.'s brief remarks
follow first; anything else not enclosed in quotation marks is what I
added afterwards for expanded clarification.

EATING DISORDERS

"People didn't have them crazy ways of eating or not eating back in
those days like they do now. Grammaw always used peppermint or
catnip tea, depending on if she wanted to crank up the hunger drive
(catnip) or to slow it down some (peppermint)." The nepelactones in
catnip appear to stimulate appetite, while certain components in peppermint seem to encourage smaller food intake and shorter satiety.

ECZEMA

"Oh shoot, that's an easy one. Jest grab yourself some jewelweed from
the field, crush it in your hand, and rub it on the skin. If that ain't
around, hunt for some plantain and do the same with it." Another effective method is to spray the skin with a *cool* solution of tincture of
witch hazel (available in drugstores and supermarkets).

ELBOW PAIN

"You mean like the kind that rich white folks get when they go out
playing golf or tennis?" [I flashed a quick smile and nodded in agreement.] "Grammaw made a special liniment out of pure turpentine and
Jack Daniels, which she always used to rub on sore places like this or
the knee or shoulder or lower back, depending on where the pain
was." The remedy is very similar to one I saw being used by some hill-
billies in the Ozarks years ago. But instead of commercial whiskey they
used their own home-made brand of moonshine. For every pint of
hard liquor they added one teaspoon of *turpentine.* NEVER use paint

thinner for this. It is a good idea to test a very small section of skin with a few drops of this liniment to see if there is any allergic reaction to it. Wait for an hour after doing this and if there is no discomfort of any kind, then you may safely apply it over a larger area for soothing relief.

EMPHYSEMA

"My uncle had that much of his life. Mom would make him a pot of marshmallow tea and take it over to his place and have him drink it warm. It always seemed to make him breathe easier after that." Marshmallow root is very mucilaginous and extremely good for injured lung tissue. When making the tea (one cup of dried, cut roots to one quart of water) always be sure to simmer the contents on low heat, covered, for about ten minutes before setting aside and steeping another 15 minutes.

ENCEPHALITIS

"That sounds contagious. Is it catchy? *Raw* garlic and onion, always consumed with a little honey, was what Mom recommended for anything catchy that she didn't understand too well." Chewing a peeled garlic clove followed by a swallow of one-half teaspoon of pure honey is probably the best way to take this.

ENDOMETRIOSIS

"That's white women's disease; no colored women I ever knew had this. Grammaw always said getting pregnant for a woman was the Lord's way of preventing things like this." One must consider the background culture from which such folk philosophy originates. When this is done the statement doesn't seem racist or sexist as when taken for full value. A medical examination is required to make sure it really is endometriosis since this disease is capable of mimicking a number of other female health problems. Hormonal herbs such as alfalfa, red clover, dong quai (dongguei), and ginseng may be especially helpful here in capsule form (two to three daily of any one of them but not all). I spoke with a female yoga instructor who informed me that she has assisted quite a few "preforties" women in successfully coping with this problem by guiding them through some simple stretching exercises that involve use of the legs and pelvic area quite a bit.

EPILEPSY

"Surest thing for this grammaw told us was to use snuff. She had a couple of cases where the people were unconscious, and she poked a little snuff up their nostrils and they came right out of their fainting spell lickety-split. Black pepper also works the same."

ERECTION PROBLEMS

"For guys it shouldn't be that hard. The mind should be emptied of all distractions and complete attention given to the woman. I found when I was a younger man that if I ate some real spicy food an hour before having sex that there was no problem in me 'getting my nature up.'" Apparently the capsaicin in red pepper expands the tiny blood vessels in a man's organ to allow for enhanced blood flow, which then increases erection dramatically.

ERYSIPELAS

"Goldenseal root . . . my mom used this internally on several folks who had it and it cleared right up." Apparently antibacterial herbs like this or echinacea or garlic will help kill the group A streptococcus responsible for this bacterial cellulitis.

EYE FLOATERS

"Close the eyes and rest them for an hour. Floaters go away after that."

EYESTRAIN

"Lay down and put a cold wet washrag over the eyes. This will remove the strain. Mom did this sometimes and it always seemed to help her."

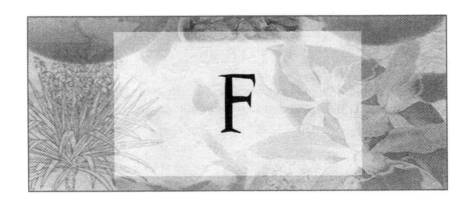

FACIAL PARALYSIS

A Hospital Treatment

In 1980 I was one of four faculty advisers for 29 medical students who went to the People's Republic of China under the sponsorship of the American Medical Students' Association. We were one of the first groups of Westerners permitted into that Communist country shortly after U.S. President Richard Nixon's so called "Ping Pong diplomacy" paved the way for such things to happen. Now, of course, it's relatively easy to go to China but back then it was still exceedingly difficult.

One of the places I remember our group visiting was the Suzhou Chinese Traditional Medical Hospital in Suzhou, Jiangsu Province (directly west of Shanghai and reached in one-and-a-half hours by steam locomotive). There we saw first hand the marvelous healing results from the simple applications of many Chinese folk remedies. Dr. Lin Xi, who then managed the Department of Herbal Therapeutics, showed us how he and his staff treated people suffering from facial paralysis.

A Chinese woman in her midthirties suffered temporary paralysis of the right side of her face and jaw, making speaking and chewing very difficult. Red radish, radish plant, and radish seed were all employed in different ways to bring about a correction of this problem. A strong tea was made from the dried seeds (one teaspoon) and plant (two tablespoons) by simmering them in water (one-and-a-quarter pints), covered, for up to 12 minutes. After the solution had sufficiently cooled, the patient was instructed to drink one cup every four hours. The red radish itself was made into a juice along with some of the fresh plant leaves, and this was given to her also to drink from a glass. Several radishes were also pulverized and then laid on a clean cloth; this poultice was then applied to that side of the patient's face that was paralyzed. Continued treatment of this condition in other instances, we were told, usually resulted in the disappearance of facial paralysis within a week.

FAINTING

Quick Action

While I, three other doctors, and 29 third- and fourth-year medical students from America were in the People's Republic of China in the summer of 1980 we were able to visit a large teaching hospital in the city of Suzhou in Jiangsu Province just west of Shanghai. Among the many different forms of materia medica common to Chinese traditional folk medicine, we were shown some things for which lotus is used. Among these is fainting.

Lotus is an aquatic, perennial herb. The *oujie* (lotus rhizome) grows horizontally, is stout, and consists of nodes. When the rhizomes are collected in the late fall and early winter, the nodes are cut out, cleaned, dried in the sun, and the fibrous roots then removed. A tea is made from them by boiling a small handful of dried nodes in one pint of water, covered, for eight minutes.

The resulting liquid is dark red, emits a slightly "moldy" odor, and tastes somewhat astringent. Some of the warm infusion is placed in a cup directly beneath the nostrils of the person who has fainted, and it generally revives that individual within a minute or less. The person is also given the tea to drink immediately after awakening so as not to faint again.

FEAR

Bravery Through Lotus Leaf

At a medical school and hospital in Suzhou, China (west of Shanghai), *heye* tea is frequently used to help timid people overcome their personal fears. The dried leaves of the lotus plant are made into a simple tea and then given to such patients to drink morning and night, one glass each time. Not only does it dispel imagined fears, but it also helps to allay vertigo and heat exhaustion encountered during the hot and humid summer months.

Dancing Fears Away

In a Monday, September 13, 1999, issue of The Washington Post was a feature story by reporter Jon Jeter entitled, "Congolese Dance Their Cares Away." The article began by highlighting the 1996 coup that rid the Democratic Republic of Congo of its longtime dictator Mobutu Sese Seko. But his replacement, military strongman Laurent Kabila, has left the people even poorer than they were before.

So the question most frequently asked these days isn't "When will things get better?" but rather "Care to dance?" The journalist interviewed some of the nearly 300 people crowded into a Kinshasa nightclub called the Station Miilhouse. One woman by the name of Emerance Tshela told Jeter, "I go out to dance more now than I did before the war started because I find relief in music. A lot of people do. It soothes us."

The music she was referring to, of course, is *soukous*. This brand of Congolese pop music is a fusion of Cuban rumba and African dance music. It is generally performed by five or six musicians and relies heavily on guitars and horns. Like its American counterpart jazz, which was created by freed slaves borrowing from vast cultural sources, Congolese music is a potluck of African culture and its cross-fertilization with the French and Caribbean cultures during their colonial periods.

One band leader, Lutumba Masiya Simaro, informed Jeter that his people couldn't go without their music for very long. "We take it in like we do the air—it is our life, our sustenance . . . it gives us vitality of spirit!"

Civil-servant Jean Pierre Manile, who dances with his wife nearly every weekend at the Station Miilhouse, told the reporter, "As long as we draw breath, we will find a way to dance in Kinshasa."

He Faced Up to His Worst Fears

Ron Curby is a sales manager for a business-equipment-products company in Salt Lake City. In mid-September 1999 he came into the Anthropological Research Center, which I've been the director of for over two decades, and delivered some canisters of toner powder for one of the four photocopy machines we have on the premises. It was the first time we had ever met, though he was familiar with our ten-year account with his firm. A few minutes into our short chat, I inquired about the appearance of a presumed burn covering most of the left side of his face.

He told me it was a birthmark known as port wine that had given him nothing but trouble during the first part of his life. "Kids used to tease me terribly in elementary and junior high school," he said, "not knowing what it was. It was even worse in high school, where some kids actually thought I had an incurable disease of some kind. I was looked upon as some sort of 'monster' by some of the student body. No girls would ever dare date me for fear of being ostracized by their friends. Those were pretty lonely and frustrating years for me as I look back on it now."

Ron said that it was only when he joined the U.S. Army that he was finally able to come to grips with the very thing he had been trying to avoid all of these years. "I had a sergeant who told me in no uncertain terms that I had to stop focusing on my birthmark and begin paying attention to my personality instead. He encouraged me to develop the type of personality that would win people over and cause them to like me for who I was instead of what I had. I took his strong advice to heart and concentrated on developing this part of my character. It really worked, and things started paying off for me in big dividends.

"I decided to get into a type of business where I could meet people face to face and look them in the eyes as I spoke. That's essentially how I got into sales. Now, whenever I talk with people, their focus is on me as a person, the message I have for them, and the way I present it. They may notice the birthmark in passing, but it no longer consumes their time or attention as it use to. My army sergeant was right and I'm mighty glad I took his orders to heart. My life has been a lot happier ever since."

FEVER

"Mud Fruit" Cure

The lotus is a watery perennial herb growing in shallow lakes and ponds all over mainland China as well as in Taiwan. I have been to both countries several times in past years and witnessed a number of helpful uses for this plant by many practicing herbalists and doctors. Some of them have already been mentioned under previous entries (facial paralysis, fainting, and fear).

Shilianzi is the Chinese medical name for the dried ripe fruits of *Nelumbo nucifera*. These fruits are collected from mud deposits at the bottom of shallow lakes and ponds where the lotus is extensively culti-vated. This "mud fruit" is grayish or dark brown in color, glaucous, with a circular scar of the style at the top and a scar of pedicel at the base. The pericarp is somewhat hard. The fruit is odorless and astrin-gent but slightly sweet.

It is ground into powder and added to water, milk, or juice to help reduce fevers. The dried *shilianzi* can also be broken into smaller pieces with the aid of a hammer or nutcracker. After this, some of it (two tablespoons) can be placed in a little water (about a pint) and gently boiled, *uncovered*, on low heat for ten minutes. When it cools, the tea is strained and given to feverish patients to drink every four hours. Usually their fevers will break within a few hours after drinking a six-ounce glass of this warm tea.

FIBROMYALGIA

Crossover Benefits

In the plant kingdom there are botanicals that have "crossover" bene-fits. This means that while an herb may be specifically intended for one thing, it has equal and valid application for a very different type of malady.

Take the case of motherwort as a prime example of this. In China *yimucao* is ordinarily used for different female problems with good suc-cess. But those same sun-dried flowers and stems works just as well in relieving the darting pains associated with fibromyalgia when drunk as a tea twice daily.

FINGER INJURY

Smashed Fingers Healed

One of the most remarkable episodes of recovery from smashed fingers without the need for splints or surgery appeared some years ago in *The Saints' Herald* (January 22 and 29, 1935; pp. 112, 143), the official publication of The Reorganized Church of Jesus Christ of Latter-Day Saints with its headquarters in Independence, Missouri. The account was taken from "The Memoirs of Joseph Smith III," first president of this largest offshoot of the Mormon Church. The year was 1843 and at age eleven Smith's family still resided in Nauvoo, Illinois.

"Mother's duty was to take her family back to Nauvoo and it was not long until we were on the road . . . The carriage [we rode in] was a new one, built by a man . . . connected with a new firm in Nauvoo. I have reason to remember this vehicle because of an accident I suffered on the second day of our homeward travel [from Lee County, Illinois].

"We had stopped by the roadside for lunch and to bait the horses. Upon getting back into my seat after the brief interval, I thoughtlessly put my hand around one of the carriage posts, and as the driver closed the door, two of my fingers were pretty badly crushed. The wounds bled freely and Mother [Emma Smith] bound them up with some cloths from her bag, and we traveled on.

"My fingers became very painful, and after a while we stopped at a farmhouse. Mother unwrapped them, soaking the temporary dressing off with warm water and re-wrapped them with fresh cloths. Taking from her trunk a little bottle of whiskey and wormwood, she turned the tips of my fingers upward, and poured the liquid upon them, into the dressings—at which, for the first time in my life I promptly fainted! It seemed as if she had poured the strong medicine directly upon my heart, so sharply it stung and so quick was its circulatory effect.

"When I returned to consciousness I was lying on a lounge against the wall and Mother was bathing my face most solicitously. . . .

I soon recovered and we proceeded on our journey, reaching home in good time and without further mishap."

FLATULENCE

Ways to Avoid Getting Gas

Passing gas may be good for a few laughs in the movies, for the crowds worked over by standup comedians, or as a college-class prank. More often than not, though, it is considered to be socially rude and not what people of finer upbringing do in public. It's also symptomatic of problems within the digestive tract itself. Certain herbs will help to allay most of it, such as peppermint, spearmint, and ginger, a little yogurt, or live acidophilus like that found in Bio-K+ (see Product Appendix).

But it isn't always what you have to take *afterwards* to clear up the problem, but rather preventive measures followed *before* it ever occurs. Don't hurry when eating a meal or snack. Take small bites and chew each one carefully and thoroughly before swallowing. Try not to talk very much while eating. Avoid drinking fluids, if possible, so stomach gastric juices don't become diluted. And try to separate animal protein from carbohydrates—consume them at separate meals but not together. Worst case scenario for a really B-A-D gas attack: steak, mashed potatoes and gravy, dinner roll, dessert, and coffee.

FLU

Onion Milk

Tuesday evening, September 14, 1999 I received a phone call at home from a Persian lady in San Diego named Pary Yahiapoor. She had just read my book *Double the Power of Your Immune System* and had called to thank me for it. She said, "I'm Persian and my English is somewhat limited. I have other health books but can't understand them. Yours I can, though, because you write very simply *and from your soul!"* I mentioned to her the present work, which was then in progress. She voluntarily contributed the following remedy for my book.

"We have a very old Persian remedy that goes back for many centuries, I'm told. It is commonly used throughout Iran to treat flu, colds, and coughs.

"Take one medium onion. It can be white, yellow, or purple; the color doesn't matter. Grate it into a stainless-steel pot. Then add three cups of goat's milk. Simmer uncovered on low heat for maybe 15 to 20 minutes. Set aside to cool a bit. Strain one cup of the *warm* onion milk and slowly sip. Drink another one-half cup every three to four hours after that. Once you get use to it the onions can be taken with milk and chewed before being swallowed."

Pary insisted that this remedy is fool-proof. "I can personally guarantee that *any* cold, flu, or cough will disappear overnight after taking a few cups of this. You have my word on that!" She then signed off by saying, "I intend to keep your [immune system] book by my bedside where it will become like my [health] bible. May Allah bless you in all the good you're doing for others."

FLUID RETENTION

Voodoo Priestess Recommendation

Voodoo is practiced throughout the Caribbean and is very popular in New Orleans. Miriam Chamani is the priestess of the Voodoo Spiritual Temple located at 826 North Rampart Street (504.522.9627). She is one of the better known voodoo practitioners in the city. The priestess came onto the radar of many New Orleans-area residents in early 1999 when her temple became the repository for the ashes of Chicken Man, so named because of his willingness to demonstrate the sacrificial voodoo rite involving biting the head off a live chicken.

Priestess Miriam—as most people call her—was 56 at the time of our interview. She practices a type of voodoo that is a curious amalgamation of African rituals and Roman Catholicism. Frequently she gets advice from a spiritual guide named Simbi, who sometimes takes the form of a mermaid in dreams.

Once when an overweight client consulted her in regard to her edema condition, the priestess conferred with you-know-who and early the next morning got her answer through the dream state. Her mermaid counselor suggested that her client eat one whole pink grapefruit every morning, drink lemonade or lime juice at noon, and drink a glass of grapefruit juice in the evening. Her client did this and within two weeks had lost 27 pounds, most of which had been due to fluid retention.

Baptist Minister Helped

But the story doesn't end here. Sometime later I had a Southern Baptist minister from a large and well-respected congregation in Texas call me to inquire about a similar condition. He suffered from fluid retention badly and experienced constant pain in his hands and wrists and feet and ankles.

I suggested the voodoo remedy, but didn't inform him as to its source; nor did I label it as "voodoo" either, telling him only that it was from the Caribbean. He followed my counsel and phoned back almost a month later very elated that his edema had cleared up. His verbal rejoicing included, "Praise the Lord for such a thing! You must be a man of God, Dr. Heinerman, to have received such wonderful inspiration as this. I'm fully cured of my problem!"

He was so enthralled to be well again that I didn't have the heart to send his soaring spirit crashing to hell by telling him that a pagan priestess had been the *true* source through her dreamy mermaid Simbi.

Maintaining Fluid Balance

Those who are engaged in daily physical workouts of some kind need to make sure they are maintaining proper fluid balance, David R. Lamb, an exercise scientist at Ohio State University, said in a recent interview. Drinking 16 ounces of fluid at bedtime and another 16 ounces first thing in the morning is an effective habit for preventing mild dehydration (something that an estimated 45 percent of Americans currently suffer from).

And while water is the logical choice, juices may also become part of this routine. He recommends fruit juices in the morning and vegetable juices in the evening. The human body needs carbohydrates (which convert to glucose) upon arising for energy and minerals such as sodium and potassium to maintain electrolyte stability. A simple snack of some type of fruit (carbohydrates) with a few soda crackers and celery sticks (sodium and potassium) will fill both needs.

The standard practice is to consume 16 to 32 ounces of fluid one hour before a workout, then 8 to 16 ounces about 20 minutes before the activity commences. During exercise, 5 to 12 ounces every 15 to 20 minutes is recommended by him. Lamb said that water-rich foods are great for maintaining normal fluid balance and to prevent dehydration. These include watery fruits such as cantaloupe, watermelon, and strawberries, along with vegetables, cucumbers, yogurt, and cottage cheese. In fact, in the latter three a person is getting adequate sodium and potassium ions for replacing electrolytes used during physical workouts.

The so-called sports drinks that are wildly popular these days due to their flavor varieties actually drive thirst so that more fluids are craved. This may help to remind a person to drink more in order to prevent becoming dehydrated, but it can also have a negative impact on the kidneys, pancreas, and blood pressure. Water is by far the most logical choice—it's simple, inexpensive, readily available, and good for you.

FOOD AND DRUG INTERACTIONS

Things to Look For

In the many years that I've been practicing and writing about folk medicine and food therapy, I've come to acquire certain wisdom with regard to using prescription drugs and over-the-counter medications. While there are obvious alternative substitutes for many of them, some are still necessary to take and, in fact, DO save people's lives.

Within recent years there has also been an accumulation of evidence in medical and pharmaceutical journals listing which foods to avoid when taking certain drugs. I have many of these reports in my extensive files for periodic referencing. So as not to burden the reader with a lot of heavy science, I've decided to keep things simple and combine my own acquired wisdom with what the journals have reported on this topic.

Not much attention is given to food–drug interactions, but improper combinations of both can be serious if not fatal, as the following three examples illustrate. A young attorney heavily in debt argued frequently with his spouse and partner. He suffered from migraines and to find relief took aspirin with orange juice on a fairly regular basis. In six weeks he was hospitalized for bleeding ulcers. The combined acidity of the citrus juice and aspirin eroded the mucosal tissue that protected his gut and resulted in the acute ulcer attack.

A highly charged, overweight business executive went on one of those many "crash diets," consuming copious amounts of dark leafy greens. He promptly suffered a stroke. What happened here was that his excessive consumption of vitamin K-rich foods induced blood clotting. Since he had already suffered a *prior* stroke, he was taking the medication Coumadin, a blood-thinner, which worked at cross-purposes with his otherwise healthy diet.

A depressed housewife who enjoyed drinking beer and wine as well as snacking on cheese and sausages attended a party at which she consumed a lot of these beverages and foods. Hours later she became nauseous, collapsed, and died. She had been taking an anti-depressant, Marplan, one of a class of drugs called MAO-inhibitors. The cheese and alcoholic beverages that she regularly consumed contained large quantities of tyramine, which turned lethal when combined with the MAO antidepressant.

New clinical evidence has shown that certain foods and nutritional supplements can inactivate or exaggerate the effects of some medications. For example, calcium—whether from milk, antacids, or supplements—binds to molecules of the antibiotic tetracycline, preventing the drug from being fully absorbed by the bloodstream. On the other hand, grapefruit and grapefruit juice actually increases the body's ability to absorb certain drugs. What this means is if you take a grapefruit chaser with felodipine for hypertension and heart disease, terfenadine for allergies, cyclosporine for preventing rejection of transplanted organs, or saquinavir for AIDS, you would be unwittingly exceeding the recommended dosages.

By the same token, high-fiber foods such as cooked oatmeal, bran muffins, buckwheat pancakes, rye toast, steamed brown rice, and nonbutter, unsalted popcorn can have just the opposite effect of grapefruit: They can decrease the amount of a drug absorbed by the bloodstream. Fiber has been found to interfere with the absorption of the heart drug digoxin and tricyclic antidepressants. Fiber can also complicate the absorption of iron supplements in the system. Those who suffer from anemia or are prone to regular fatigue and depend on iron to give them daily energy boosts should take their iron supplements on an empty stomach and several hours away from any fiber-loaded meal.

Besides food content, the way in which food is prepared can alter the performance of drugs in the body. Spices stimulate the drug-metabolizing enzymes found in the liver, thereby accelerating the absorption of medications and some medicinal herbs, whereas sulfur-bearing foods such as cabbage enhance those found in the intestines. Charbroiled meat such as beef, pork, or chicken can reduce the actual time that certain drugs are meant to stay in the body, which speaks well of boiling or baking in such instances.

Just as food can affect the way drugs behave in the human system, so, too, can drugs affect the manner in which the body uses food, possibly altering its nutritional status. Drugs may be responsible for changes in appetite; in gastrointestinal digestion and absorption; and in nutrient metabolism, excretion, and requirement. Although nutrient depletion of the body occurs gradually, the risk of developing vitamin and/or mineral deficiencies increases when a particular medication is used over a long period of time. Moreover, certain population groups are more susceptible to deficiencies than are others: children, who need a larger proportion of nutrients in relation to body size in order to facilitate normal growth; the elderly, in whom drugs behave differently as a result of age-related body changes; those with marginal diets; and individuals with chronic illnesses.

No Clear-Cut Rules

Aside from the things already mentioned, there are really no hard-and-fast rules that dictate what foods not to eat with which drugs. Also, the fact that every individual has a different metabolic rate of absorption will produce endless variations of food–drug interactions. Gender and ethnicity also play some minor roles in these outcomes, but not as extensively.

There are a few things, though, that you can do to protect yourself from unwelcomed and unexpected food–drug interactions. First, if in doubt about *any* medication, simply take it on an *empty* stomach and at least 4 hours between snacks or meals. Second, stick with *neutral* or bland foods such as applesauce, pears and pear juice, bananas, mangos, baked squash or pumpkin, or mashed potatoes (without skins) when eating and taking medications at the approximate same times. Third, talk to your primary-care physician and pharmacist relative to any potential interactions they may know of between their prescriptions and some of your food favorites.

Finally, you may log on to various computer web sites for further data regarding food–drug interactions: Healthtouch at www.healthtouch.com; Institute for Safe Medication Practices at www.ismp.org; Pharmaceutical Information Network at www.pharminfo.com; USDA at www.fda.gov; and U.S. Pharmacopoeia at www.usp.org.

FOOD POISONING

Activated Charcoal

For many years Drs. Calvin and Agatha Thrash, though trained and licensed as medical doctors, practiced their own brand of medicine along natural lines. They employed such diverse measures as hydrotherapy, massage, diet, medicinal herbs, and charcoal for helping sick people become well again. Eventually they established a nonprofit natural-health-education institution in Alabama where they could teach their patients and other interested parties the concepts they espoused.

I was one of the lucky ones, fortunate enough to have spent some time in their clinic as well as their school, learning some of the different methods they used to bring about healthy recoveries. While all of their remedies were effective in one way or another, none stood out in my mind so much as their nearly constant use of activated charcoal.

Charcoal has been used in homeopathic medicine for several centuries and was listed in the U.S. Pharmacopoeia as an official drug for over a century. It was removed from the book, however, in 1950, having fallen out of favor with physicians and into general disuse by the public. Even today it is somewhat difficult to obtain because most drugstores and pharmacies do not carry it on their shelves, although it is still quite popular elsewhere in the world.

The light and fluffy black powder of charcoal or its ink-black tablets have served as efficient antidotes to general poisoning and even food poisoning. The best wood sources for making charcoal is the bark of willow, eucalyptus, pine, oak, juniper, ash, elm, spruce, and various nut and fruit trees. However, charcoal may also be obtained from the burning of citrus, banana, and potato peelings as well as empty nut shells. Charred toast and other scorched kitchen foods make the worst charcoal and aren't good for you.

As Calvin Thrash, M.D., explained to me one time, "Certain electrostatic properties develop in activated charcoal during its production, which favor the binding of most poisons. When the gases, resins, proteins, fats, and other unwanted materials in wood are burned out, the heat generated and the change in chemistry causes the development of a charge on the charcoal granules that attracts most poisonous substances. Once tree bark, vegetable and fruit peelings, or nut shells have been sufficiently burned, the charcoal is then subjected to the action of an oxidizing gas such as steam or air at elevated temperatures. This process enhances the adsorptive power of charcoal by developing an extensive network of fine pores in the material. Following this activation, the surface area of one cubic centimeter is 1,000 square meters! This expanded surface is due to the fact that charcoal particles have thousands of crevices, pits, grooves, and holes that, when opened out, make quite a large surface area. The physical and chemical properties from the original material and the condition of the carbonization process itself determine the properties of activated charcoal."

Making Your Own Charcoal at Home

Since activated charcoal is so difficult to obtain anymore due to doctor apathy and consumer ignorance, it may become necessary to make your own at home, or if you live in an apartment, condominium, or trailer, then at the house of a friend or relative. When doing so, put pieces of wood in a fireplace or grill, char the wood well, then cut the charred portions from the wood with a sharp knife, machete, or hatchet. Then grind these pieces in a Vita-Mix blender to a fine powder, using the container blade intended for grinding wheat to flour (see Product Appendix under Vita-Mix).

This type of charcoal will require three to four times the dosages ordinarily recommended for the activated kind. The ultimate in making your own charcoal begins with a wood fire out of doors. After the wood is burning brightly, it should be covered with a large piece of tin with dirt pulled over the tin to make a dome to exclude air. As the heat continues to burn the wood with decreased oxygen, the soft parts of wood are burned out first and the hard parts remain, yielding a decent batch of charcoal. The charred parts of the wood should then be pounded to coarse granules in a cloth bag using a hammer and then ground in a Vita-Mix unit to pulverize to a fine powder. WARNING: *Never* use food-grilling briquettes as a source of charcoal. Various fillers and chemicals are applied to hold the charcoal together and to ensure rapid igniting. But in the body *they are harmful!*

Administering Charcoal

The first-aid treatment of choice for chemical, plant, or food poisoning should always be charcoal. Use two heaping tablespoons of the activated kind or up to eight tablespoons of the homemade variety in four to six ounces of water. Stir and drink promptly. This should do the trick and remove most of the painful stomach cramping, nausea, diarrhea, fever, and generally sick feeling that is common to food poisoning.

In the event that more is required later on, proceed to mix one heaping teaspoonful of activated charcoal (or four times this amount of the homemade type) in three ounces of water. Drink a glass of this every hour thereafter for four hours straight until a black stool is produced and a general feeling of relief and wellness sets in. (Activated charcoal may be ordered from Anthropological Research Center. See Product Appendix for address.)

FOOT PAIN

Easy Relief

Simple foot pain that doesn't require a trip to a podiatrist can be relieved several different ways. Roll the sole of the foot across an empty glass soda bottle on a carpeted surface for five minutes at a time. A rolling pin may be substituted if so desired. Soaking the foot in a pan of hot water containing a handful of Epsom salts and a cup of white vinegar also delivers quick relief and feels mighty darned good besides.

Arching the front half of the foot back and holding it there for 15 seconds before returning to its normal position again sometimes helps. Also have someone rub the sole of your sore foot with the flat part of his or her hands in an up-down motion from toes to heel with the fingers interlocked across the top portion of the foot, while the subject is sitting or lying down.

FRACTURES

Things to Do to Ease the Pain

Any type of a serious bone fracture requires immediate medical treatment in the emergency room of a general hospital or doctors' clinic. No self-treatment should be attempted, but certain things can be done to help ease the pain and reduce swelling.

Apply ice in a zippered plastic bag to the injury. A cool compress will also do nicely. And, if possible, soak the fractured limb in cold water for a while. Elevating a bone fracture in the legs or arms above the level of your heart will minimize swelling and reduce pain considerably.

Protein shakes, bonemeal, brewer's yeast, dessicated liver powder, a calcium/magnesium supplement (see Product Appendix under Trace Minerals), alfalfa, horsetail, and slippery-elm capsules, chlorophyll powder (see Product Appendix under Wakunaga for Kyo-Green), stinging nettle, kelp tablets, and cooked oatmeal are supplements and foods to be used to speed up bone healing. (See also *"Broken Bones."*)

FROSTBITE

What a Famous Cartoonist Did

The American cartoonist Walter Crawford Kelly was known for his famous cartoon characters inhabiting the Okefenokee Swamp extending from Southeast Georgia into Northern Florida. Two of the most famous were the opossum *Pogo* (after whom the comic strip was named) and Albert Alligator.

During the war years he worked as a civilian in the foreign-language unit of the Armed Forces Institute, illustrating language manuals. One winter day he was out in the cold longer than he should have been without boots or gloves to protect his hands and feet. As a result his toes and fingers became frostbitten.

Remembering an old remedy his grandmother used in his childhood, Kelly went to a local drugstore and purchased a small jar of Ben Gay. From a nearby lumber store he bought a small can of genuine turpentine. He scooped out a level teaspoon of Ben Gay and scraped it into a small dish. He then carefully counted out *no more* than five drops of turpentine and added this to the liniment. After mixing both ingredients together with a butter knife, he proceeded to rub a tiny amount over each finger and toe. After this he covered his hands with a warm pair of cotton gloves and slipped on two clean pairs of woolen stockings. By the following morning the effects of the frostbite had completely disappeared from these body extremities.

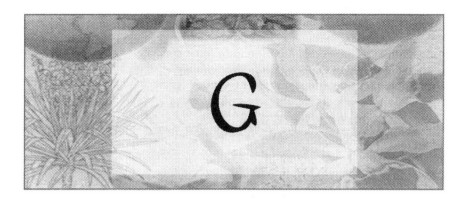

GALLSTONES

A Vegetable Medley or Is It Melody?

Walt Kelly (1913–1973), a gifted American cartoonist, created a comic book for Western Printing & Lithographing in 1943 entitled *Bumbazine and Albert the Alligator,* about a young boy (Bumbazine) and his pet alligator in the Okefenokee Swamp, which eventually became the genesis for his serialized newspaper comic strip *Pogo.*

It proved to be a big hit with the American public because of its silly slapstick, imaginative fancy, and sharp political wit. A number of books followed over the course of time, one of them being *Song of the Pogo* (New York: Simon & Schuster, 1956). Kelly, who had once suffered from an attack of gallstones, was advised by his aged grandmother to eat certain cooked and raw vegetables for a period of time. This he did, and within a matter of days he expelled a number of stones and was never troubled with them thereafter.

He decided to put this vegetable medley into a nonsensical melody that he aptly titled "Parsnoops." One of his swamp characters, Milady Bruharrow, was gossiping over the backyard fence with a neighbor and telling her how this cleverly composed song would be played by their local band conductor. "This conductor of ours was the fella what stands up in front of the orchester and waves his arms and keeps birds and bugs away so the fellas can play good on them hot summer nights when a body can't sleep."

The lyrics to this silly song are as follows (I've italicized each of the vegetables that Kelly ate to get rid of his gallstones):

Parsnoops
Oh, the *parsnips* were snipping their snappers,
While the *parsley* was parceling the *peas*,
And parsing a sentence from handle to hand
Was a hornet with the bees.
The *turnips* were passing the time of the day
In the night of the moon on the porch,
With the shade from the shadows
So shortfully shrift
That the *scallions* were screeched in the scorch.

GASTRITIS, GASTROENTERITIS, GIARDIASIS

Problem Similarities

Gastritis (stomach-lining inflammation), gastroenteritis ("stomach flu"), and giardiasis ("giardia" or digestive-tract infection) share some common similarities: abdominal pain, severe cramping, vomiting, diarrhea, fever, belching, bloating, headache, backache, and extreme fatigue. During the settling of the great American West in the mid-nineteenth century, hundreds of thousands of pioneer men, women, and children periodically suffered from several or more of these symptoms. In most cases it was attributed to rank water, spoiled food, sudden climate adjustments, and mosquitoes.

These illnesses went by different names: Some called them "mountain fever"; others termed them "spotted fever"; a few preferred longer titles such as "high-altitude mosquito-borne malaria" (which wasn't true malaria at all). Many people were laid low by these symptom-shared problems but usually recovered within a few days' time; it was seldom that anyone ever died from them, except a few infants or elderly people on occasion.

The Worth of Pioneer Journals

Of the numerous people who followed newspaper editor Horace Greely's advice to "go West," only the Mormons, it seems, were the most prodigious in producing journals of their travels. This is not to infer that others didn't do the same, but only that the Latter-Day

Saints did more of it than anyone else and became "masters at record-keeping" as several historians have observed.

In tracing their famous trek westward from Illinois to the Valley of the Great Salt Lake in 1847, different Mormon pioneers recorded episodes of sickness with symptoms not unlike those mentioned earlier. Norton Jacob, a member of the first pioneer vanguard into the Salt Lake valley under the direction of Brigham Young, reported in his diary on Saturday, July 3rd that he was "suffering excessively with pain . . . [and] with a high fever." One of the Church hierarchy, Heber C. Kimball, advised him to be "rebaptized for the restoration of health," which was soon done by some other men and had the desired effect of breaking his fever.

Composition Tea and Warming Herbs

Many other pioneer travelers, however, chose to rely upon medicinal herbs to make them well again. In his 1846 and 1847 Mormon Trail journals, Thomas Bullock mentioned feeling "sick from over exertion" and manifesting some of the symptoms cited here. He recounts being made well again "by Composition Tea & chewing Ginger Root."

Wilford Woodruff, a Mormon Church apostle and in the same 1847 company as Jacob and Bullock, wrote this in his journal under the date of July 9, 1847: "I took to my bed at 10 o'clock with distressing pain in my head [and] back & all through the system. Attended with Cold Chills & hot flashes through the body . . . We traveled 13 miles over as bad road as we had had on the journey which makes it exceedingly painful to the sick. The day seemed exceedingly long to me. When we stopped at night I took composition [tea and] cayenne . . . I had better nights [after that]."

Composition Tea was originally formulated by one Samuel Thomson in the 1830s to help correct digestive disturbances. His form of eclectic medicine spread like wildfire and became immensely popular both in the eastern cities as well as the primitive American frontier. He had three different types of composition powders, each of which could be added to hot water with a little sugar for different gastrointestinal troubles. I've arranged the preparations so readers can see differences among them.

First Preparation	Second Preparation	Third Preparation
Bayberry (2 lbs.)	Bayberry (1 lb.)	Bayberry (2 lbs.)
Ginger (1 lb.)	Ginger (1 lb.)	Ginger (2 lbs.)
Cayenne (2 oz.)	Poplar (1 lb.)	Poplar (1 lb.)
Cloves (2 oz.)	Hemlock (1 lb.)	Oak bark (1 lb.)
Pulverize/mix well	Red or White Oak (1/2 lb.)	Cayenne (3 oz.)
	Cayenne (3 oz.)	Cloves (2 oz.)
	Cloves (2 oz.)	Finely pulverize/
	Pulverize/mix well	mix well

He recommended that his patients take "a tea-spoonful in a cup of hot water, sweetened" every few hours. "It is a valuable medicine," he goes on to state, "and may be safely employed in all cases. It is good for relax[ing] pain in the stomach and bowels. And to remove all obstructions caused by cold." And then this follows as an incentive for guaranteeing wellness in his *Botanic Family Physician* guidebook (Albany, NY: J. Munsell, 1841; p. 710): "A few doses of this, the patient being in bed, with a steaming stone at the feet will usually throw off disease in its first stages."

Being highly distrustful of medical doctors back then, a number of early Mormon leaders and their converts chose this form of medicine over other kinds because they believed it was more natural and worked without causing injury to the body. Brigham Young, who became the second leader of the Mormon Church following Joseph Smith's assassination by an angry mob in Carthage, Illinois, adapted Thomson's formulas into his own Composition Tea (which carried his name with it) and started recommending it over the pulpit to his people in occasional sermons.

Brigham Young's Composition Tea

4 oz. powdered bayberry
4 oz. powdered poplar bark
4 oz. powdered hemlock
2 oz. ground ginger

2 oz. ground cloves
2 oz. ground cinnamon
1 oz. cayenne pepper (capsicum)

DIRECTIONS: Take a small bit on a spoon, put in 1 cup of hot water, with plenty of sugar and cream. Take in leisure. *(Missouri Historical Society Bulletin,* April 1963, p. 299)

It should be observed that about half of the ingredient are pungent or aromatic spices, which when ingested produce a warming sensation within the gut. They basically increase blood flow, which helps in the distribution of the berries and barks.

Testimonies of Wellness

Twenty-four years ago (from 1999) my first health book came into print in December 1875: *Joseph Smith and Herbal Medicine* (Manti, UT: Mountain Valley Publishing). On page 177 I listed "Brigham's recipe for this delightful concoction of pleasant herbs." The book went through two editions very quickly, but the third edition was shredded and destroyed on orders from some of the Mormon Church hierarchy who were terribly upset by some of the harsh antimedical rhetoric that I frequently employed throughout the text. After that numbing experience, I decided to write *no more* for a specific Mormon audience and went on to write 55 additional health books for non-Mormon readers worldwide. It is a decision I've never regretted.

But from that first small publishing effort of mine came a steady stream of testimonial letters that eventually tapered down in succeeding years. Many who wrote spoke highly of "Brigham Young's Composition Tea," having tried it for themselves for a number of different digestive-tract disturbances. However, on my advice given in that first book, they *omitted the hemlock* due to its volatile and sometimes poisonous nature.

A letter dated New Year's Day of 1998 from Harold H. Humpherys of Tucson, Arizona, complimented me on one of my Prentice Hall titles *(Encyclopedia of Nuts, Berries and Seed)*. Then in the next paragraph he stated this: "I should also mention another book that I am in the midst of reading and finding very fascinating is *Joseph Smith and Herbal Medicine*. I discovered this book in a box of books of my father that I received after his death. Have you thought about updating and republishing this book? I believe it would be well received by those of us who are becoming converts to the benefits of herbs."

Mr. Humpherys then proceeded to share with me his own experience involving Brigham's Composition Tea. "I was suffering from a severe attack of gastroenteritis, probably due to something I ate in a public restaurant which may have been spoiled. I was in a lot of pain and hurting mighty badly. I looked through your book *[Joseph Smith and Herbal Medicine]* and discovered that Composition Tea of Brigham Young's. I made some up and followed the instructions given. In less than seven hours my troubles had totally gone and I felt like a new man again. I have found that I can rely on your judgment for the health information I need. But I can't say that about every health author I read in some book or magazine article. I compliment you on what you have done to raise the standard of health care so high."

GLAUCOMA

"A Good Trick"

Helen Chadwick of Lexington, Nebraska, wrote me a seven-page letter a while back in which she graciously thanked me for writing "some of your wonderful books put out by Prentice Hall." She also passed on several handy remedies for me to include in future books.

"Here is a good trick to get rid of glaucoma. My eye doctor told me how [to] check for gla[u]coma. Take your thumb and first finger and press on the eye ball, with the lid closed, as you would a rubber ball. If it is spongy like a rubber ball you are OK.

"If the eye ball feels hard it has pressure in it. The drainage system is plugged. The eye ball may be as much as twice the size of the other one. In which case you give that eye the treatment until it becomes the same size as the other eye ball.

"The treatment consists of massaging the problem eye ball with the lid closed, with your thumb and first finger. Rub underneath and *around* the eye socket with your thumb, but gently rub the eye ball with the first finger for a few minutes every day.

"Check the eyes occasionally to keep in good condition. Believe me it works. I've been diagnosed TWICE with glaucoma and did this to it each time. And my glaucoma DISAPPEARED!" *Note:* The American Glaucoma Society describes the disease as a "sneak thief of sight" because the common "open angle" type progresses so slowly that an individual may never notice any problem until vision loss has become significant. And since glaucoma is so serious, you should check with your ophthalmologist for available options besides doing the preceding simple exercise.

The Chinese Approach

Chinese medicine teaches that the eyes and the liver are interrelated. If vision is failing, then the liver should be given specific attention in terms of cleansing and nourishment. Dandelion root and stinging nettle teas are the best for detoxifying this important body organ. Drink two to three cups of either or one of each tea daily for up to 60 days. Nutritionally, choline (350 mg. twice daily) and cold-pressed flaxseed oil (1 tbsp. or 500 mg. capsule, twice daily) will help maintain proper liver function. Look to carrot juice and chlorophyll sources such as alfalfa and parsley as well as orange-yellow foods (some citrus, squashes, and pumpkin) for healthy vision.

GLUE EAR

A Simple Procedure

Common sense suggests that when self-treatment of an ear problem is to be initiated, the person doing so understand what is involved. Speaking with an eye–ear–nose–throat specialist before implementing the following remedy may be a good idea.

Mullein, lobelia, wintergreen, and yarrow are good herbs to use. They should always be in liquid form and *warm* before being administered in very *tiny* amounts through the ear canal. Mullein, wintergreen, and yarrow work best as teas. To one-and-a-half cups boiling water add one-quarter teaspoon of any of this herbal trio, stir, cover and set aside to steep for 15 minutes. While still somewhat warm, strain out a teaspoonful of the liquid and then fill a glass dropper half full with it. Tilt the head sideways, insert the dropper, and gently squeeze a small amount of tea into the ear canal. Keep head in tilted position for 30 minutes; by then the tea should have helped loosen things up a bit. The ear canal can then be swabbed out with several cotton tips that have been moistened with a little olive oil first.

Lobelia tincture or fluid extract may be purchased from a health-food store. Use that which is nonalcoholic. Heat a small amount in a teaspoon with a cigarette lighter or over a flame such as a burning candle. When nicely warmed, put into the ear canal with a glass dropper and retain for 30 minutes.

Greek Festival Promotes Natural Healing

For 23 years Salt Lake City's oldest, largest, and most popular late-summer ethnic block party has attracted thousands of curious and hungry visitors who've come to the Holy Trinity Greek Orthodox Church for the food, fun, festivity, and in 1999, some folk medicine. The event was born in 1974 and was an immediate hit. In 1998 it drew 50,000 visitors; a year later some 59,000 were drawn to it by the sweet smoke from lambs rotating on four spits over hot coals or just by the merriment of many others in general.

I was there on Saturday, September 11, having walked the several blocks distance from my downtown research center. I joined a conversation around one of the barbecue pits where the pork soulvakia was cooking and nibbled on some feta cheese in the process. One of the men gave me a thorough lookover before asking if I had been on television recently. I stated in the affirmative, having been on a local talk show of one of the independent stations located in the Salt Lake valley.

Upon learning this, he replied, "Now I remember where I know you from." He then beckoned me to follow him. "There's someone I think you should meet." We walked over to a table serving squid as the main course and baklava for dessert, where I was introduced to Constance Andopoulos, then visiting our city from her native Athens. "This is a guy who knows a lot about herbs," my unnamed new friend told her. We shook hands and he left us to ourselves.

I learned from Constance that she is somewhat of a folk healer herself and enjoys a certain popularity throughout parts of her country. "Over here," she laughed, "you *believe* a remedy might work, but in my Greece we *make* it work!" She gave me her remedies for the following four conditions, which I purposely brought up, seeing as how I would be working on them in my office later that evening. I felt she might be able to contribute something to each of them.

GONORRHEA

She was unfamiliar with the American colloquial expression for it as "the clap," but gave a quick, simple reply that indicated she had some experience in treating it. "We boil crushed olive pits first for a few minutes before adding the olive leaves and simmering, covered with a lid, for a few more minutes. The tea is strained when cool and drunk several times a day. Also the private parts of a man or woman are washed or douched with the same thing." A little olive oil is sometimes used afterwards on those private parts for additional comfort.

GOUT

"Take four figs and boil them in a pint of water until half the water remains. Let it stand and cool before drinking. Repeat as much as is needed."

GRAY HAIR

She looked at my gray hair and playfully teased, "You should be able to use this one right away." She then explained that black cumin, the remedy to which she was referring, was very popular for flavoring Russian rye bread, certain Turkish breads, and a few dark Greek breads as well. "Crush one-half cup cumin seeds and one-quarter cup sesame seeds" with a hammer, brick, smooth rock, or stone rolling mill. "Boil in two cups of water on medium heat until only one cup remains. Rinse the hair with that every day after showering *and leave it in* until the next time you bathe. Do this for 60 to 90 days and gray hair is gone for good."

GUM INFLAMMATION

"Wet your forefinger with the tongue and dip it into some powdered fenugreek seed. Rub this along the gums morning and evening. Inflammation vanishes just like . . . !" she said while snapping her fingers together.

I stayed to enjoy some roast lamb, learning as I did that 26 whole lambs and 50 legs had been prepared for this year's grand event. In fact, the lamb wasn't b-a-a-a-d at all!

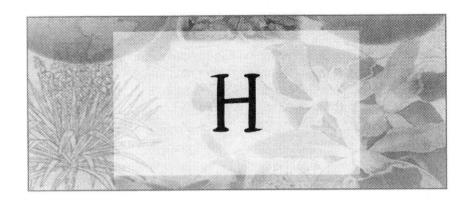

HAIR LOSS

Physician, Heal Thyself

The weekend of September 11–12, 1999, found me at the Holiday Inn in Cincinnati, Ohio with Mark Petersen of ShapeRite, lecturing to a room full of distributors on the healthful merits of fruits, vegetables, and the company's Bountiful Harvest (see Product Appendix under ShapeRite). During the course of my remarks, I remember saying this: "How credible do you think my words would be to all of you if I came here to push the merits of a new wonder cream or lotion for curing baldness?" I then ran my right hand over the top of my bald pate and bent my head slightly forward to further emphasize my point. "With this much baldness in the middle, would I truly be believable?"

Everyone laughed and shook their heads in the negative. "Of course I wouldn't be," I continued. "Because of HOW I look, my words would essentially fall on deaf ears. The same principle applies with equal force to each and every one of you. If you are out there in the public arena recruiting new distributors for your own line and talking to them about health, but do so holding a lit cigarette or are 50 pounds overweight, how credible do you think you or your message will be? Far too many people involved with different networking health products companies these days present poor images of the wellness messages they're trying to put over. Be sure that you are the epitome of health first before you try to change others over to your personal points of view. There is great wisdom in that ancient adage of 'Physician, heal thyself FIRST before thou tryest to heal others.'"

Bring Some Blood to the Top

While I haven't found the cure for baldness, at least I've discovered a few things that will help to *slow* the loss of further hair. Upon arising each morning, sit on the edge of your bed. Bend your head down toward your knees and vigorously massage your scalp for five minutes. Also, do a dry brush rub on your head using a *natural* bristle brush. Both stimulate circulation to bring more blood to the scalp to help nourish hair follicles.

HALLUCINATIONS

Hopi Ways

In past years I have spent some time on the Hopi Indian Reservation located *within* the boundaries of the much larger Navajo Reservation in northern Arizona. My first venture into the centuries-old village of Old Oraibi on top of Third Mesa was something of a cultural shock, to say the least. Greeting me a short distance from the pueblo dwellings, which archaeologists have determined were built around A.D. 1290, was a big plywood board sign painted white and mounted on two upright cedar posts with huge black letters reading: "WHITE PEOPLE NOT WELCOMED HERE!"

I drove away discouraged, but not for long. I drove to another Hopi community on top of the mesa, Bacobi, some five miles away and there met with a few friendlier individuals who paved the way for me to eventually visit the other, more ancient village. Just a mere handful of people were still living in Old Oraibi at the time of my first and only visit there. What had previously been a population numbering into the hundreds was less than 40 souls when I came. Several dissensions within the village in past decades had resulted in dissatisfied parties relocating elsewhere—the newer communities of Hotavila, Bacobi, Moenkopi, and New Oraibi were the results of these splinter groups' resettlements. Hence, Old Oraibi was in a pretty disintegrated state when I arrived.

Blue-Corn Drink

An old wrinkled medicine woman who looked as if she were a hundred years old (but in actuality was only 61 years of age), spoke with me through an interpreter. To get rid of hallucinations encountered during a fever or from drugs, she would give her patients some blue-corn water to drink. Blue corn is an Indian specialty and is what blue-corn chips are made from. The corn is removed from the husks, sun-dried, and put away in jars for later use. One half of a tin cup of this dried blue corn is boiled in three cups of water for a while (probably 25 minutes). It is set aside to cool before being strained. The *cold* liquid is given to the patient four to five times daily until all hallucinations cease.

Since then I've had a chance to test this out on a few others who've experienced similar feverish or drug-induced delusions with fairly good success. By what mechanism the corn accomplishes this, remains a mystery, though.

HAND PAIN

Liberal vs. Conservative

The Hopi villages on top of Third Mesa in northern Arizona present a rather sharp contrast between liberal and conservative thinking. New Oraibi is the most progressive, while Hotavila, located down the road a short six miles, is the most conservative. Hotavila still lacked tin-roofed houses in the mid-1970s, but New Oraibi had at least nine of them. However, the residents of Hotavila had the last laugh, as their earthen-roofed homes were considerably cooler than were those of their more liberal brethren in the other place.

The older homes in Hotavila were built in rows running in straight lines so as to form courts and streets. But in New Oraibi no such arrangement could be found. Many houses there seem to have been built without regard to the placing of the other structures; many are much larger, however, but stand in greater isolation. There is a weaker sense of community spirit in New Oraibi than in Hotavila. New Oraibi homes were furnished with carpets, refrigerators, couches, chairs, TVs, beds, tables, chairs, and cupboards, while Hotavila residences were rather spartan in appearance.

Saltwater Soak

One of the older gentlemen in Hotavila had hurt his right hand in some way. An old male shaman boiled a quart of water over the fire and added one-and-a-half cups of ordinary table salt. He stirred it thoroughly with a stick and then removed the pot when the water was quite warm. He had the other fellow stick his hand into this saltwater solution and keep it there for a while. (I tested the water with my fingers and found it to be somewhat hot but not at all scalding.) After soaking it for about half an hour, the older gentleman withdrew his hand, wiped it off, and got to his feet telling the tribal doctor all the pain had disappeared.

I've recommended this same simple remedy to those who've twisted an ankle or hurt their hands or feet in some way. Most of those who tried it reported a complete cessation of pain within minutes. It really is quite a miraculous cure that costs only pennies, is totally safe and easy to do, and, best of all, works like a charm every time!

HANGOVER
(See "ALCOHOLISM")

HAY FEVER

Hot Coffee Cures Ka-choos

A number of years ago I spent several weeks visiting different Hopi villages located on several mesa in the northern part of Arizona. I found the village of Mishongnovi to be closer to the conservative and community-minded Hotavila than it was to the more liberal and selfish New Oraibi. The ceremonial system was still intact, the native arts and industries provided the means of livelihood, and there had been no sharp changes of any kind within the previous 25 years.

In Mishongnovi the family was matrilineal, female ownership of houses existed, and the maternal uncle had the relationship to the children. Yet in other ways, the economic life of both villages remained identical. What differences there were were more of native culture rather than differences in the degree of Americanization.

While staying at Mishongnovi with one family, I was bothered by the dust that seemed to collect everywhere on a daily basis. This kept me sneezing up a storm until one afternoon the woman of the house brewed me up some strong black coffee, which I drank hot every few hours. My hay fever ceased almost immediately after that. But the downside to this experience was that while everyone else in the village snored away and counted sheep in their dreams, I was outside in the cool of the night air, viewing the clear and breathtaking heavens and counting, as it were, just about every star I could see!

HEADACHE

Coyote Clan Cure

Some years ago I drove my pickup truck to Black Mesa in the north-eastern part of Arizona. I saw the high, dark, flat formation rising above the desert floor in front of me and stretching over nearly all of the western horizon. Black Mesa is about 60 miles in length and 30 miles wide. About a dozen different Hopi villages are scattered over the three mesa fingers that jut out from Black Mesa.

I went to Mishongnovi on Second Mesa, among some of those I visited. There I met the town crier Starlie Lomayaktewa, whose business it was to publicly declare all important events relating to the village on any given day or week of the month. He was a member of the Coyote Clan and, at that time, served as acting chief of the village. This meant that he was responsible for the group's religious life, sort of like a "father figure" to all his people.

When I knocked on his door he shouted from within, "Come in," which I did. The house was filled with a number of people. There were no formal introductions. He said, looking toward me in sober tones, "You must be the anthropologist we've heard about. Sit down." He then spoke in his native tongue to some women present who fetched me something to eat.

Later that evening, probably because I ate in a hurry and didn't chew my food, I had a king-sized headache that didn't want to go away. I told my host about it and he handed me a small piece of brownish-colored root and instructed me to chew on that a while. The very sweet taste and mildly aromatic odor told my senses at once that it was licorice root. After about 45 minutes of constant chewing, I began to feel my throbbing headache ebb away.

Being curious as to how he came by way of this, since licorice root is from Europe and Asia and not at all part of Hopi indigenous medicine, I inquired as to its source. In his same poker-face expression, Starlie tersely stated, "We trade blue corn for it at white man's health-food store in Phoenix." Later he said that they sometimes will make a tea from licorice root to help with headaches. I was astonished to learn of this new use for a very old herb. None of the herb books I'm acquainted with list it for this condition, which I mentioned to Starlie. With his same dignified, unsmiling countenance, he matter-of-factly declared, "Maybe Hopi are smarter than whites or Chinese."

HEARING LOSS

An Islamic Remedy

Several of my informants of some years ago told me about fenugreek-seed tea being used in parts of Iran, Iraq, and Syria for the treatment of deafness. The seeds would be made into a warm tea and consumed several times a day for periods of a few months or more. They claimed that hearing was restored in the early stages of deafness.

Since then I've probably had six or eight different opportunities in which to recommend this to others, both old and young, who were having difficulty hearing or distinguishing certain sounds. Of those who actually tried the remedy—five in all, I believe—four of them reported back by letter or postcard in time that their hearing had substantially improved because of this treatment. Unfortunately, there are no other data than this to present at this time, except to say that the remedy is safe and seems to work most of the time in *moderate* hearing loss only, always as a tea consumed *orally* (never put into the ears), but ineffective in capsule form.

HEART ATTACK

The Davy Crockett Craze

In 1955 Walt Disney trotted out a weekly adventure fantasy entitled, *Davy Crockett, the King of the Wild Frontier.* The half-hour program became an instant hit with kids and set the marketplace on its ear.

From May to December 1955, coonskin was nothing but pure gold. During the seven-month boom, an estimated 4 million records and 14 million books were sold to a new generation of little pioneers. The demand for Crockett caps sent furriers scuttling after used raccoon coats and boosted the wholesale price of raccoon tails from 25 cents to as high as $8 a pound—a very tidy sum in those times.

Dime stores such as Woolworth's and S.H. Kress devoted up to 70 feet of counterspace to some three thousand items—powder horns and rifles, bath towels, telephones, ukeles, lunch boxes, and ladies' panties. I remember when I was in the third grade and attended the old Maeser School in Provo, Utah, that most of the other boys brought with them their Davy Crockett lunch boxes every day, while my brother and I had to content ourselves with brown-bag sack lunches instead. Some of the other kids made fun of us because we weren't part of this Davy Crockett crowd. How could we have been, seeing as how we never had television in our home until I was well into my twenties?

By Christmas of that year, however, the craze had evaporated. Davy T-shirts had been reduced from $1.29 to 35 cents, and still weren't moving. While it lasted, though, an estimated $100 million had changed hands in the name of the embattled backwoodsman, forever immortalized on the boob-tube by actor Fess Parker. Not surprisingly, Mrs. Margie Flowers Cohn of Okawville, Illinois, officially certified as Crockett's closest living descendant, never even realized a nickel's worth of this fortune.

Heart-Attack Saver

One of Mrs. Cohn's close relatives attended an herb lecture I gave in nearby Germantown, Clinton County, Illinois, for Nature's Sunshine Products. She gave me a little background information as to the personal history of Margie Cohn and then told me about the woman's relationship to the historical Davy Crockett. My informant said that young Davy really was a juvenile delinquent and kept running away from home a number of times to seek his fortune in the world. And nobody ever believed him when he claimed he had shot 105 bears in nine months, because folks knew the teenager couldn't even count that high.

But one thing Crockett did do was to hand down through his descendants an old Indian remedy for revitalizing the heart when it started to give someone serious problems. The liquid tonic consisted of one-half teaspoon each of powdered cayenne pepper and ginger root and one teaspoon of chopped garlic added to a quart of "fire water," a euphemistic term for hard liquor. The contents would be shaken each day and left to set in a cool, dark place for two to three weeks. Two or three tablespoons of the tonic would be taken every few hours if serious chest pains, nausea, dizziness, and fainting developed. Many potentially fatal heart attacks were thus remedied by this "heart-attack saver." *Note:* A heart attack is always life-threatening and demands prompt medical attention in a hospital emergency room. No attempt at self-treatment should be made if symptoms appear to lead to fatality.

HEARTBURN, HEATSTROKE

Cooling Fruit Juice

When I was in the Philippines in the early part of the 1990s gathering more folk remedies as well as "wife hunting" (no luck there!), I discovered some simple fruit juices for relieving heartburn and overcoming heatstroke. Those thusly affected need to drink *cool* papaya, mango, guava, or pear juice. Any of these will do, and they work almost instantaneously to soothe burning guts, chest, and throat, and reducing elevated body temperature due to sunstroke.

HEEL PAIN

A Gypsy Treatment

The gypsies are believed to have originated from somewhere in northwest India, which they left for Persia in the A.D. first millennium. Gypsies usually travel in small caravans and make their living as metalworkers, singers, dancers, musicians, horse dealers, and auto mechanics. Gypsy women are famous as fortune-tellers. Most gypsies are dark-complexioned, short, and lightly built.

In the course of their wanderings, gypsies have sometimes mixed with nongypsy neighbors and have occasionally settled down, but have managed to cling tenaciously to their own customs and identities. Their physical type has largely remained unaltered; their bands are still governed by elders. Although these people are traditionally sorcerers and necromancers, they generally adopt the religion of their country of residence; the greatest number are either Roman Catholic or Orthodox Eastern Christian.

Among their numerous folk remedies is one for heel pain. A few bay leaves (probably ten) are boiled in two quarts of vinegar, uncovered, for 35 minutes. When the tea is still rather hot (but not scalding to the skin), it is strained through cloth into a larger pan and the sore heel soaked in this until the liquid turns cool. It can then be reheated several more times and used for repeated soakings. The heel pain usually disappears after the second soaking.

HEMORRHOIDS

Rectal Insert Helps

There are an estimated five million gypsies in the world today. They speak Romany, which belongs to the Indo-Iranian family and is closely related to the languages of northwest India, while their blood groupings have been found to coincide with those of southern Himalayan tribes.

An old "sure-cure" gypsy treatment for hemorrhoids is this: Add one tablespoon each of marjoram and thyme (cut, dried herbs and not their powders) to a pint of boiling herb. Cover with a lid and gently simmer on low heat for five minutes. Set aside and steep for another 15 minutes. Strain and bottle and refrigerate. Soak a small, clean piece of folded cotton cloth or several cotton balls bunched together in a small portion of this reheated, *lukewarm* solution and then insert this material directly up the rectum and leave there for a while. The itching will cease and the inflammation will subside.

HEPATITIS

Necessity Is the Mother of Invention

During the years of the terrible Holocaust in Nazi Germany, besides six million Jews, approximately 500,000 gypsies were arrested by the Gestapo and sent to the gas chambers and concentration camps, where they eventually died miserable deaths. Some of the lucky ones, however, managed to survive, but barely. Sanitation conditions were horrible. Prisoners were denied soap with which to clean themselves and toilet paper was an unheard-of thing. Many people contracted hepatitis because they were unable to adequately cleanse their hands after using the toilet and were forced to eat their meager rations with fecal-contaminated fingers. A great number died as a result of this.

A few gypsies who contracted hepatitis pulled through their ordeal by picking stinging nettle and chickweed, which grew in wild abundance in and around some concentration camps, made a brew of both herbs, and drank it regularly instead of water.

HERNIA

Self-Treatment Only for the Stout-Hearted

A hernia is serious business, and the responsible thing to do is obviously to consult with a physician immediately so that surgery can get it rectified. But not everyone is inclined to join this mad lemming rush over the cliff and into the dangerous waters of hospital care. My aged father, Jacob Heinerman, who turned 86 in January 2000, and I are two such people. Both of us have experienced our own individual hernias and have dealt with them in the following ways.

My father has suffered from a double hernia for 50 years of his life. He was always worn trusses around his hips to hold both of them in and has taken a daily steady supply of vitamins and minerals to help his body better cope with them. As a rule he has managed very nicely. But about a year ago, he briefly "bought the farm," as it were, when one of them accidentally popped out in the middle of the night when he sneezed (he removes his trusses when he retires to bed so he can sleep better).

He awoke my brother Joseph, who sleeps in the same room with him but in a different bed, and had him assist in trying to push the hernia back through the muscle tear and into its original place. But they were unsuccessful in their attempts to do so. Finally, my brother came into my room directly opposite theirs, woke me up at 2:30 A.M., and hurriedly explained the situation to me.

I immediately got up, put my glasses and slippers on, and walked into their bedroom, where I found our father in serious trouble and looking very pale to say the least. I carefully examined the area of the difficulty and instructed him to lean a certain way while I tenderly manipulated the turkey egg-sized hernia back through the tissue tear again. It took some patience and a little finger dexterity to do this, but it was nicely accomplished within a couple of minutes, much to my father's and brother's relief.

After that, I had my dad start drinking a combination of slippery-elm bark and marshmallow root to help promote tissue knitting. While the left side still remains a problem, he reports that the right hernia seems to have partially corrected itself. These are the same teas that I drank nearly every day for five years from the age of nine to thirteen for my own right groin hernia, while wearing a truss the whole time to hold it in place. Eventually, my young body was able to heal itself, and I no longer required the rupture belt or drinking the tea.

Bear in mind, though, that "what is good for the goose may not always be good for the gander" simply meaning that we grew up in a *constant culture* of natural healing where herbs were used regularly. Also, my dad's mother, Grandmother Barbara Liebhardt Heinerman, was a seventh- or eighth-generation folk healer from Europe and possessed "a healing intuition" about her, which I ultimately inherited. Our lengthy and intense distrust of the medical profession necessitated that we find other ways to take care of our own health problems, when such alternative treatments were terribly unpopular with most doctors and the general public. But, it is my STRONG recommendation that anyone suffering from a hernia opt for emergency medical treatment if his or her faith and understanding of natural remedies is limited.

HERPES

Stress Is a Triggering Factor

Much has been written on the subject of herpes. It infects close to 500,000 Americans annually. Eight out of ten people in America today have the herpes virus in them; if you had chickenpox as a youngster, then you still have the herpes virus inside of you, although it's probably in a dormant state. Under an electron microscope, herpes looks like a greasy virus. It hides deep within the ganglion nerves of the spine, upper torso, and upper thighs.

But any kind of severe mental or emotional trauma can trigger it in a heartbeat. Also, a fairly constant diet of junk food weakens the immune system just enough to turn it loose. Therefore, two methods of prevention are to always have a happy heart and cheerful disposition and to practice good nutrition at all times.

Home Remedies to Try

In the event there is an outbreak on the skin of herpes, here are some simple remedies to try for relief:

- Take white-willow-bark capsules or drink peppermint tea to reduce pain and any fever.
- Apply cool compresses of witch-hazel tincture (available at pharmacies and supermarkets) to skin lesions six times a day.
- Apply over-the-counter anesthetic creams purchased from pharmacies—Anbesol and Campho-Phenique are two of the best.
- Numb the area with an ice pack. Put an ice cube in a zippered plastic sandwich bag and wrap the bag in a cloth handkerchief. Apply this to the skin for 15 minutes, then remove for seven minutes before reapplying it.
- Avoid wearing tight-fitting underwear or pants.
- Make sure your underclothing is made of 100 percent cotton, since air can penetrate more easily to help dry the sores and minimize their pain and irritation.
- Always keep the genitals clean and dry. Pat rather than rub yourself dry after bathing or use a hand-held air dryer on the coolest

setting. Use a separate towel for the genitals to prevent spreading the lesions to other parts of the body.

HIATAL HERNIA
(See "HEARTBURN/HEATSTROKE")

HICCUPS

Take Some Tepid Suds

Just about everyone has a cure of some sort for hiccups; the problem is most of them don't work! Here is a "sure-cure" thing if you start hiccuping for no reason at all: Room temperature or slightly heated *warm beer*, slowly sipped, will never fail to work. Try it for yourself or on a friend, and see if I'm not correct. (You can reach me through Anthropological Research Center listed in the Product Appendix; I'd love to hear from you on this one.)

HIGH BLOOD PRESSURE

A Plan to Make Your Pressure Plummet

Watch your weight. If you are 20 percent over the ideal weight for your height and bone structure, then you could become a likely candidate for hypertension. Losing just 10 percent of this excess weight will be doing your heart and body a huge favor.

Stay away from salty foods and ordinary table salt. Flavor your food with herbal seasonings instead, such as basil, thyme, oregano, tarragon, kelp, and sea salt (which is considerably different from table salt). Trace Minerals Research of Roy, Utah sells a nice low-sodium liquid mineral ConcenTrace from the Great Salt Lake which can be sprayed on any type of food (see Product Appendix).

If you are a social drinker, cut down on your intake of alcohol: Allow yourself no more than two drinks a day. Commercial beers and most wines should be avoided: a little red wine is permissible. Dark ales are the healthiest, but should also be moderately consumed.

Potassium is the one mineral for helping to control existing hypertension. Your potassium–sodium ratio should always be 6:2, meaning for every two grams of ingested sodium, you need six grams of potassium to offset any harm the other might do in elevating your blood pressure. Dark leafy greens, potatoes (with skin intact), fresh fruit, and fresh water fish are loaded with this valuable mineral.

Aerobic exercise is useful here. Try rope jumping, skipping, trampoline bouncing, swimming, or horseback riding. Even a 30-minute walk every day will control your blood pressure unbelievably well.

Think vegetarian. Studies have shown that those who don't eat meat (except fish), invariably have 10 to 15 mm Hg. lower for both systolic and diastolic pressures.

Talk less and be happier. Yacking a lot and being in an irritated mood can really drive blood pressure through the roof. Learn to shut up occasionally and make peace with yourself and those around you.

Interact with a friendly dog or cat (unless otherwise allergic to canines). It is a medical fact that older men and women who have dogs or cats to keep them company, see their blood pressures decline as a result of this animal companionship.

Finally, learn to pray more often. This can be done irrespective of your personal religious beliefs. Doctors who are on the cutting edge of prayer science found that those who regularly invoke the name of a deity (in a reverential and thoughtful way, of course) seem to enjoy better cardiac health and normal blood pressure.

HIGH CHOLESTEROL

Raise Your Fiber and Double Your Sulfur

High-fiber cereal grains, vegetables, and nuts, along with sulfur-rich fruits and vegetables are the key to controlling your daily serum cholesterol levels. Whole-wheat bread, bran muffins, buckwheat pancakes, cooked oatmeal, rye or pumpernickel toast, and figs, garlic, onion, leeks, scallions, cabbage, kale, kohlrabi, Brussels sprouts, cauliflower, horseradish, mustard greens, red radish, broccoli, and watercress are the foods to be considered for this.

HIP PAIN

Besides chiropractic adjustments, massage and yoga exercises, try the remedies listed under *"Hand Pain"* and *"Heel Pain"* by soaking the hips in a small tub of hot saltwater or bay vinegar (called a sitz bath in Europe).

HIVES

Dairy-Cream Soother

The quickest, easiest, and cheapest way to treat hives is to sponge over them some *cool* dairy cream or half-and-half several times a day. Whole cow's or goat's milk and buttermilk may also be used effectively for this.

HOARSENESS AND LARYNGITIS

A Stop on the Road to Heaven

The great American humorist and author Mark Twain (Samuel Longhorn Clemens in reality) once said that Americans on their way to heaven make a brief stop in Bermuda and think they've already arrived. Those were shared impressions when I first set foot on its friendly shores sometime in 1983. Over the ensuing week that followed, I sailed her bays and inlets, watched some of my friends dive along her coral reefs (I never learned how to swim), explored her sea-carved cliffs, lay torpid as a lizard on her talc-soft beaches, left portions of my ego on her rugged, windy links, and pedaled a bike down nearly every flowered lane of her nine parishes.

After this, I think I came to know her a bit better. Only 21 square miles in area, Bermuda has unbelievable riches crowded into very little room. No one of her parishes (each named for some English gentleman linked to her British history) quite resembles another; Paget's prim beauty looks at Sandy's rural ways, and St. George, former seat of Bermuda's Government, thinks of them both as Johnnies-come-lately.

Yet, for all her diversity, Bermuda is, in my humble estimation, small enough to be grasped and comprehended as a whole.

Warm Papaya Juice Does the Trick

I became hoarse late one afternoon after talking nonstop for six hours with a host of friends whom I had come with. I was beside myself as to what should be done, since I had an important speaking engagement later that evening. One of the local residents recommended *heated* papaya juice (in an eight-ounce glass) along with a little cognac (one teaspoon) stirred in for good measure. I tried this "Bermuda tawdy" as they call it, and within 30 minutes experienced nearly a full recovery of my voice for a strong vocal performance in that night's health lecture.

HODGKIN'S DISEASE

Shakespeare's "Bermoothes"

The first person ever to set foot on the islands constituting Bermuda was the Spanish navigator Juan de Bermúdez (1503–1511), after whom they were probably named. But these islands remained uninhabited, despite assorted visits by both Spaniards and Englishmen, until Sir George Somers and a group of colonists on their way to Virginia were shipwrecked there in 1609.

This incident was known to the renowned English playwright William Shakespeare when he wrote *The Tempest*. The bard included the highly unpredictable weather the islands are known to have when he wrote about the "still-vex'd Bermoothes." He charged Prospero and his sprite Ariel with having "bedimm'd the noontide sun, call'd forth the mutinous winds, and 'twixt the green sea and the azur'd vault set roaring war."

Seaweed Success

In the early-to-mid 1980s I worked for a networking health-supplements company in Florida. The company sponsored a week-long cruise to Bermuda for a number of its top distributors. I was invited along to give some health lectures in the evening, which I readily accepted.

An old gentleman by the name of Mulligan Fox claimed to have been descended from some of the early ninteenth-century privateers who frequently looted storm-tossed ships that piled up on Bermuda's innumerable reefs. He suggested the use of seaweed and certain seafood, especially shrimp, for the "curing" (as he swore) of Hodgkin's disease. He said there had been considerable success with such iodine-rich foods among those who came there seeking relief from this affliction. It was his opinion that the thyroid was somehow involved in this malignancy and that *natural iodine from seafood* could halt its rapid progress. I ran this by an oncologist friend of mine a few years later and he scoffed at the idea, calling it "ludicrous and preposterous."

Well, it wasn't too long after that that I had a chance to test this Bermuda remedy for myself to see if there was anything to it beyond presumed folklore. A woman in her fifties was diagnosed as having full-blown Hodgkin's disease and given only a short time to live. Her husband contacted me by phone through one of my many Prentice Hall health books (my unlisted home phone number is in the back appendices of most of them).

I gave him the same information that Mulligan had freely shared but in greater detail. He promptly put his wife on a diet of cooked seaweed, boiled shrimp, and further supplemented her with eight capsules of kelp every day. There were a number of other foods she subsisted on as well, but I remember those as being the most prominent in her eating regimen. Within 60 days ALL traces of Hodgkin's disease had totally disappeared. Her husband was ecstatic and wanted to pay me a goodly sum of money in gratitude for the data provided, but I refused it, saying that "as I had freely received so had I freely given," and that there was no charge for assisting them in their particular health dilemma.

HOT FLASHES

Virtually Absent in Other Cultures

In a number of other societies that I've lived in and studied around the world, I was amazed to find that the condition of hot flashes so common in our culture was virtually absent in them. I attributed this to several things. First, the women of those other cultures ate very little junk food and drank very little soda pop or colas. More important, they didn't have the hectic lifestyles and technological stresses imposed upon working women in America and Europe by our sophisticated materialism and ambitious drives to succeed. If modern women in the West could ever learn to take things easier, move at a slower pace, and eat better, they would have *fewer* hot flashes.

HYPOGLYCEMIA

B.T. Express

Bermuda lies 650 miles from America, more than 3,000 from Europe, and is, in fact, one of the most isolated spots on earth. Oddly, it has become more famous for something other than its luscious setting and idyllic climate. I'm referring, of course, to that triangular terror of which many myths and legends have been perpetuated—the *Bermuda Triangle*. Its boundaries are mysterious, believed by the "experts" to extend from northern Bermuda to southern Florida, down to a point through the Bahamas past Puerto Rico, then back again to Bermuda.

The Bermuda Triangle has lain in wait since humans first learned how to travel by water and air. But it didn't become the popular media prostitute we now know it to be until around 1945, when it started to snatch airplanes from the sky and ships from the sea with an uncanny vengeance. Since that date, hundreds of vessels have vanished, thousands of lives have been lost—suddenly, mysteriously, and completely. No wreckage, no bodies, no oil slick, no warning.

The B.T.'s most famous incident is the one concerning Flight 19 on December 5, 1945. (Festively, most of the disappearances occur in the months surrounding Christmas.) Five Avenger torpedo bombers, minding their own business on a routine navigational exercise, took off from Fort Lauderdale Naval Air Station, flew over the Bermuda Triangle, and, within two hours, vanished not so simply into not-so-thin air. (The cunning Triangle conveniently cuts off radio communication, causes compasses to spin erratically, churns patches of otherwise calm ocean, and envelops ships and planes in a hazy yellow, green, or blue cloud—as well as other reported excesses of cinematic overkill—before dispatching its prey.)

A twin-engine Martin Mariner patrol plane with a crew of 13 was sent to rescue the five Avenger bombers of Flight 19, but it, too, disappeared. Naturally, what else would you expect?

A subsequent exhaustive search mission (307 planes, four destroyers, 18 Coast Guard vessels, numerous submarines, hundreds of helpful local planes, yachts, and boats, not to mention the RAF and a Royal Navy unit) combed 380,000 square miles of land and sea (the Atlantic, the Caribbean, the Gulf of Mexico, the Florida mainland) but turned up nothing. Of course, they wouldn't!

In fact, the crafts involved in the rescue mission ran the risk of succumbing to the same fate—the Bermuda Triangle is an equal-opportunity purloiner. Nothing flying or floating through the dreaded region is safe. Over the decades since then, battleships, schooners, sailboats, speedboats, jets, cargo planes, private charters, military bombers, fishing boats, dinghies, lifeboats, rafts, and even the odd rubber duck have been launched into limbo. There are many damn good anecdotes to this effect that can cause your hair to stand on end and your skin to experience a prickly sensation after listening to a bunch of them.

Like most serial killers, though, the B.T. has a playful, charming side: Sometimes it leaves the ship and takes only the passengers and crew. And it has a very peculiar pet peeve: It won't take animals of *any* kind—they've always been found stranded on crewless ships adrift at sea.

Surviving B.T.-Induced Hypoglycemia

One of the well-known contributing factors to hypoglycemia is emotional anxiety and sudden climatic change. Bruce Gernon, Senior and Junior, experienced both, and lived to tell about their weird ordeal. In December 1970, this father and son casually flew their Beechcraft Bonanza into a nightmare from which they eventually recovered. They had planned a rather routine trip from the Bahamas to Palm Beach, Florida. However, in midflight, the plane was suddenly enveloped in a thick, ugly cloud, which by now you should already know is par for that course (thick, ugly clouds being a mainstay of the old Triangle). But this one turned into a glowing, clockwise-rotating tunnel. The plane shot through it at an incredible speed, and the Gernons felt weightless. Not to mention helpless.

The father described it to me some years later. He indicated that both he and his son became "sick to our stomachs." They suddenly felt a tremendous loss of unexplained physical energy, which neither could account for. "We barely had enough strength to keep our heads up and to remain conscious. We were scared out of our wits. I reached around the seat behind me and groped through a tote bag brought along filled with snacks and beverages in case we got hungry. I hauled out two small cans of V-8 juice and some pretzels. We opened these items and drank and munched on them as best we could. We were surprised to find our overwhelming fatigue melting away as our energy rebounded. We felt renewed and revitalized!"

At the end of the tunnel they entered the traditional greenish-white haze. Naturally, their compasses flipped out, their navigational equipment took a hiatus, and any ground communication was out of the question. Eventually and miraculously, the haze lifted and the Gernons were able to land their small aircraft in Palm Beach. But, strangely, they arrived 30 minutes earlier than they should have and had used 12 fewer gallons of gas than usual. So in this particular instance, the Bermuda Triangle was a convenient and thrifty route to take.

After hearing the elder Gernon's fantastic report, I started recommending V-8 juice, pretzels, and salsa and tortilla chips to those experiencing sudden drops in their blood-sugar levels. Invariably, they always tend to rebound after consuming such things. I also advise some of them to stay away from the B.T.

Coincidental or Nonsense?

Is all this stuff coincidental? Or is it mere nonsense? Is there some logical, scientific explanation?

There are theories. Magnetic fields. Clear-air turbulence. Time warps. Vortices. Aliens. Sea monsters. The CIA. Lucifer and Company. Was Flight 19's Lieutenant Charles Taylor strung out on drugs or chewing some "whacky tabaccky" when he radioed into headquarters, "Don't come after me . . . they look like they are from outer space"? Just whom did he mean by "they"?

HYPOTHERMIA

The Grave Yields Its Secrets

All over the world, traces may be seen of the prehistoric past, of the dwellings and the graves of ancient man. But in nearly every case it is only through skeletons or scattered bones, sculptures, or other handiwork that we can form our picture of early man. To see our distant ancestors as real human beings, we are forced to rely on our imagination in most instances.

But not so in Denmark! In this little land exceptional conditions of preservation have permitted us to see Bronze Age and Iron Age Man, not of course, living, but in some cases so wonderfully preserved as to appear to be separated from our own era not by the millennia that have, in fact, truly elapsed, but only by a few hours' sleep, as it were.

Two large groups of discoveries provide these unique relics: Bronze Age burials from about 3,000 years ago and peat-bog finds from the Iron Age at about the commencement of our Christian Era. Some of the bodies found in these peat bogs of Jutland have been preserved to such an astounding degree that they show not the slightest desiccation and lie with rounded limbs as if asleep.

There are an estimated 50,000 large mounds of the Bronze Age that lie scattered over the 16,576 square miles of Denmark. In these grave mounds lie the chieftains of the Bronze Age and their families, buried in coffins of hollowed oak trees and clad, not as elsewhere in the world, in special grave clothes, but in the everyday clothing they wore during life.

In Jutland, in cases where an iron-oxide formation, "hardpan," formed around the coffin soon after burial and hermetically sealed its contents, the hollowed oak trunk still survives in its original rounded form and preserves within its walls the woven clothing, the hair, the skin, even the eyebrows of the dead. When the lid is lifted, the thin layer of skin that remains still shows the expression of the face.

A Coffin Antidote for Hypothermia in the Netherworld

One of the best preserved oak coffins discovered (in February 1921) was that from Egtved near Kolding in southeast Jutland. There, lying at full length on her back, was a young woman in her mid-thirties with fair hair of page-boy cut, dressed in a short-sleeved jumper and a skirt of knee-length tassels.

A braided hair ribbon lay behind her head, and around her waist she wore a belt with an ornamental disk, decorated with spiral patterns. She had a comb of horn, and on her wrists were two beautiful bronze bracelets. In front of her face a little box, of linden raffia, contained a leather pricker and a spare hair ribbon.

By her feet stood a birch-bark jug that had contained cranberry wine, made bitter with bog myrtle and sweetened with honey. It had been purposely placed there after being gently *warmed* over a fire to serve as an exhilarating drink for the dead girl in helping her to resist the legendary hypothermia that her soul would be experiencing as she made her way to the realms of the departed.

Now after seeing and listening to all of this myself from a Danish archaeologist colleague, I wondered whether or not such a beverage for the dead might not have some useful function for the living as well in regard to the same problem. So, I readjusted things a bit and incorporated cranberry juice (one cup), some brandy (one-quarter cup), a dash of wormwood powder (one-eighth teaspoon), and some honey (one-quarter teaspoon). After everything was thoroughly mixed together I then briefly heated the solution over a medium-setting gas range flame. I poured it into a tall glass and then opened the front door of my house in the middle of winter and called for a friend (who had reluctantly volunteered for this strange experiment) to come in out of a heavy snowstorm, which he did with surprising quickness. After stomping and brushing off the excess snow on his boots, coat, and cap, he removed his gloves and declared himself cold enough to try my "Underworld Hypothermia Tonic."

What people won't do in the name of science, especially if they're being paid $100 to participate in such a quirky stunt as this. I waited patiently for him to drain the contents, as it took several minutes while he drank, smacked his lips, and then quaffed some more. Finally, he handed me back the empty glass and stated without hesitation, "John, I do believe this concoction has thoroughly warmed my innards like nothing I've ever tried!" Based solely on this single test, I, thereafter, began recommending it for hypothermia, and always with good results.

HYPOTHYROIDISM

The Kampo Approach

Kampo is a unique Japanese system of herbal medicine, which was borrowed in principle from Chinese traditional medicine, but especially adapted to the former culture. Kampo herbs give the person the exact energy he or she needs to return to the fundamentally sound, vibrant, and robust state of health people were meant to enjoy.

One of the most important kampo formulas for treating low thyroid activity is a combination of Oriental scullcap (one tablespoon), cinnamon bark (one teaspoon), and wild-cherry bark (one teaspoon). If making a tea, use the dried, coarsely cut, crude herb parts for this: Brew them in one pint boiling water for three minutes, covered, and then set aside to steep for another 50 minutes; strain and drink when cool. If capsules are to be taken, then the powders of these three herbal ingredients may be used instead. Drink one cup twice daily or take two capsules morning and night with meals.

Kampo medicine requires that immune-stimulant herbs such as aloe, American ginseng, astragalous, bamboo, burdock, chrysanthemum, ginger, Oriental ginseng, kelp, motherwort, Siberian ginseng, echinacea, and wheat grass be avoided during this period of time. Kampo doctors, with whom I spoke through an interpreter, vouched for the safety and efficacy of this formula.

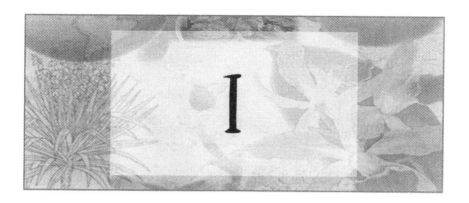

IMPETIGO

Simple Treatment

This skin affliction is common in newborn babies and very young children and is distinguished by shallow sores that form a crusty surface with a characteristic "honey" color. The weepy blisters and crusty surface of impetigo are due to a strep infection. The problem is rare in adults and older kids.

The easiest way of coping with this is to gently remove the crust with soap (I prefer Dial brand) and water (preferably distilled). It may be necessary to apply some wet gauze dressings to the crusts to soften them before their removal. Afterwards apply some hydrogen peroxide with cotton tips or cotton balls to disinfect the areas. Then put some type of commercial antibiotic ointment on, such as Neosporin.

One may also empty a few capsules of echinacea or goldenseal powders, mix them with a little Vaseline, and apply to the skin with a wooden tongue depressor. This will work nearly as well as the over-the-counter antibiotic.

IMPOTENCY

Maintaining an Erection Naturally

The itinerant street minstrel whom I met in Dallas, Texas, some years ago, Samuel Johnson Williams or just plain S.W., has his own colorful description for this problem: "Gettin' your nature up!" For which he recommended consumption of spicy food laced with plenty of cayenne pepper an hour before sexual activity was to begin. (See under Eating Disorders—Eyestrain for more information.)

But, in reality, "impotence" is really a misnomer. It somehow implies that a man has lost all personal sexual vitality and that he is an utter failure in that department, which could be nothing further from the truth. The term "erection problem" is more correct because that is all this condition entails—an inability to raise or maintain an erection during arousal and sexual intercourse.

There are certain contributing factors that hinder a healthy erection in a normal man. Alcohol is the chief cause of erection impairment. One drink may be useful to induce lovemaking, but *no more* after that. Drugs that induce drowsiness or exert tranquilizing effects impair erection. These range from narcotics, hypnotics, tranquilizers, and antipsychotics to some hypertension, antiulcer, and antidepressant medications. Aging is also bound to have some modest effect on a man's ability to experience a full, firm erection as he gets older. Mental anxiety and emotional stress also cause a man's sex organ to go limp when he doesn't want it to. The same thing may be said for depression, too. A man should be in a positive frame of mind and have a joyful or happy heart when about to engage in sexual pleasure; otherwise he's apt to become very discouraged while in the act.

There is an old hillbilly saying among the mountain folk of Kentucky and Tennessee to the effect, "Don't expect your penis to stand up if you can't do so yourself!" This is to say that any acute illness, from a simple cold to a more serious disease, can cause loss of interest in lovemaking and erection impairment. Mountain folk maintain that physical lovemaking involves a great deal of energy and that a man's stamina must be in top shape for peak performance in sexual activities.

A few helpful "do's" and "don'ts" may be in good order here:

- Begin slowly; don't hurry lovemaking; let nature take its course.
- Don't be preoccupied with the state of your penis during sex; focus your attention on your partner instead and let the other take care of itself as the business of pleasure proceeds along.
- Vary your sexual routine somewhat, but keep it simple and avoid anything that is degrading or perverted.

- Take two tablespoons of Rex Wheat Germ Oil an hour before sex. (See Product Appendix under Anthropological Research Center.)

Certain nutrients and herbs will also help to promote a meaningful sexual experience for the man and his mate. They include some of the B-complex vitamins, chromium, zinc, selenium, ginseng, ginger, sarsaparilla, yohimbine, fenugreek, and royal jelly. To take these things individually wouldn't be very practical, since there are just too many of them to swallow at any given time. But taking them all together in a particular formula especially designed for erection problems would be the most logical thing to do. Synergy Worldwide, an Orem, Utah-based nutrition company, has developed a wonderful product called Euphoria that includes all of these and many more items and helps a man to achieve satisfying sexual fulfillment in concert with his companion. (See Product Appendix under Synergy Worldwide.)

INDIGESTION

From My Grandma to You

The best remedy that my aged Hungarian grandmother Barbara Liebhardt Heinerman always used for stomach complaints was peppermint tea by itself or in combination with chamomile tea. Sometimes she even used the chamomile alone with good success. She would always drink one or two cups of either herbal tea, *warm*, with meals. Her folk wisdom in this matter has proven itself true in the decades since her demise, and thousands of people have benefited from this knowledge she passed on to me and that I've included in previous health books.

Another outstanding remedy for food-related or digestive-connected headaches is acidophilus. I've enjoyed using the Kyodophilus brand from Wakunaga of America (see Product Appendix) for this. My recommendation is to take two to three capsules at one time with a full glass of water. The headache will usually disappear within 10 to 15 minutes. This product should be kept refrigerated once the bottle is opened. Drinking a little buttermilk or eating a small dish of yogurt also helps.

Learn to chew your food slowly. Don't eat under stress. Keep your meals simple. Don't overeat. Consume starches and proteins at different meals.

INFECTION

The Man Who Created Tarzan

Edgar Rice Burroughs (1876–1950), the creator of the world-famous jungle hero Tarzan and the John Carter/Mars series, was blessed with a powerful imagination and writing gift at an early age, but refused to develop it in his early manhood. Instead he tried his hand in the business world at a number of different enterprises, though always unsuccessfully, and ended up broke. Finally, in the summer of 1911, with 35 years of his adult life gone, he paused and meditated upon the numerous failures he had experienced in the corporate world in rapid succession. "My business venture," he wrote, "went the way of all other enterprises and I was left without money, without a job, and with a wife and two babies" (the Fine Arts Supplement Section of the *Chicago Examiner*, April 4, 1918).

At last, having tried and failed at everything else, he was ready to put his ideas on paper. First came the romantic hero John Carter, a character creation whose background and physical accomplishments were a super version of his own. Burroughs's Carter was a cross between Indiana Jones and Buck Rogers who suddenly and mysteriously found himself transported from the hot Arizona desert and the hostile Indians he was at that moment fighting to the angry red planet of Mars where he faced a race of huge green Martians whose young were hatched in glass incubators from eggs two-and-one-half feet in diameter.

Science-fiction writer Ray Bradbury, who himself grew up as a boy on the Burroughs jungle and space epics, had this to say about the other man's writings. "Mr. Burroughs influenced several dozen million scores of boys all across the world [for about] sixty years." Bradbury asserted that Burroughs outranked Rudyard Kipling, Jules Verne, and a host of other fantasy writers because of "the sheer romantic impossibilities" contained in all of his fast-moving stories, which could delight the heart of "any ten-year-old boy."

Recovering from Blood Infection

While much is known about Burroughs's life, very few are currently aware that he and his new bride Emma Hulbert moved to Salt Lake City in the spring of 1904 and spent approximately six months there, residing in some rented rooms at 111 North First West. Burroughs was hired on as a "depot policeman" by the Oregon Railroad Company. His job, as he later described it in Bob Davis's column in the *New York Sun*, July 20, 1940, "was in the railroad yards where after nightfall I rambled and fanned bums off the freight cars and the blind baggage of the Butte Express."

In his unpublished *Autobiography*, Edgar Rice observed that he was kept busy "rushing bums out of the railroad yards and off the passenger trains. It was not very exciting for the bums and eggs were seldom as hard boiled as they are painted and only upon one or two occasions did I even have to flash my gun." He considered drunks to be the worst offenders. "If you have never tried to eject a drunk from a day coach," he wrote, "you have no idea how many arms and legs a man can have."

On one such occasion, a large burly Irishman, who was definitely feeling the bravery of his whiskey that day, stabbed Burroughs in the arm with a fountain pen as the man was forcibly kicked off a train. The ink in his veins brought on blood poisoning, which might have proved itself fatal had Burroughs not used common sense in treating the problem right away.

Burroughs had learned some things about herbs from the short time he spent with the Seventh U.S. Cavalry at Fort Grant in Arizona Territory between 1896 and 1897, hopelessly chasing the wily renegade Indian, the Apache Kid. He instructed his wife to procure for him some yucca powder, while he peeled a large onion and cut off a few slices, which he then placed over the infected site and securely bound it to his arm with strips of an old sheet. The onion drew out most of the poison, and he would replace old slices with fresh ones every few hours. He mixed one teaspoon yucca powder with one-half teaspoon goldenseal powder in with a little canned milk and then swallowed this concoction in a hurry on account of its rather nasty taste. Both herbs seem to have helped in neutralizing the effects of whatever black ink remained inside him.

He recovered quickly enough and continued on about his duties as a railroad cop for another few months until his job ended. In their plans to return to their home state of Michigan, Edgar and Emma encountered their most serious obstacle: They had no money for the railroad fare. At this time the couple dreamt up a brilliant scheme. All they possessed of value was the household furniture, dragged along with them "all over Idaho and Utah." This they would auction off, hoping to obtain enough money for the journey to Chicago.

About the results Edgar wrote in his *Autobiography:* "That auction was a howling success. I never imagined people would buy such utterly useless things and pay real money for them. The only decent things that we had brought little or nothing, but the junk brought about ten times what it was worth, and so we got home again, traveling first class [all the way]." Early on, the Burroughs had discovered the magical economic power generally attached to the all-American "garage sale." "What is one man's junk is another man's treasure," certainly applied well in this case.

INFERTILITY

Midget Stuntman Fertility "Secret"

Throughout the 1930s and early 1940s, Metro-Goldwyn-Meyer (MGM) film studios made a series of Tarzan epics featuring the duo of Johnny Weissmuller and Maureen O'Sullivan in the leads as Tarzan and Jane. For its 1939 movie, first titled *Tarzan in Exile*, MGM, through screenwriter Cyril Hume, initiated a daring plot. Tarzan and Jane discover a young boy whose parents have died in a plane crash. They raise the boy, played by five-year-old Johnny Sheffield, and, as the plot develops, their temporary son is revealed to be the heir to a fortune; at the story's end he returns to civilization. The movie was finally released under the revised title of *Tarzan Finds a Son.*

On August 22, 1939, Burroughs received an interesting letter from Harry Monty, who had done all the doubling and stunt work for Tarzan's young "son" in the film. Monty offered the following interesting details: "I am 32 years old, 53 inches tall, weight 89 pounds and am known professionally as the Midget Strong Man with the most Muscular Perfect Physique of any small person in the World. I have worked many years on the stage doing strong acts, muscular posing, feats of strength, aerial work, and am an all around gymnast . . ." Though he hadn't read any of the Tarzan books himself, he eventually met Burroughs at the latter's estate in Tarzana, California.

Sometime during their lengthy visit, the conversation turned to infertility, the subject being broached by the feisty little midget. He informed Burroughs that for a number of years he and his wife had been unable to have any children together. Careful physical examinations of both by doctors eventually determined that the problem lay with him and not her.

Monty sought the advice of an old Romanian gypsy immigrant recently arrived in the Golden State. She advised him to make a strong tea of hops and to drink two cups of the warm brew every night faithfully for 45 days. During this time he was to have no sexual relations with his wife. He was also to avoid taking hot baths. Furthermore, he was told to counsel his wife to remain on her back for an hour with her knees drawn up and a feather pillow placed under her hips following sexual intercourse.

The gypsy woman's recommendations were followed to the letter, and eleven-and-a-half months later his wife gave birth to a lovely infant daughter whom they named after their benefactor.

INFLUENZA
(see "FLU")

INGROWN TOENAILS

Tarzan's Astonishing Popularity

An article that appeared in *The Boys' Outfitter,* June 1934, and titled "Tarzan Enters the Boys' Department," described the tremendous popularity of the vine-swinging jungle man. More than 34 million copies of the Tarzan books had been sold to date, and the Tarzan strips, launched in 1929, were now appearing in 253 newspapers worldwide.

Tarzan, the Ape Man marked the first appearances of Johnny Weissmuller and Maureen O'Sullivan. Weismuller was described as cutting a "great" Tarzan figure on the silver screen with his wonderful "youth, a marvelous physique, and a magnetic personality."

The Tarzan fever that had gripped the public was visibly demonstrated in the record-breaking attendance throughout the country. Burroughs mentioned to a friend on May 9, 1932, about the eager crowds in Los Angeles for the movie's initial debut: "The rush was so great Saturday and Sunday that they advertized in this morning's paper that they are forced to put on seven shows a day, starting at about nine in the morning."

Tarzan's Toe Cure

During the filming at "Lot No. 2" at the MGM studio, Weissmuller complained of experiencing pain in his big toe due to an ingrown nail. A Beverly Hills podiatrist was immediately called for some quick consultation on the situation. The studio couldn't afford to delay filming important action scenes, and it certainly wouldn't look good for the jungle man to be limping around when he should be moving in bold strides.

The unnamed doctor examined Weissmuller's foot, then proceeded to clean out the infected toe with an alcoholic tincture. After this he applied a little eucalyptus oil, which he apparently sometimes used in his practice. Within minutes the pain was gone and filming resumed!

INSECT BITES AND STINGS

Mud Always Works

In previous health books I've mentioned an odd assortment of remedies for relieving the itching and reducing the swelling and pain suffered from insect bites and stings. Among these have been the application of cucumber slices, saliva, meat tenderizer, and tropical-fruit pulp such as papaya, guava, or mango. Also, the "juice" or spittle from chewing tobacco is equally effective for this. In India they use human or animal urine to obtain the same results.

Having been in my share of jungles around the world in years past (though never personally encountering the loin-clothed, vine-swinging hero himself), I believe that I'm somewhat of an expert when it comes to effectively dealing with skin irritations of this type.

I've always resorted to smearing mud on any such bites and stings and leaving it there to dry. Within a minute or less the hot, jabbing sensations of pain and the incredible itching have markedly subsided. Nothing else that I know of relieves as well as cool mud.

INSOMNIA

Jane's Nightly Toddy

During the filming of the various Tarzan movies in which Maureen O'Sullivan appeared with her co-star Johnny Weissmuller, production schedules were often long and hectic. As a result, normal sleep patterns were often interrupted, and some of the production crew suffered from periodic insomnia. Maureen O'Sullivan was one of these who tossed and turned a lot during the late night hours and found it very difficult to get a good night's rest.

She decided to make herself some warm chamomile tea and would drink two cups of this 30 minutes before retiring. It worked fairly well, but did even better for her when she added a tablespoon of heated rum to every cup of tea she drank. After that, she always slept like a charm.

INTESTINAL PARASITES

Herbs That Work

Doctors who specialize in tropical diseases in various countries have told me that some of the best herbs to use against intestinal parasites are those plants that contain the awful-tasting alkaloid berberine: *Argemone mexicana*, *Chasmanthera dependens*, *Hydrastic canadensis*, and *Mahonia aquifolium*. While the first two plants are somewhat difficult to obtain, the latter pair, goldenseal root and wild Oregon-grape rootstock are readily available in powders or as dried, cut tea material.

I prefer mixing equal parts of goldenseal or Oregon grape with wormwood powder before encapsulating them by hand. Two capsules can then be taken on an empty stomach for the best discharge of parasites. If making a tea, add one tablespoon each of goldenseal or Oregon grape and wormwood in one quart boiling water. Cover, reduce heat, and simmer ten minutes. Then set aside and steep for 20 minutes. Strain and drink cool, one cup between meals several times daily.

Be advised, however, that berberine is decidedly hypoglycemic and could, therefore, drag down already low blood-sugar levels. Garlic and onion are useful substitutes in the event the terrible taste of these other herbs is profoundly overwhelming, but they, too, are strongly hypoglycemic. Such herbs will eliminate parasites, though, in an amazing hurry.

IRRITABLE BOWEL SYNDROME

Soothing Slickness

The herbs fenugreek seed, marshmallow root, and slippery-elm bark are the three best remedies I always turn to for relieving the agonizing symptoms of irritable bowel syndrome, colitis, and diverticulitis. These herbs may be consumed in tea form or taken as capsules with a meal. They are invaluable but safe and can be trusted to do the job effectively.

IRRITATION

Ways to Make Yourself More Pleasant

Just about everyone at some time or another has become irritated at something or someone that causes us a great deal of vexation. In all too many instances, unfortunately, the majority "fly off the handle" and say and do things that they later on regret and usually end up having to apologize for.

But there are healthier and more prudent means of coping with such crises when they inevitably arise. One of these is to sing a song or hum yourself a favorite tune. It's amazing how the gentle sounds of music can soothe the "savage beast" in the worst of us. The Old Testament informs us that whenever King Saul raged (due to an evil spirit in him), then David the Shepherd Boy would play his harp, which would restore the other to his former state of sensibility.

Deep breathing is another way of stifling one's anger. It seems that the additional intake of oxygen somehow defuses the biochemical hostility that can build up if we let it. Walking and breathing at the same time certainly helps cool down hot-headed tempers.

Drinking water also is of some benefit. I don't know exactly how this works in the system, but I know for a fact that IT WORKS! Always be sure the water is slightly cool but never ice cold. Gently sip it and drink more than one eight-ounce glass if necessary. It helps, of course, if such liquid is an unsweetened herbal beverage like chamomile or peppermint tea.

Refocusing your attention to something else is critical in achieving calmness. Quiet meditation or silent prayer is beneficial for this. A spirit of peace prevails, and the atmosphere is less charged with static emotions and thoughts.

Seeking for humility and meekness are absolute criteria for becoming a peacemaker. There is no room for arrogance and conceit; such lofty pride only perpetuates an argument and fans the flames of discontent.

ITCHING

A Solvable Solution

On November 1, 1994, I stood in Christie's Park Avenue gallery in New York City with a few hundred other spectators and watched as a contingent of Italian bankers attempted to bring back to their country a 72-page notebook containing more than three hundred illustrations and scientific writings compiled from 1506 to 1510 by Leonardo da Vinci. The contest to acquire this landmark of creativity, called Codex Hammer since 1980 in honor of its most recent owner, the late chairman of Occidental Petroleum, Armand Hammer, provided some tense but thrilling excitement for the Italians, including a few other spectators.

Along with them, I noticed how some of us began fidgeting as auctioneer Stephen C. Massey opened the bidding at $5.5 million. Several scratched their necks, a few others stroked their faces, and still others rubbed their palms together to relieve the nervous itching that ensued. Some tried to be less obvious and scratch their ankles or calves with a shoe from the other leg. But it was apparent that a number of us were *itching* in anticipation of the high amount for which this great manuscript treasure would go as well as just who would get it.

My hands and face itched so badly I retreated from the gallery and made my way to the men's bathroom, where I washed my troubled skin with lots of cold water. It felt good going on, so I decided to leave it on and not wipe any off. The coldness of the water immediately made the itching disappear.

I returned to the gallery just in time to see this incredible document go to a private collector bidding anonymously by telephone for a staggering $30.8 million, a record for a book or manuscript sold at auction.

The next day it was announced in *The New York Times* that computer billionaire Bill Gates had been the secret purchaser of this notebook, written in Leonardo's distinctive backward style and containing such speculations as why the sky is blue and why fossils can be found on mountaintops and predicts the invention of the submarine and the steam engine several centuries *before* they were actually developed.

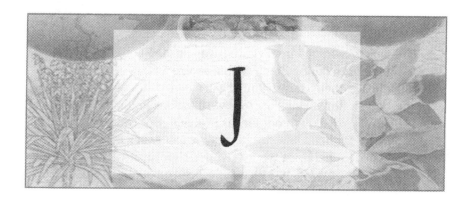

JAUNDICE

The Sewers of Paris

Some years ago I had the good fortune to visit Paris, France, for one-and-a-half days. Being on a very short time schedule, I had to decide between the Arc de Triomphe de l'Etoile built to commemorate the victories of Napoleon I, the 984-foot-high Eiffel Tower, or the Louvre, France's foremost grand architectural museum of art. As I was contemplating which of the trio I would choose, I overheard someone say, almost as a joking aside, "Why not the sewers of Paris?"

This immediately piqued my interest, and all of a sudden the others became terribly boring to me. "Let's go where the rats are!" I cheerfully responded to hosts, who, it must be admitted now, were rather taken aback by my astonishing announcement. There are 1,300 miles of such sewers running beneath the streets of this huge, sprawling metropolis. Each year, about a thousand sewer workers evacuate 500,000 cubic feet of filthy waste matter. Murkiness, showers of putrid water, slimy walls, and abrupt rises in the water level can make a sewer worker's job quite difficult.

Dandelion Wine and Curried Rice

During my visit with others to some of these sewers, we had the good fortune to watch a crew of workers in action as they cleaned off the walls and ceilings with their machines. They stopped to take a break, and I had a chance to speak to one of them with the assistance of my interpreter.

229

The fellow whom I interviewed was named Louis Vignon, aged 34. He told about coming down with a severe case of jaundice several years before we met. He attributed part of his disease to the nasty work he had to do. Various doctors with whom he consulted recommended heavy drug treatment for his problem. But the idea of putting a lot of synthetic chemicals into his body wasn't very appealing. So he conferred with an herbalist who suggested that he drink a small wineglass of dandelion wine every evening before bed and that he eat a small bowl of curried rice three times a week by itself. This he commenced doing, and about two months later his jaundice had virtually disappeared. (If you're unable to procure dandelion wine, you can make a near equivalent for your own health needs. Purchase a bottle of expensive French white wine; be willing to spend in the neighborhood of $100 for it. Gather about one pound of yellow dandelion blossoms from an unsprayed area by clipping off the tops with a pair of shears or scissors. Wash these in a colander under cold water and drain thoroughly. Place on some paper towels and pat the excess moisture from the flowers. Then carefully snip them into small pieces into a crockery jar and cover with French wine. Put a lid on top and store in a cool, dry place for two to three weeks, stirring the contents with a wooden spoon every two days. Strain, bottle, and cork for later use. Discard the blossoms.)

JET LAG

Rats and More

One of the most interesting places I've ever visited were the underground sewer tunnels that run beneath the streets of Paris. When I descended 20 feet below ground, the first museum exhibit I saw was *a stuffed rat*. My guide informed our small group that for every inhabitant in Paris, there are three rats, which stomach even the strongest poisons incredibly well. They certainly are well fed. Each day these rats devour an estimated 100 tons, or one third, of the sewers' entire waste.

A lady from Australia complained to her companion of suffering from jet lag. I encouraged her to not drink any caffeinated beverages or soda pop at least two hours before returning home and certainly none on the flight back. She wrote me six months later, sending along a money order in U.S. funds for the purchase of several of my health encyclopedias. She penned a notation thanking me for the advice, saying she had been on several more trips since then and had never suffered from any more jet lag.

JOCK ITCH

A Subterranean Cemetery

Quite awhile back I happened to be in Paris for a short stay and elected to join some others in a visit beneath the huge sewers that seem to go on forever in many different directions. After an hour-long tour, we were all happy to come up again for a breath of regular Paris smog, which though highly polluted felt a lot better than the miserable dank dampness we were forced to inhale below for so long.

Our guide informed us that "to really see the innermost depths of our city, you must go to the catacombs!" They are located 66 feet underground and contain the skeletal remains of about six million people. Oh joy! I thought to myself but went along with the others to see this medieval curiosity just for the heck of it.

It all started in the Middle Ages when people were buried in or near cathedrals. This brought money to the Catholic Church but was most unhealthy, as the cemeteries were always in the center of town. It became a nightmare for the neighbors of the largest graveyard in Paris, this being none other than the Saints-Innocents. Its one and seven-tenths acres welcomed corpses from about 20 different parishes, as well as unidentified bodies and unlucky victims of various plagues.

In 1418 the Black Death contributed some 50,000 corpses alone. In 1572, tens of thousands of victims of the Saint Bartholomew's Day massacre were crammed into Saints-Innocents. There was a call for the closure of this cemetery. About two million bodies, stacked sometimes 30 feet deep, had raised the ground level by more than six feet. The cemetery had become a horrible breeding ground for infection, and it gave off an awful putrid smell, strong enough it was said to turn milk or wine sour. However, the powerful clergy opposed closing the city's cemeteries.

In 1780 a communal grave cracked open and spewed forth rotting corpses into neighboring cellars. That was the proverbial straw that broke the camel's back. City officials promptly shut down the cemetery, and burial in Paris was thereafter forbidden. The mass graves were then emptied into the disused Tombe-Issoire quarries. Each night for nearly one-and-a-half years, macabre envoys transferred the bones. This was extended to include another 17 cemeteries and 300 places of worship. The bones were thrown down a 57-foot shaft, where a stairway now leads down from the street into the catacombs.

A Young Man's Problem

One of our small party witnessing such a bizarre exhibit happened to be a happy-go-lucky, 15-year-old American teenager named Jeremy, who was accompanied by his parents on this unique occasion. While in conversation with her son on the subject of my profession, she raised this question: "My son has suffered from jock itch for a couple of weeks; what can I do to help him get over it?"

I explained to her that it was important for her boy to always keep his skin dry in that area of his body. I noted that any accumulation of moisture would only aggravate it more. I advised her mixing two tablespoons of baking soda with one teaspoon of goldenseal powder and then dusting his skin *and* underwear with it *every day* for two weeks. She did this and reported back sometime later that his condition had entirely cleared up.

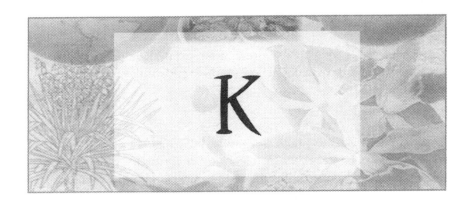

KIDNEY FAILURE/KIDNEY STONES

Skeletons in the Paris Closet

During a short Paris visit some years back, I toured an underground graveyard with my French hosts and some other people. From the Denfert-Rochereau Square, just south of Paris's Latin Quarter, we made our way down the 91 steps into the catacombs. In 1787 the powdered and painted mademoiselles of the royal French court were among the first to view this underground burial chamber by the light of burning torches. Today, 160,000 visitors come each year to get a peek at the dead.

After the staircase came a seemingly endless series of galleries where skeletons are stored by the dump-truck loads. Some of us walked rather gingerly, reflecting on the fact that these catacombs occupy more than 100,000 square feet of space. We were told by our guide that a fellow named Philibert Aspairt gained unsought fame when he tried to find his way through these hundreds of miles of galleries. In 1793 he became lost in this incredible maze; his skeleton was discovered some 11 years later, being identified by his keys and the clothing he had worn.

About 30 percent of the area under Paris has been quarried. For a long time, quarrying was uncontrolled, which eventually led to a mishap. In 1774, one thousand feet of rue d'Enfer (Hell Street then, but Denfert-Rochereau now) collapsed into an abyss 100 feet in depth. The public became alarmed that the rest of Paris was in serious danger of collapsing. As one French writer aptly put it: "The stones seen above ground in magnificent buildings are the very ones missing from

233

under our feet!" To support these underground galleries, elaborate archways were constructed at considerable government expense.

Kidney Remedy

In private conversation with our guide, I learned about a useful remedy that had been in his family for several generations. It was designed to help promote better kidney function as well as eliminate stones. The recipe calls for boiling a small handful of cracked walnut shells in one-and-a-half pints of water for five minutes. To this would then be added one-and-a-half teaspoons catnip herb and two tablespoons rose petals. The mixture is stirred, covered with a lid, and set aside to steep for 40 minutes. Three cups are taken daily in between meals for as long as needed.

In the course of time, I had several opportunities to recommend this to various individuals who consulted with me on specific kidney problems. I included parsley herb, though it wasn't in the original formula. But I felt that its presence was important and could only give the tea greater health benefits. Those who took this formula regularly, after informing their doctors of what they were doing, reported greater kidney activity and little or no kidney stones after several months on it.

KNEE PAIN

Grimacing Skulls and Brittle Femurs

The time occupied in writing this section of the book occurred around Halloween of 1999. It seemed fitting and appropriate, therefore, to include something of the macabre here. I am reminded of how I took care of my injured knee after touring the infamous catacombs of Paris, France, some years back.

I was standing about 60 feet below ground in a damp, poorly lit gallery piled high with hundreds of thousands of bones. Since my shoes were already quite muddy from the wet ground, trying to stay upright was a bit tricky in places. Without looking where I stepped next, I slipped in a puddle but managed to grab hold of a heavy bronze door before falling. However, in doing so, I inadvertently swung my right leg around quite hard and smashed my kneecap into the thick metal door. Pain suddenly shot up and down my leg and a deeply throbbing hurt set in. With the assistance of my French friends, I was able to hobble along for the short duration of our tour.

Behind this door lay a corridor with walls built entirely of *human* bones—grimacing skulls and brittle femurs and tibiae arranged in neat rows and in the shape of crosses and wreaths, which presented an altogether extremely morbid scene. Slabs were engraved with an odd assortment of Bible verses and poems to reflect people's meditation on the meaning of life and death.

Self-Treatment in My Hotel Room

After emerging into the daylight again from these eerie catacombs, my friends took me back to the Marseilles Hotel where I was staying. I asked one of them to procure for me from a nearby drugstore some Epsom salts (or its French equivalent). When that was brought back, I had the bathtub filled half full of hot water, to which was then added two cups of Epsom salts. After one of my friends stirred the water well with her hand, I asked her husband to assist me in undressing and get into a pair of swimming trunks. He then helped me step into the tub with my good leg and slide the rest of my body down in the water, although this was quite painful for me to do.

I lay back and enjoyed my hourlong soak. The heated water felt good and the addition of the Epsom salts lessened the pain. I was able to get out on my own (though with some difficulty), and after drying off with a towel, I proceeded to apply six to eight drops of peppermint oil (which I always carried with me in those days) to my injured kneecap. I gingerly rubbed it over the skin and then loosely covered the area with a dry towel in order to retain as much of the warming influence as possible. I slept pretty well that night, except when I turned over on my right side, and by the next morning most of my pain was gone.

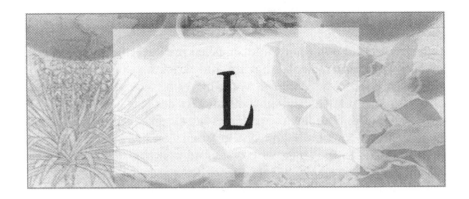

LABOR AND DELIVERY PROBLEMS

Costly Sneeze at an Art Auction

A young thirty-something woman who works in the American Painting and Sculpture Department of Christie's, the renowned auction house at Rockefeller Plaza in New York City, related the following true tale to me recently by phone. "We had an important auction in November 1999 that involved a number of pieces depicting nineteenth century scenes of the early American frontier. Among the more important ones were Albert Bierstadt's "Buffalo Hunt, Yosemite" and two fine works by Frederic Remington from a private collection: 'Pretty Mother of the Night—White Otter Is No Longer a Boy' and 'The Wolves Sniffed Along the Trail, but Came No Nearer.'" My informant said that the first piece depicted two nearly naked Indians on ponies riding the desert and looking up at the night sky together, which went for almost $3 million; the other one showed the backside of a near-naked Indian walking through the sagebrush at night with a pack of wolves following at a respectable distance behind him (this sold for slightly under $2 million).

Among the elegantly attired and well-heeled crowd on hand for the bidding was a distinguished-looking gentleman accompanied by his wife. It was apparent that he had a severe head cold because he made considerable use of several silk handkerchiefs during most of the auction. As the bidding proceeded, something in the air must have tickled this patron's sensitive nose and he suddenly let forth with a rather loud and violent sneeze that was totally unexpected and astonished everyone, including the man himself. He quickly retrieved his

236

handkerchief from the top pocket of his dress jacket and while doing so, sneezed again. This promptly caused his right hand, which then held the handkerchief, to jerk upwards into the air a bit before he could bring it down to cover his nose and mouth.

The moment the auctioneer spotted his hand and handkerchief go up, he pounded down his gavel with a resonating smack and declared in a loud voice, "S-O-L-D to the gentleman in the seventh row, middle section, seat number nine, for $1.87 million dollars!" The auctioneer then proceeded to open the next bid, Sanford Robinson Gifford's ocean scene, "Manchester Beach, Massachusetts," at $400,000. The man who sneezed twice sat speechless with a dumbfounded look on his face. He had inadvertently bought a very expensive piece of nice artwork, which he never wanted in the first place. To soothe his agitated feelings, his wife leaned over and gently whispered in his ear that they could hang the thing in his study (she shared this information with my informant when the auction finished).

Herbs for Birthing

The main purpose, though, for this anonymous Christie's employee calling me was in reference to a female friend who was due to give birth in several weeks. Her friend's doctors had informed the woman that she faced the potential risk of serious delivery problems (which were never specified). My caller wanted to know what could be done to assure her friend's having a safe birthing. She had got my number out of one of my health books.

First, I recommended an immediate change in her friend's diet based on information given to me some years ago by an old Hawaiian *kahuna pale keiki* (midwife) on the island of Maui. She was to abstain from ALL pork products, salty foods, and fatty fare (including anything fried or deep-fried). Instead she was to start subsisting more on cooked yams and baked sweet potatoes, as well as ripe bananas, broiled fish, leafy greens, and fruit juices (papaya, mango, guava, and pear). She was also to avoid highly seasoned foods EXCEPT in the last few days of her due date. Then and ONLY THEN was she to dine out at various Mexican restaurants and consume as much beef and cheese enchiladas, beef tacos, and Spanish rice as her heart desired. "This latter eating experience generally results in quick and easy delivery," I said.

Second, I gave her an efficient Pregnancy Formula that came from Northern California herbalist Kathy Keville back in March 1980: two teaspoons red-raspberry leaves, one teaspoon lemongrass, one teaspoon oatstraw, one teaspoon peppermint leaves, and one-half teaspoon alfalfa herb. Steep these in one-and-a-half pints boiling water for 20 minutes; strain and "drink whenever convenient throughout the pregnancy," as Kathy told me.

Well, it wasn't long before I got a call from my auction house fan: She happily reported that her friend delivered "a healthy eight-pound girl without a single thing going wrong!"

Traditional Medicine in Malaŵi

Some years ago I had the good fortune of journeying to the landlocked southeast African country of Malaŵi in company with two pharmacologists, one from the University of Glasgow in Scotland and the other from the University of Natal in Durban, South Africa. For several weeks we toured the length (520 miles) and breadth (5 to 100 miles) of this economically progressive and politically stable republic.

The nation occupies a narrow, curving strip of land along the Great Rift Valley. Almost 20 percent of its total area is dominated by lake surface (mostly Lake Nyasa known in Malaŵi as Lake Malaŵi). We found it to be one of the most water-rich countries on the entire African continent. Ambitious hydroelectric projects of every description were underway or in the planning stages when we were there. Having attained independence in July 1964, it has done an outstanding job of attracting foreign capital investments and has made enormous strides in the exploitation of many of its natural resources.

In spite of the impact of modernization, Malaŵi's traditional culture has survived largely intact. One of its most distinctive features is the variety of traditional songs and dances that use the drum as the major musical instrument. Among the most notable of these dances, I found, were the *ingoma* and *gule wa mkulu* for men, and the *chimtali* and *visekese* for women. This Muslim-Christian nation of approximately 6.2 million also has a variety of traditional arts and crafts, including beautiful sculptures in wood and elephant ivory.

Traditional (folk) medicine was still alive and doing well when my colleagues and I arrived. Working with our hosts at the University of Malaŵi in Zomba and at the Kamuzu Central Hospital in the capital of Lilongwe further to the north, we managed to catalog a number of important plants used by folk healers in villages scattered all over the country. Here, I should perhaps define their locations better. On the plateaus, which support the bulk of the population, the most common village sites are at the margins of *madambo*, which are usually contiguous with streams or rivers and are characterized by woodland, grassland, and fertile alluvial soils. In highland areas, scattered villages are usually situated near perennial mountain streams and pockets of thin but arable land. We found native residences to consist of both the old and new: the traditional round, mud-walled, grass-roofed huts as well as government-sponsored rectangular brick buildings with corrugated iron roofs.

The majority of herbal medicine (as we found it then) was practiced mainly by middle-aged to elderly women, who generally incorporated *muti*—the power of magic—into nearly every aspect of their healing arts. What some might term witchcraft, was, in fact, a curious blending of native "faith healing" and actual medical herbalism. Some of our principal informants were Johanna Ramalepa (aged 49), her sister Matsie Masela (aged 65), and Lizzie Makgabo (age unknown). They permitted us to look on in silence while they treated the sick.

Traditional healer Makgabo, for instance, would check the sick patient's vital signs first—that is, hand to the forehead for skin temperature; looking carefully at both eyeballs with the lids held back by two fingers; closely examining a stuck-out tongue and smelling mouth breath at the same time; poking here with a forefinger or jabbing there in the patient's body with a thumb and asking if such-and-such hurt or was painful; studying the person's immediately discharged warm urine in an old pan; and scrutinizing with a stick fresh human feces. After doing all of these fairly elementary and pretty common medical diagnoses, Lizzie then resorted to something that was definitely very unscientific. She emptied a set of small bones from various animals (chicken, duck, antelope, monkey, and *mlamba* or catfish) into a wooden goblet, placed her hand over the top, shook the container vigorously with both hands, then squatted down on her haunches and threw the contents out onto the dirt floor of her little hut. She spent the next several minutes quietly surveying the manner in which they lay; we later learned that depending on how they fall determines a lot the course of treatment she would be employing.

Invariably all of the patients we witnessed being treated by these three women eventually got over their particular problems. Plants, of course, formed a big part of the whole healing procedures. The most common method in which these herbs were administered, either singly or in combination, were as liquids—warm teas or cool broths, depending on whether body temperatures of their patients were below or above normal. (No oral or rectal thermometers were ever used, just the palms or backs of the healers' hands.)

We were astonished as scientists to later discover just how many of these medicinal herbs were fairly common in other parts of the world. As for those plants that were purely indigenous to Malaŵi itself, I found suitable American or European replacements for them that worked equally effectively for the same problems mentioned here. The reader can be assured that all of these remedies have been tried, tested, and found to work quite well for the health situations in which they've been continuously used.

LACTOSE INTOLERANCE

Lizzie's older sister, Matsie, always used *mabanga* (kola nut) for this. One-half cup of warm tea twice daily *before* milk consumption would overcome this problem. In the event kola nut isn't handy, just drink one-half cup hot, black coffee *or* one-half can cola drink *before* consuming milk or milk products. It may seem strange, but I swear it works.

LEARNING DISABILITIES

Johanna made a broth of *soukou-nou-baba* or basil leaves and tiny pinches of black pepper and table salt. One or two cups of *hot* broth would tend to stimulate the mind and increase mental function considerably. *Note:* If you suffer from hypertension, omit the salt.

LEG PAIN

All three made strong tea from *badarendjabouya* (lemonbalm or citronelle) and *na'na'akhdar* (spearmint), which they gave their patients *warm* to drink, but *hot* to soak their aching limbs in.

LEUKEMIA
(Also see "CANCER")

Mbaazi or *dried* peas and the *dried* pea leaves and stalks made into a simple broth and flavored with a little pond algae (chlorella) is an impressive treatment for this cancer of the blood.

LICE

The treatment is really quite easy, but some parents may hesitate before using this *natural* substance: Our three folk healers routinely massaged *very small* amounts of *genuine* turpentine onto the scalps of their younger patients thus afflicted; we saw *with our own eyes* every single case clear up in less than 36 hours!

LIGHT SENSITIVITY

Believe it or not, eating the fruit of *nkalanga* or drinking a juice made of it or a tea made from *nkalanga* leaves would correct this in nothing flat. And what, pray tell, is *nkalanga*—why nothing more or less than sweet, delicious, iron-rich figs.

LIVER DISEASE

A combination of the sweet fruit pulp of *ol massamburai* (tamarind) and dandelion greens and flowers (substituted for another hard-to-get African herb) works exceptionally well in helping a diseased liver recuperate rather nicely. Blend the *fresh* dandelion parts (thoroughly washed, of course) and tamarind fruit in a Vita-Mix blender for about two minutes, adding a wee bit of water, if necessary, to thin it out if the mixture proves to be too thick to pour.

LOSS OF SEXUAL INTEREST
(Also see "ERECTION PROBLEMS" and "IMPOTENCY")

Lizzie Makgabo gives all of her male patients a bottle of *warm* beer to drink, with a pinch of cayenne pepper or ginger-root powder included for good measure. Johanna Ramalepa uses *warm* beer, too, but adds a pinch of cinnamon powder instead, which she claims the ladies like a lot better. As for the elderly Matsie Masela, she just laughed when we posed the identical question and replied that at her age "there was no sense in reactivating it."

LOW BLOOD PRESSURE

A tea made of flowers of *zu'rur* and consumed every three to four hours would help to elevate blood pressure to a healthier level. Not bad knowing that *hawthorn* is also good for this.

LUPUS ERYTHEMATOSUS

The root and leaves of *'awarwar* (mullein) are a very popular remedy for this condition. The medicine is taken as a *cool* tea twice daily on an empty stomach.

LUNG CANCER
(Also see "CANCER")

Watercress by any other name is a common vegetable green throughout much of the world. And in Malaŵi we discover that *harriqa* was just as important when drunk as a warm tea for cancer of the respiratory system as it was in meals when served up raw or in soups.

LYME DISEASE

Many of the symptoms associated with this American tick-bite problem may be found in a near-equivalent African version of the same thing. Our three informants always employed *shiba* (wormwood) for this: They made it into a tea with a pinch of salt and a small squeeze of lime juice added for good measure. We were surprised how well it worked.

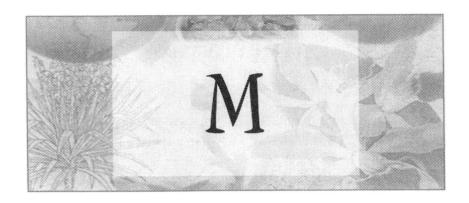

MACULAR DEGENERATION

Pet ER

The patient was hustled into the emergency room with a wild and frantic look in his eye. "I think he's in shock," one of the medical technicians stated. Clamps were put to both of the patient's ears to register his blood pressure. Another machine measured blood-oxygen content.

"He looks pretty good to me," pronounced the doctor after feeling around the patient's body with his hands. "But let's give something to calm him down anyway."

The patient in question went by only one name, Seth, and was still curled up into a tight fetal position, making him look like a wet orange Nerf basketball. "It's a classic case of a Rottweiler attacking a cat," the veterinarian said as he turned in my direction.

Welcome to the usually hectic, often life-and-death world of the all-night pet doctor. The Salt Lake Valley, where I reside, has three such clinics operating on a 24-hour basis, each with an on-site vet.

Reversing an Eye Disorder

The medical technician with whom I spoke afterwards in another room told me what she had been giving her elderly father of late for his macular degeneration, which comes in two forms: exudative ("wet") and atrophic ("dry"). She had him on the following supplements: *fresh* marigold flower petals (one teaspoon daily) mixed with a spinach salad (for the lutein benefits, obviously); shark cartilage (three 750-mg. capsules daily with meals); one glass of carrot juice every two days (for the beta-carotene); rutin and hesperidin bioflavonoids (one tablet of each daily with meals); zinc sulfate (100 mg.) and copper (2 mg.) daily; bilberry (80 mg. twice daily of a standardized preparation containing 25 percent anthocyanidins); and ginkgo biloba (40–60 mg. with a minimum of 24 percent ginkgo heterosides, twice daily).

Within four months her dad's vision had dramatically improved.

MALARIA

Hope from the Philippines

Some years ago I went to the Philippines for work and pleasure: to undertake an evaluation of the medicinal plants used over there and also to find me a wife, perhaps. My local female contact, a devout Mormon Church employee at the time, was Gloria Cruz, who always held to the same strict, high moral standards as I do. In many ways we were quite compatible, but in the all-important area of faith, I discovered, quite sadly, that hers wasn't up to par. Gloria let fear rule her life, and no amount of discussion on the matter could dissuade her away from that position. So, we remained just good friends thereafter and, at the close of 1999 I'm still an available bachelor at the age of 53 and continue to look for a younger mate somewhere in the world with whom I can share my life, thoughts, and feelings.

But I found many useful applications for plants over there that I never imagined were possible. Take, for example, the treatment of malaria. It consists of giving the feverish patient *lúyang-diláu* in fish chowder and many different kinds of rice dishes. In fact, turmeric powder is not only an efficient medicine for this, but also makes a delightful food condiment as well.

MANIC DEPRESSION

Vitamin and Mineral Therapy

Over the years I've recommended just two vitamins and one mineral to those cases afflicted with this mental disturbance. I encourage them to take a high-potency vitamin B-complex (three tablets) and some

Rex Wheat Germ Oil (one tablespoon) every day, along with 600 mgs. of magnesium.

They're also instructed to listen to the many witty and charming songs from a number of the Disney movies and even to learn to hum or whistle some of the tunes themselves. I find these songs invariably put people in a better frame of mind than they were before.

MEASLES

Grandmother Knows Best

When I was old enough to start kindergarten, my Hungarian grandmother was still alive and fast approaching 100 years of age. Some of the other children in our neighborhood contracted measles from school. I was one of the fortunate ones who didn't. Though quite young at the time, I still remember her recommending to the mothers of these other sick children that they give them some warm mullein tea sweetened with a little honey to drink several times a day and to bathe their skin with cool yarrow tea.

The few moms who followed her sage advice discovered that their kids got well a lot sooner than the children of those who ignored her counsel on account of her advanced age and peasant upbringing.

MELANOMA

A Navajo Cure

In previous health books, such as *Miracle Healing Herbs* (Paramus, NJ: Prentice Hall, 1998) I've recommended the generous use of chaparral tea consumed in copious amounts (four to five cups per day). This is an old Navajo remedy for diseased animals but works equally well for skin cancer. There is some limited published scientific evidence to the effect that this desert shrub of the American West and Southwest truly lives up to its strong anticancer reputation. The tea must be simmered for 30 minutes and allowed to set overnight for 10–12 *hours* before using in order to be fully effective.

MENINGITIS

Chinese Treatment

In 1980 I accompanied the American Medical Students Association to the People's Republic of China. For two weeks we toured a number of clinics, hospitals, and medicinal herb factories to see firsthand how effective traditional Chinese medicine was. We discovered in our travels that many doctors prescribed *raw* garlic to those patients suffering from some form of meningitis. About ten of the small cloves per day was the standard recommendation. About 78 percent of those on this garlic therapy experienced full or partial recovery from their affliction. With the remaining 22 percent there was little or no change in their conditions.

MENOPAUSE

Secrets to Pleasant Menopause

Many books have been written by women for women on the subject of menopause. Invariably they list hundreds of things to do and to take in order to cope with this "change-of-life" phase. During the many years I've spent traveling around the Orient, I've noticed one astonishing thing—most Oriental women don't experience the symptoms of menopause the same way their Western counterparts do. This got me to thinking and looking harder at what they might be doing right that American and European women could benefit from.

I made several amazing discoveries in the course of my careful research. For one thing, Oriental women seldom consume refined sugar, chocolate, alcohol, coffee, or red meat, all of which worsen menopausal symptoms. Second, Oriental women consume a great deal of soy foods, which are rich in phytoestrogens. These plant estrogens appear to function much like natural estrogens in many ways. If Western women would eat just two ounces of soy products (tofu, miso, aburage, koridofu, and soybeans) each day that would be enough to reduce most of their menopausal griefs.

Other foods high in phytoestrogens include yams, sweet potatoes, split peas, sunflower and sesame seeds, kidney and adzuki beans, brown and wild rice, red clover, barley, oats, apples, beets, cabbage, cauliflower, watercress, mustard and turnip greens, parsley, fennel, and olives and olive oil.

If a woman suffers from hot flashes she should increase her intake of seaweeds such as kelp, dulse, bladderwrack, nori, and the hajiki.

MENSTRUATION DIFFICULTIES

What to Do About Cramping

One of the most common menstrual problems is cramping. A woman is advised to stay away from alcohol, coffee, colas, and sugary foods, all of which promote inflammation and increase cramping terribly. Gas-producing foods also should be restricted; these include sugary and greasy foods.

A woman's diet should be high in roughage. Such fiber-rich foods include green vegetables (cooked and raw), root vegetables (carrots, parsnips, rutabagas, potatoes), and cereal grains (oatmeal, whole-wheat bread, bran muffin).

Fish oil is good to take for cramping. Something as simple as a tablespoon of cod liver oil every morning—with food if you can't stand the taste—will work wonders in this regard. Also consuming fresh- or saltwater fish (steamed, broiled, or baked, but never fried) helps a lot.

A good calcium–magnesium supplement is advisable. The ShapeRite Co. of Sandy, Utah, features one of the best on the market. Take four capsules every morning with food. (See Product Appendix for more information.)

Excessive bleeding is another frequent problem during the menstrual cycle. Vitamin C with bioflavonoids (1,000 mg. daily) and fish-oil vitamin A (50,000 I.U.) will slow this down in a hurry. Also, one tablespoon of Rex Wheat Germ Oil will reduce nervous irritation and the craving for junk foods. (See Product Appendix under Anthropological Research Center.)

Fatigue can be successfully corrected with vitamin B-12. Take 250 mcg. of sublingual vitamin B-12 once a day for up to ten days. After this reduce your intake to just 1,000 mcgs. weekly.

Useful herbs for menstruation difficulties include dong quai (two capsules daily), red-raspberry-leaf tea (one cup *warm* tea twice daily), ginger root (hot tea compress placed on the lower abdomen to relax tight muscles), and chamomile tea to preserve your sanity.

MENTAL ILLNESS

Steps for Mental Improvement

The classic steps in getting well mentally and emotionally are these: (1) Eat three regular meals or five smaller meals throughout the day. This keeps your blood sugar levels up at all times. (2) Drink ample fluids, especially water, throughout the day. I've noticed that a majority of mentally disturbed folks are always in a state of semi-dehydration for some strange reason. (3) Supplement regularly, focusing on B-complex and vitamin E, as well as calcium, magnesium, potassium, boron, and lithium. The omega fatty acids are also of prime importance here. Such nutrients feed the brain and help keep thought patterns from becoming squirrelly. (4) Seek for inner peace, be satisfied with what you have, and don't get greedy for more than what you really need. (5) Maintain regularity of the bowels. Constipation is no joking matter. A buildup of waste materials within the colon can and *does* affect brainwave behavior to some extent.

Finally, think on this item a while, if needed, to become fully convinced that *it is true*. The ancients believed and some primitive societies in modern times still subscribe to the idea that *evil spirits* are the cause of much of our mental, emotional, and physical woes. Modern medical science, of course, scoffs at this presumed "antiquated notion" and relegates it to the back closet of weird concepts. But I can tell you in all candor as a social scientist that such a thing isn't as farfetched as health professionals would like to have the public think it is. The keys to winning this "invisible war" of the mind and heart is to *always* think good thoughts and feel good feelings, both toward yourself, others around you, and the environment in which you live.

MEXICAN-RESTAURANT SYNDROME

Be Careful of What You Eat

This particular restaurant syndrome could also be called Chinese or Vietnamese or just about anything else for that matter. It consists of nausea, chills, stomach cramps, vomiting, diarrhea, and general fatigue after eating ethnic food in a specialty restaurant where perfect hygiene and proper food storage and preparation aren't actively practiced.

To stop the nausea, drink papaya or pear juice. To get rid of the chills, drink warm ginger tea. To allay abdominal cramps, drink warm peppermint tea. And to stop diarrhea, mix three tablespoons of corn starch in 8 ounces of water, stir thoroughly and drink quickly. Vomiting, though, is good, for it empties the gut of whatever is present that's making you sick. Drink some warm beef broth or clear fish chowder to regain your energy.

MIGRAINE

Crime Scene Clean-Up

One of the weirdest janitorial jobs I ever became acquainted with was from an individual who works for a California outfit called Crime Scene Cleaners, Inc. They are cleaning contractors hired to do especially difficult work and that is to clean up murder and suicide scenes. My informant acknowledged that "this job isn't for the weak-hearted by any means" and confessed to having had some problems with it in the beginning, but now is doing fine. "The pay is terrific, so you eventually learn to get over it and focus your attention on positive things instead."

Special care must be given to materials covered with human blood. "Grisly items such as bloody sheets, pillows, blankets, and mattresses that have been part of a brutal murder or terrible suicide have to be burned by law," the person said. "All of these things are considered bio-hazardous materials just like those coming out of a hospital." And there are special chemicals to clean floors, walls, and doors where blood may have been splattered. "We always pull carpets up and haul them away to be burned. They are replaced with new ones."

Migraine Makeover

My informant then turned the conversation toward personal health matters. The individual reported having suffered migraines for the previous six months and asked me for help. I answered that headaches could be the results of muscle tension, a hidden infection, disturbances in the blood vessels in the head, or imbalances in blood–sugar levels. Once the exact cause could be isolated then treatment procedures would be easier to do.

But, since neither of us really knew what the determining factor in his case could be, we settled for some general remedial information. I mentioned that white-willow bark or valerian capsules (three at a time on an empty stomach) might be substituted for regular aspirin or nonaspirin ibuprofen. For more severe headaches, though, I recommend a combination of hops, catnip, and valerian powders in capsule form. I advised the person to purchase these respective herb powders from a health-food store and then mix one teaspoon of each together before filling OO size capsules and taking four of them at one time.

I gave some dietary advice, which was essentially to stay away from chocolate, foods containing MSG (mostly Chinese food), and hot dogs and other processed meats (because of their chemical preservatives). I cautioned about "hidden MSG" (monosodium glutamate) in processed-food products listing hydrolyzed protein, autolyzed yeast, sodium caseinate, and calcium caseinate on their labels. I urged more stricter label reading before buying food products.

I explained that other herbs, such as feverfew, ginger, peppermint, and skullcap were ideal for warding off future migraines. Any of these could be made into individual teas and taken warm in one-cup doses as needed.

Minerals are especially important in the regulation of headaches. A good calcium–magnesium formula, such as the one sold by ShapeRite (three capsules at once) always helps to relax tense muscles, tight nerves, and constricted blood vessels. Chromium is very useful for maintaining normal blood–sugar levels; Trace Minerals Research has such a product that is sold in many health-food stores (one to two tablets twice daily). (See Product Appendix under respective company names for more details.)

Other helpful therapies for finding relief or a permanent solution to the problem include acupressure, massage, aromatherapy, thyroid hormone therapy, melatonin therapy, yoga, meditation, progressive relaxation, guided imagery, biofeedback training, acupuncture, psychiatric cognitive restructuring, electrotherapy, colon (enema) therapy, Epsom salts bath soak, and Tiger Balm liniment rubs on the spine, neck, and temples. Regular eating, sleeping, exercising, and toilet functions will prevent migraine recurrences.

The crime-scene cleaning expert promised to follow some of these recommendations and report back the results which was done about three weeks later. I was never told which specifics were followed, only that my advice worked and the person was now free of headaches.

ISRAELI NATURAL MEDICINE AT WORK FOR YOU

In the course of putting this work together, I had the good fortune to occasionally meet skilled practitioners who had become sufficiently trained in the medical and pharmacological sciences to do greater justice and give more credence to the natural folk medicines they preferred using over conventional drugs in their regular practices. Among these are Lazarus Malakoff, Ph.D., M.sc.Pharm. (natural pharmacist), and Earon Yoseph, M.D. (homeopathic physician and phytotherapist).

This pair of distinguished-looking and intelligent gentlemen were visiting a large health-food-industry convention in the Baltimore Convention Center in the fall of 1998; they had traveled by airplane all the way from their native homeland of Israel for this big event. During their three-day stay, they leisurely strolled up and down the many aisles in the huge exhibit halls casually searching for any kind of new or different health product they might take back with them to use in their own clinical practice.

Noticing a rather long line stretching around a particular corner of the Trace Minerals display, they decided to join the crowd for the free book giveaway. Eventually they and I met over the table where I sat dutifully shaking hands and autographing copies of one of my Prentice Hall titles. They happened to come at a very good time since my three-hour signing event was winding down. When the last few books were gone, I joined them for a lengthy dinner engagement at an exclusive restaurant in the Inner Harbor, known for its wonderful cuisine. Following dessert, we remained seated for another two-and-a-half hours and freely participated in a roundtable discussion on all types of health-related matters.

Our personality chemistries meshed perfectly together, and we discovered in each other things to learn and gain from. I had the foresight to bring along in my coat pocket a small, spiral-bound, flip-top notebook into which I made numerous entries of things they used for the 11 problems cited in this combined section. They, in turn, scribbled down on paper I provided data given by me of remedies I use for diseases that interested them. (At the time I was working in the "M" section of this manuscript and had brought this list of specific ailments with me to keep myself busy when time permitted.)

The only apparent conflict (if it can even be called that) I could see in our free exchange of health information was their extensive reliance on homeopathic preparations. This is something I've always been very unwilling to recommend to others. My opposition to this form of treatment stems largely from inspiration obtained some years earlier while in a period of meditative reflection on the subject. At some point during my moments of musing there came into my consciousness this crystal-clear idea from Providence: "John, homeopathy is *not* a system of medicine ordained of me." That and nothing more. I've adhered to that higher wisdom ever since.

However, out of respect to my new-found friends and readers of this work, I am including the homeopathic remedies that Drs. Malakoff and Yoseph freely prescribe to many of their patients. These remedies *do work for the conditions in the following pages*, although I would never use any of them myself due to prejudice and distrust.

MISCARRIAGE

Pharmacist Malakoff and physician Yoseph instruct all of their female clients who have had previous miscarriages and are hoping to have successful pregnancies next time to avoid certain substances that are known to hurt the fetus in some way: alcohol, tobacco, caffeinated beverages, chocolate, illicit drugs, over-the-counter (OTC) and prescription medications, and salty foods. Salt is a strong diuretic, they maintain, and the frequent consumption of salty foods dramatically increases the risk of early uterine contractions that lead to miscarriage. They also warn their subjects to avoid using any herbs or herbal combinations that are known diuretics.

Oddly, they include the very homeopathic preparations so frequently used in their practice. They permit the judicious use of tissue-cell salts but strictly forbid *any* remedies in potencies less than 6c, such as one that might be of 3c strength. They believe that minerals are very important in the prevention of miscarriages and prescribe a liquid mineral solution harvested from the Dead Sea in their homeland. Their expectant patients put 20 drops of liquid minerals in water or juice and drink this twice a day with meals. (A comparable product from the Great Salt Lake is sold by Trace Minerals Research under the brand name of ConcenTrace; see Product Appendix for details.)

Both are big fans of essential fatty acids (EFAs) and fish and olive oils. They favor women seeking to get pregnant taking sufficient EFAs every morning. The better fish oils are from freshwater fish (salmon, trout) as opposed to saltwater varieties (tuna, swordfish). If nothing else is available, a tablespoon of cod-liver oil every morning is adequate. The same amount should be taken of extra-virgin olive oil, too, they insist.

MOLES

Moles can be a bit tricky, they declared. Careful observation and a thorough physical examination is necessary in order to determine if they might be impending signs of skin cancer. If not, then thuja (arbor vitae) may be used: Take six c every 12 hours for up to three weeks. They advise leaving moles alone and instead working from within to make them eventually fall off or disappear.

MONONUCLEOSIS

Two homeopathic preparations are given here: Take six c of pulsatilla (meadow anemone) every two hours for up to four doses to combat the infection; and 30c of kali phos. (potassium phosphate) twice a day for up to 14 days to overcome mental and physical exhaustion.

MOOD CHANGES

Drs. Malakoff and Yoseph prescribe calcium carbonate (30c twice daily for two weeks) to allay panic attacks, extreme fear, anxiety, and undue concern of public embarrassment. With this they give potassium phosphate (30c twice daily for 14 days) to help patients cope with irritability, the urge sometimes to scream, fear of losing control over a situation, nervous anticipation, and sensitivity to touch. (Calc. carb. is made from mother-of-pearl oyster shell and kali phos. is prepared chemically by adding diluted phosphoric acid to a solution of potassium carbonate derived from burned wood potash.)

Several other homeopathic preparations periodically employed by them for different mood changes include:

Compulsive-obsessive behavior—Argentum nitricum (six c every 30 minutes for up to 10 doses, then four times daily for two weeks

Anger/insecurity/violent behavior—Lycopodium (club moss) (six c every 30 minutes for up to 10 doses)

Depression/self-pity/unprovoked crying—Pulsatilla (meadow anemone) six c three times daily for two weeks

Both Israeli practitioners believe that diet plays a huge role in determining the outcome of positive or negative mood swings. While interviewing every one of their patients, they ask them if they use sugars. "So far," Dr. Malakoff said, "100 percent of our patients suffering from personality disorders use this substance to some degree. We feel—no, *we know*—that sugar is the single greatest culprit involved. So, we take them off *all* sugar and within just a few days the mood transformation is unbelievable. Sugar is responsible for just about all of the mood gyrations we've seen over the years in our practice. Take it out of the diet and a person becomes mentally normal and emotionally stable again."

MOTION SICKNESS

While Tabacum or Indian tobacco is the standard homeopathic remedy to alleviate nausea, vomiting, vertigo, chilly perspiration, and anxiety due to travel motion, Malakoff and Yoseph like to combine this with ginger root. Thus, they have their patients take six c every 15 minutes for up to 10 doses of Tabacum and three capsules of gingerroot powder twice daily. They claim the two together are far more effective than using either one separately.

MULTIPLE PERSONALITIES

The three of us really had an animated and engaging discussion with this one. Though not fully persuaded as I was, they were willing to concede some truth to the quaint folk belief and ancient wisdom piece that basically ascribes demonic possession or evil-spirit influences to multiple-personalities disorder. Being moderately orthodox Jews themselves, however, they acknowledged faith and prayer in Something Divine as being powerful tools in dealing with such a complex and highly disturbing psychiatric problem as this. And, along with me, they have encouraged the listening of pleasant symphonic music as a means of holding the mind to just one's true personality for as long as possible.

MULTIPLE SCLEROSIS

Malakoff and Yoseph informed me that their current trip to the United States was the third or fourth one for them. They believed that by visiting the Natural Products Expo East in Baltimore periodically, it would increase their own awareness of what new health products had become available since their last trip.

In a previous visit they had become acquainted with a certain manufacturer of cold-pressed flaxseed oil and evening-primrose oil. They ordered unspecified quantities of both and began using them in their practice on problems such as multiple sclerosis. Within a reasonable period of time (never stated) they became impressed with the many positive results in some of their MS patients.

Their standard recommendation for most was this: one teaspoon flaxseed oil twice daily (morning and evening) and three capsules evening-primrose oil morning, midday, and at night.

MUMPS

They encourage parents to have their children resting in rooms that have free access to sunlight and plenty of fresh air. Also, the children are to be given spring or purified water free of chlorine or fluoride. They think that warmth, good air, and pure water will do a lot in making a sick child well again, even if no other measures are taken. To allay the fever and swelling of mumps, they prescribe Ferrum Phosphate made from iron phosphate at 30c every hour for up to ten doses. They advise worried parents to place cool packs on their sick children's forehead, chest, and abdomen to reduce any lingering fevers.

MUSCLE CRAMPS

For leg cramps they recommend Cuprum met. or powdered copper ore at six c four times a day for two weeks. For cramps from muscle fatigue, they prescribe arnica, an old and well-established European herb in use since medieval times at six c four times daily for 14 days. I mentioned to them two American-made products that are currently being marketed in Japan with great success for muscle cramps: Super Food and Body Guard from Synergy Worldwide. The former is a comprehensive food-nutrient formula while the latter is pure shark-liver oil rich in alklglycerols. They expressed a keen interest in knowing more about them. (See Product Appendix.)

MUSCLE-TONE LOSS

The following homeopathic remedies are standard prescriptions for muscle atrophy: Calcium fluor (calcium fluoride, a tissue salt), two tablets are taken every 30 minutes for up to five hours, then a reduced dosage three times a day is continued thereafter for up to 14 days; Mag. phos. (magnesium phosphate, another tissue salt), four tablets

every 30 minutes for four hours, then reduced to three times a day;
and Zinc met. (zinc sulfide), six c four times daily for up to two weeks.

On the nutritional supplement side of things, I referred them to
the ionic mineral product ConcenTrace, the source of which is the
Great Salt Lake, and mentioned that it is quite high in calcium, magnesium, and zinc, among other things. I spoke of my own experience
with this in helping weak muscles regain their normal strength and
agility (14 drops in eight ounces of water, twice or thrice daily). (See
Product Appendix under Trace Minerals Research.)

MUSCULAR DYSTROPHY

They reported seeing cases from time to time of this genetic wasting
disease. Their best success has been working with children under the
age of 12; boys seem to respond to therapy better than girls do.
They've had very little success with young adults. Their therapeutic
approach is somewhat multifaceted and includes daily massages by
hand and with a vibrator; daily doses (two tablespoons) of olive oil; vitamins (unspecified) and Dead Sea minerals; limited swimming exercises; and other physical therapies.

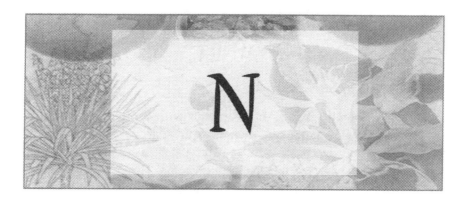

NAIL PROBLEMS

An Amish Application

In my many years of researching natural remedies around the world, I've spent my share of time among the Amish, who are principally centered in Indiana, Ohio, and Pennsylvania. To this day they remain somewhat of a novelty to outsiders and gawking tourists who are fascinated with the strange way they dress and their sole means of local transportation, the horse and buggy.

Some years ago I spent a couple of weeks traveling through various states with an old Amish folk healer by the name of Enos Yoder. He hired a driver and van to haul us around from one place to another as we gave numerous health lectures to old order Amish and Mennonites.

In one such large home located near Nappanee, Indiana, where about 65 earnest souls were gathered for the "Good Word" (as Enos put it), there were several women who suffered from different nail problems. I recommended to them silicon in the form of horsetail (also called shavegrass), three capsules daily with a meal, and a good calcium–magnesium supplement, two tablets daily.

About a month after our trip, Enos reported to me by mail the results he had heard back from my recommendation. The ladies' nails were now in much healthier condition, and they were happy with the results.

NAUSEA

A Cool Antidote

Catnip tea is one of the all-time favorites with the old-order Amish (horse-and-buggies only) and Beachy Amish (cars permitted). For nausea and vomiting, several cups of the *cool* tea are sipped to correct stomach heebie-jeebies. *Cool* peppermint or spearmint tea works just as effectively. The teas are safe for old and young alike, and there are no unpleasant reactions to them. The only lasting effect is relief and a grateful tummy.

NECK PAIN

Neck Pain or Pain in the Neck?

Amish dress styles haven't changed since the seventeenth century in Europe. Girls wear long dresses about eight inches from the floor. They never wear plaids, prints, or polka dots—just plain, drab colors such as brown, dark green, dark blue, or somber black. Up to eight years old, girls wear a pinafore called a *Schlupp Schötzli* over their dresses. Older girls wear aprons and capes fastened with straight pins—zippers and buttons are considered to be worldly and, therefore, indecent to have on clothing.

Some of the older girls wear white prayer caps like their mothers as well as the traditional black stockings and shoes that tie. Amish women never wear jewelry, makeup, lipstick, or perfume. They also *never* cut their hair. And they would never wear red since that is the Devil's favorite color to entice innocent souls into forbidden ways and the lusts of the flesh.

While traveling through Amish communities scattered from Indiana to Delaware some years ago with Enos Yoder, an Amish folk healer, I had the opportunity to treat several middle-aged Amish women for neck pain. I used some Mentholatum Deep-Heat Rub for this and gently massaged it into one lady's neck before covering it with a piece of flannel cloth supplied by a family member. Within minutes she declared all of her pain to be gone.

As I was working on the other woman, her husband walked in from the barn without removing his boots. She promptly hopped out of the kitchen chair in which she sat and went up to him and gave him a good scolding in their Pennsylvania-Dutch dialect. She shook her finger in front of his face lest he forget that she meant business. I leaned over to Enos, who was seated and watching this with some amusement, and whispered in his ear, "Not only does she have a pain in the neck, but she also *is one!*" The other lady then returned to her chair and I finished my treatment, feeling sorry for the poor husband, who undoubtedly felt his wife's wrath that afternoon.

NERVE PAIN

Some Herbal Oil Treatments

The Amish are an interesting group, and it has been my privilege to work and move among them in past years in the course of studying their quaint folk ways as well as helping some of them with myriad health problems.

Amish men and boys wear plain-colored shirts and pants with no hip pockets, cuffs, or zippers. In place of a fly, there is a large flap that hooks on both sides and works quite efficiently when "nature calls." A special kind of coat with split tail is always worn for church, and most Amish men and boys may be seen wearing the plain black, wide-brimmed hat of which I am the proud owner of one purchased as a gift by my friend Enos Yoder. Boys remain clean-shaven until they marry, at which time beards start sprouting, but mustaches remain forbidden because they are looked upon as a part of male vanity and tend to convey a sinister appearance to those who wear them.

I've watched my Amish folk-healer friend work on numerous men, both older and younger, who've suffered from sciatica or some other painful nerve inflammation. He will put a few drops of eucalyptus oil, peppermint oil, melaleuca oil, or Australian tea-tree oil on the skin surface and then commence rubbing it in with his thumb and forefingers. Relief is always guaranteed within ten minutes or less and lasts for hours thereafter.

NERVOUS STOMACH

Amish Ways

The old-order Amish of Indiana, Ohio, Pennsylvania, and elsewhere have some tried-and-true methods for curing a nervous stomach. Warm chamomile tea is consumed with meals. Good thoughts and feelings replace bad ones in the mind and heart. Foot reflexology is practiced to some extent, and tired feet are soaked in hot vinegar water, which somehow is able to calm an agitated gut, believe it or not. Smaller meals are *quietly* consumed and thoroughly chewed before being swallowed.

NERVOUSNESS

Trilingual Amish

For people who go only to the eighth grade and learn just the most basic of the three R's—reading, 'riting, and 'rithmetic—the Amish are quite fluent in language skills. They actually speak two distinctive languages in spite of their limited education. First is their own Pennsylvania Dutch, which is a dialect of *Hoch Deutsch* (High German) that is still spoken today in the Rhineland area of Germany. They also use English when speaking to non-Amish folks and politely refer to all outsiders as "English people."

It isn't uncommon to have an Amish man or woman switch from their peculiar dialect to English and go back and forth in both tongues at the dinner table. Their language is *Hoch Deutsch*, which is used only in worship services at a designated house every week, and in Bible reading, prayer, and hymn singing. Their scriptures are printed in the old Gothic script. I can both read and speak their form of *Hoch Deutsch*, which enables me to get along fabulously well with them and with similar groups such as the old-order Mennonites and the communal Hutterites.

Nervousness is a common problem among the Amish. Women tend to suffer from it more than men do. A cultural inhibition about vocalizing some of your emotional hang-ups contributes to this, I believe. Also their inordinate consumption of black coffee, homemade

wine and commercial beer, and soda pop causes a serious depletion of
B-complex vitamins and mineral magnesium.

But they nicely manage by taking different herbal teas throughout the day, which seem to help calm them down: skullcap, peppermint, black cohosh, blue vervain, catnip, and valerian. Some also take
nutritional supplements such as vitamins B and E and magnesium,
but not everyone.

NEURALGIA

A Family Tonic

Amish families usually average anywhere between six and ten children *or more!* The same may be said for Hutterites as well. Both groups
view birth control of *any* kind as an "absolute evil" tantamount to
"spiritual murder" by denying unborn spirits access to physical bodies.

Where the typical nuclear family in America has become split
apart by divorce, separation, wedlock, and same-gender living ar-
rangements, it is still alive and well and very much intact among the
central and eastern Amish and the western-based Hutterites.

Amish and Hutterite families resemble those of the nineteenth
century in many ways. In wintertime they will gather in what is considered to be the common kitchen area to eat popcorn, tell stories,
knit, play games, sing, or read from the German Bible. The children
are taught at an early stage, usually around four, to begin helping
with home and farm responsibilities. Boys are taught how to do men's
work in the field and various shop crafts such as blacksmithing, wood-
work, or mechanics (only for the Hutterites who drive modern tractors
and trucks). Girls are taught by their mothers how to cook, bake,
clean, sew, and do gardening.

Thus, every family member becomes productive in some way and
feels a sense of usefulness and accomplishment within the particular
community that he or she is very much a part of. Delinquency, as we
know it in the world, is virtually unknown among both groups as a
whole.

An effective Amish tonic for neuralgia can be made at home.
Coarsely cut six oranges, six lemons, and six grapefruit. Cook this citrus (peels and all) in two quarts of water, then strain. Next add one-

half cup Epsom salts. Let the water cook down to one quart, cover, set aside, and let stand overnight. Take one-quarter cup every two to three hours five times a day.

NIGHT BLINDNESS

What the Newspaper Says

For being so out of touch with the world in terms of materialistic possessions and cultural norms, the Amish are surprisingly well-informed on most world happenings and can discourse with reasonable intelligence on a broad variety of subjects.

Although their information doesn't come from magazines, radio, televisions, or the computer Internet, they do get it from other sources. The major one, of course, is a long-standing newspaper called *The Budget,* published in Sugarcreek, Ohio, and circulated to 34 states and 11 foreign countries or wherever groups of Amish or Mennonites may dwell. Another common source is the English neighbors around them, who freely discuss with them what's happening in the outside world. And Amish preachers will sometimes spike their otherwise long and boring sermons with bits and pieces of national and global events, using them as effective examples of particular points they wish to make to their respective congregations.

Some years ago I wrote a regular column in *The Budget* called "Homespun," which was chatty and informative on health-related issues. In one of the issues I regularly received there was a little piece from an Amish woman named Lenora Eck in Smicksburg, Pennsylvania. She made salads and juice from various bright-yellow flowers such as dandelion and sunflower. She said that these were good for helping people to see better at night. I borrowed this interesting remedy and began recommending it to others who suffered from night blindness. I was informed later on that in most instances these plant flowers helped quite a bit.

NOSEBLEEDS

How to Stop It

A practical Amish method to halt the bleeding is to press the nose between the finger and thumb for a few minutes with the head tilted slightly back. Also, a cold, wet, folded washcloth is placed on the nape of the neck for five minutes. These work every time.

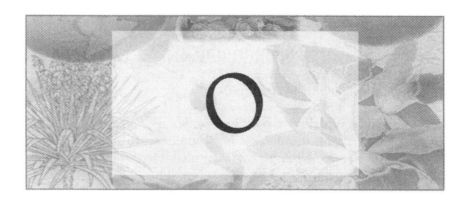

O

OSTEOARTHRITIS

Heat, Stick, Salts, and Oils

The most common form of arthritis is osteoarthritis (also known as degenerative joint disease or DJD). The second most prevalent form of arthritis is rheumatoid arthritis.

About 57 percent of adults over age 30 suffer some form of DJD. Those who perform repetitive tasks are the most prone to developing it: typists, computer-keyboard operators, carpenters, and athletes. The chief symptoms are pain and stiffness. Usually the pain is an aching associated with movement of the affected joint(s). The pain typically subsides when the aching joint is rested. Some osteoarthritis sufferers experience morning stiffness, which usually subsides as they engage in a variety of physical activities throughout the day.

I was bothered with a bit of osteoarthritis in my lower back for several months in 1999. I treated myself with a variety of remedies and gradually the pain and stiffness went away. I mentioned my methods of self-treatment to about a thousand distributors at the ShapeRite convention in the Salt Palace in Salt Lake City in October. Everyone liked just about all the remedies I mentioned except for the capsules of baby-harp-seal oil from Newfoundland that I took each day during my short period of suffering. Some of the more environmentally sensitive folks complained about this afterwards, but the greater majority enjoyed what they heard.

I explained how I applied a vibrating heating pad behind my back and used it for 25 minutes of every hour for three to four hours a day. I also soaked in a tub of hot water to which had been added some Epsom salts (one cup) and peppermint oil (50 drops). I used a big walking stick to get around, which gave me the support I needed. And I took six capsules of ShapeRite's Musculoskeletal formula along with four capsules of the baby-harp-seal oil every morning before breakfast. These greatly facilitated easier and painless physical movements for me. (In lieu of harp-seal oil, which is unavailable in the United States due to the enforcement of the Marine Mammal Protection Act, one can substitute an omega-fatty-acids or fish-oil product instead with reasonable results. Also see Product Appendix under ShapeRite for more information.)

OSTEOPOROSIS

How One Woman Reversed Her Bone Loss

Bone is living tissue. And like other tissue, the body constantly creates new bone to replace the old as it wears out. This process is known as "remodeling." In those under 35 years of age, the body draws on calcium dissolved in the blood to replace the entire skeleton about once every ten years. However, after age 39, women, who are already nine times more prone to osteoporosis than men, begin to lose more bone than they could ever replace. This bone loss commences slowly but gains speed over time.

Eleanor Lutizano had reached an age (which she refused to disclose in our interview) where she began showing classic signs of bone loss: back pain, a noticeably curved spine (the infamous "dowager's hump"), permanent height loss of one-and-a-half inches, and two minor vertebral fractures. She was supplementing her diet with a number of different calcium or calcium-magnesium products but "seemed to be getting nowhere," as she phrased it.

A certified nutritionist whom she consulted explained that the only real assimilable calcium came from food and put her on a high-calcium diet. The list of foods Eleanor had to eat for the next four months included the following, ranked according to their calcium content: Swiss cheese, cheddar cheese, canned sardines, whole peanuts and organic peanut butter, milk, yogurt, canned salmon, whole-wheat bread, almonds, sesame seeds (in the form of a paste spread on whole-wheat bread), kale, broccoli, garbanzo beans, collard greens, black beans, tofu, spinach, cottage cheese, and parsley.

She also did some regular exercise (bending, stretching, walking, aerobics, gardening, jogging, and dancing), which kept her hips and lower back in pretty good shape. After several months of this regimen, she reported a disappearance of lower-back and hip pain, a strengthening of her spine somewhat, and no more bone fractures. Tests showed that her blood was now full of mineral calcium, whereas before, she insisted, "with all those supplements that I took there wasn't much there to brag about."

OVERWEIGHT

Turning Back to a Better Plan

Obesity is one of America's leading diseases. The number of Americans considered obese jumped from about one in eight in 1991 to nearly one in five in 1998. This is based on data supplied by the U.S. Centers for Disease Control and Prevention. What worries most health professionals now is that young children and teenagers are currently experiencing an epidemic of obesity.

Sarah Liebowitz, a neurobiologist at The Rockefeller University in New York City, believes she knows why this is happening. At an Agriculture Department conference in Washington, D.C., at the beginning of November 1999, she explained why people eat what they eat. Young people especially have strong cravings for high-fat foods such as juicy hamburgers and mounds of ice cream. She believes they are responding to hormones that kick in at the onset of puberty.

The idea at work here is that the hormones trigger production of a chemical called galanin, which stimulates the desire for intake of fatty foods. This, in turn, perpetuates a vicious cycle by increasing production of even more galanin. But switching to a low-fat, high-carbohydrate diet isn't the answer either. A high-carb diet can lead to obesity, too. Additionally, it stimulates production of a chemical similar to galanin, neuropeptide Y. This actually encourages cravings for still more carbs.

A little-known but highly successful diet plan of the midnineteenth century proved to be of inestimable value to those whose ample girth and hefty size were in serious need of reduction. It was known in those times as The Oneida Eating Plan, but would eventually disappear from the public record upon the death of the genius behind its inspiration. But to appreciate the diet itself, we must first mention some things about the community from which it evolved.

The Oneida Community

John Humphrey Noyes, founder of the Oneida Community, was of upper-class birth. His mother was a relative of U.S. President Rutherford B. Hayes, and his father was a U.S. congressman and a successful businessman. John was born in 1811, one of eight children. He entered Dartmouth College and graduated in law.

In the late 1820s and early 1830s much of the eastern United States was caught up in a frenzy of religious rejuvenation. Joseph Smith, Jr., the Mormon Prophet, was from Vermont, the same state as Noyes. Both men, though at separate times in their early lives, attended religious revivals in their respective neighborhoods (Smith in Palmyra, New York, and Noyes in Putney, Vermont) and came away "alive with ideas, spiritual enlightenment, and visions of eternal truth." Each went his own way and founded organizations that persist even today—for Smith it was The Church of Jesus Christ of Latter-Day Saints and for Noyes it was, first, the Putney Perfectionists (in Vermont) and later the Oneida Community (named after the Indian tribe) in New York State.

Noyes encouraged his followers to adopt a communal way of living in which all material things were shared. Later, spousal sharing was added during the Vermont phase, which resulted in a court trial for Noyes and his escape from mob violence into New York. Those who embraced Noyes's Perfectionist ideas came from the upper-, middle-, and lower classes. They lived along the lines of Shaker communalism but believed in marriage and raising families. Like the Shakers, though, they were thrifty and industrious and proved to be excellent businesspeople as the narrative will show.

There was once recorded in a handwritten journal of Oneidan history this small but noteworthy incident, which demonstrated the strength of their communal living habits. An outsider came to visit them and was given the "royal tour" by a community member. He was escorted through the community hall known as the Mansion House.

The stranger paused, sniffed the air, and inquired, "What is the fragrance I smell here?" To which his guide casually replied, "It must be the odor of crushed selfishness, sir."

The Oneidans were more fortunate than some of their contemporaries: The Shakers were continually plagued with legal suits based on property rights, while the Mormons had to contend with rank apostates always spreading lies. But the Oneidans had neither and lived in harmony and contentment for a number of decades, while prospering economically at the same time.

The real windfall of their unbelievable financial success came from an old northwoods hunter and trapper by the name of Sewell Newhouse, who with his cantankerous wife joined the colony. Because of his prodigious strength and size, this man made his own traps by using a blacksmith's forge, anvil, and hand punch. He made an outstanding product and had no trouble selling his traps to local woodsmen. Why such a man of rough ways and gnarled character would ever join a society of spiritual and intellectual refinement is anybody's guess.

In time Newhouse revealed to John Humphrey Noyes the secret process of spring-tampering his traps. By the late 1850s the Oneidans were turning out traps by the hundreds. In 1868 alone the Community manufactured 278,000 traps, most of which were sold in the United States and Canada. Once they had "turned the corner" with their trap business, the Oneidans' other products—canned vegetables and preserved fruit, bags, silk thread—proved to be valuable sidelines. So, too, did their tourist business. As their fame spread even further, the number of visitors—with their admission fees—grew proportionately bigger.

Later on, in 1877, the Oneida Community began the manufacture of silverware. Although there were some ups and downs in the beginning, this business also proved highly successful. In 1881, when the community finally disbanded, the industrial component was perpetuated under the name of Oneida Ltd. These silversmiths have grown and prospered, and their products are in wide use and great demand today.

The Oneida Eating Plan

John Humphrey Noyes was a benevolent but strict authoritarian and oversaw every aspect of his Vermont and later New York communities. Following his religious revival experience in Vermont, he enrolled at Yale Theological Seminary, where he acquired the reputation of being somewhat of a fanatic. He traveled through New York and the New England states spreading his doctrine of Perfectionism: Man and woman could be without sin. His basic theological postulate was this: Christ had already returned to earth—by his reckoning in A.D. 70—so that redemption or liberation from sin was an accomplished fact. Given the proper environment, therefore, man and woman could lead a perfect, or sinless, life.

By his standards, *anything* involving indulgences of the flesh were sinful. But through careful and consistent "reconditioning," a person could move away from sin and into Perfectionism, where balance and harmony existed in everything. Gluttony or giving way to the wrong appetite indulgences was a terrible sin because it made a mockery of the "perfect" body that God had given to every person.

Noyes, therefore, set his mind to work and devised an eating program that was probably one of the first "diet plans" ever conceived in America. It's basic premise was to live in accordance with what nature intended for men and women to eat, rather than to eat those things one desired for pleasure.

He emphasized the use of wholesome herbs for the maintenance of the physical body, the vitality of nerve constitution, and the soundness of mind and heart. The herbs available in each of the three warm and cool seasons (spring, summer, and fall) were to be mostly consumed within their respective seasons. Hence, dandelion greens, burdock leaves, and alfalfa tops were of tremendous value in cleansing the blood and revitalizing the constitution following the long winter. Summer yielded a variety of leafy vegetables for rebuilding each of the body's different internal system: parsley for the circulatory system, cabbage for the immune system, spinach for the eliminative system (colon), mustard greens for the heart (cardiovascular system), watercress for the liver, leaf lettuce for the eyes, and endive for the brain. Autumn harvest yielded certain field herbs, meadow grasses, and pasturage for fortifying the body for the cold months ahead: catnip, mullein, red clover, yellow dock, plantain, yarrow, and echinacea.

The "fruits of the vine" were important in each of their own seasons: raspberries and strawberries in late spring; peaches, apricots, tomatoes, and cucumbers in the summer; and apples, melons, and squashes in the fall. Each category of "vine fruits" (which also included tree and bush fruits) was intended to "purify, protect, and produce" the organs and glands in the body. Noyes taught that the *real* "fruit of the vine," in this case grapes, were beneficial in whole form or as juice, but detrimental when consumed as fermented liquid (wine).

Another part of his Perfection Eating Plan involved the frequent use of tuber foods. He held forth that root vegetables, such as carrots, radishes, turnips, parsnips, rutabagas, potatoes, yams, and sweet potatoes, were full of the earth's own magnetic energy and pulled from her soil much mineral goodness. These became a mainstay of Oneidan diets for many years. They were to be received into the body with thanksgiving and joy whenever consumed.

A cornerstone of his religion-based nutrition plan was grains. He took the scriptural injunction literally that "bread is the staff of life" and made it one of the centerpieces of Oneidan diets. The darker the bread and the least amount of milling done to the flour resulted in better sustenance for active and needy bodies. While "all grain is good to eat," he wrote, "yet some are more fit for man and others more suited for beasts of the field." So, while men and women might enjoy all grains, wheat was more adapted to their physical makeups, while oxen benefited from corn, oats were helpful to plow and riding horses, pigs and chickens thrived on rye, and barley did well for all other domesticated creatures. (This portion of Noyes's food ideas paralleled closely the Mormon Prophet Joseph Smith's own Word of Wisdom. It is highly unlikely Noyes ever imitated Smith's code of health conduct, but, nevertheless, it is intriguing to think he might at least have been aware of it on one or more occasions.)

Lest food purists and earth-conscious consumers imagine that John Humphrey Noyes was vegetarian, it should be stated that he advocated the consumption of *some* animal flesh. He said that meat consumption was more justified in heavy labor and during cold weather than it was with less physical activity in warmer climate.

Noyes's own writings as well as some of the records kept by the Oneidan Community show that very good health prevailed among nearly all members and that "*not a one* is inclined to signs of being corpulent," but rather that "all tend to show slenderness of frame, quickness in step, and liveliness in personality." Outsiders who often visited this strange sect reported later of meeting "those with ruddy countenances and sparkle to their eyes, possessing a sharpness of wit."

In working with some severely obese individuals, I've tailored portions of this Oneida Eating Plan to suit their specific metabolisms with extremely good results. I heartily endorse and recommend it to anyone who is overweight.

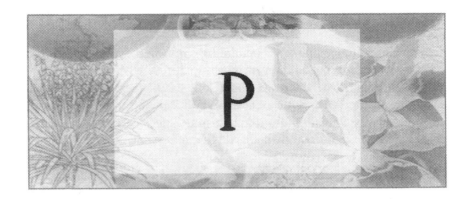

PAGET'S DISEASE

An Egyptian Approach

There are some health problems that afflict only a very small number of people and for which there seems to be no ready solution. Paget's disease is one of these—you won't find mention made of it in most self-care books on natural or alternative medicine.

However, I learned of an effective treatment for the *management*—NOT cure—of this disorder from an Egyptian folk healer in Cairo when I visited that city many years ago. Moussa Al-Akhbar had been using fenugreek seed and carob powders in a simple formula for years in the treatment of this problem with apparently good success. Due to its low incidence, however, the actual number of patients treated in nine years was just under a dozen. But several patients whom he directed me to interview said that Moussa's remedy had helped them lead fairly normal lives in spite of their condition.

Although the Egyptian made his own pills from the herbal powders, I suggest filling 00 size capsules and taking them with a full eight-ounce glass of water or juice. Three-quarters fenugreek seed powder and one-quarter carob powder are mixed together and put into gelatin capsules. Moussa had his patients taking 20 small round pills a day, which is the equivalent of three to four capsules.

PAIN

Inca Relief

In the mountainous highlands of Peru and Bolivia live a few million Quechua Indians. They eke out a sparse existence on potatoes, some wild edible greens, nuts, seeds, dried fruit, and some meat (obtained mostly from llama, alpaca, or mountain goats). These people often live in minor poverty for most of their lives but somehow manage to get by with what little they have.

Their hygiene leaves a lot to be desired, though; dirt and lice seem to accumulate on them and in their dwellings over an extended period of time. Still, they are humble and gracious to outsiders, though one would never suspect them ever to be the descendants of the once mighty and powerful Incas who ruled these parts in great civilized style centuries ago.

One of the outstanding highlights of a visit to these people was finding an herbal formula for relieving general body pain. It has to be taken *as a hot infusion* in order to work effectively. In one quart of hot water, combine one cup of mountain mullein leaves and flowers, one-half cup coltsfoot leaves, one-half cup chopped burdock root, and one-quarter cup juniper berries. Cover the pot with a lid and simmer over low heat for five minutes before setting aside to steep 20 minutes. Then strain and slowly sip one cup of hot tea on an empty stomach every four hours. Hot poultices of this tea applied to the body can also relieve pain. Precede this, however, by first rubbing into the muscles some oil of either peppermint or eucalyptus or melaleuca or tea tree. It will expedite relief more quickly once the hot tea has been ingested.

PAINFUL BREATHING

Navajo Tom's Bitter Tea

An elderly Navajo sheepherder from Window Rock, Arizona, showed me some years ago how to make a *warm* tea to facilitate painful breathing. Tom Begay filled an old and well-used coffee pot with what I judged to have been one-and-a-half cups of water from a water wagon sitting in the front of his hogan. He threw a few more chips of cedar wood on the glowing embers of some hot coals until there was a sufficiently strong fire going. He suspended the pot on a tripod over it and waited for the water to boil. One of his sheepdogs walked up to me and licked my gloved hand in a gesture of canine friendliness as if to suggest that this stranger was welcomed in those parts.

Tom removed from several coffee cans lined up on a rickety table the following herbs and mixed them together in an enamel pan in these amounts: one small handful each (one tablespoon apiece) of dried cedar bark and juniper berries; a thumb-and-finger pinch (one teaspoon) of pine needles; and a tiny pinch of Skoal (Scandinavian brand of chewing tobacco). These were tossed rather indiscriminately into the coffeepot and permitted to percolate at random for an unspecified number of minutes (probably 10–12). He then poured out some of the brew *without steeping* it first and strained the liquid through a torn remnant of an empty bean sack. When it had sufficiently cooled we drank it together.

Yes, the tea was bitter to my taste buds, but the impact sure made my lungs sit up at attention—my breathing became more vigorous after this, and I soon felt invigorated from all the extra oxygen I had taken in. This tea helps to heal inflamed lungs and make breathing considerably easier.

PAINFUL INTERCOURSE

An Old-Fashioned Approach

Pain attendant to either sex during intercourse may be due to an existing internal infection or inflammation. Sometimes the physical positioning of the bodies involved or the level of aggressiveness at which they engage in sex can result in pain. Occasionally, the diet can play a role, albeit a minor one, especially when intensely spicy foods or excess alcohol are consumed prior to intercourse.

Now certain conservative religious groups (Amish, Mennonites, Quakers, Pilgrim Holiness, German Baptists) whose sexual practices I've studied by way of respectful interviews almost invariably *never* show any indications of pain suffered during the intercourse process. A good part of it, I think, has to do with the shared cultural attitudes that such people bring to the bedroom when engaging in something like this.

With but few exceptions most of these respondents willing to discuss such private matters with this anthropologist after he had gained their confidence and trust informed him that sex, to them, was merely "a means to an end." Namely, that physical intercourse was a tool for the express purpose of procreation, to be used exclusively for the begetting of children and not for lust. Their moments of intercourse were also shorter in time and fewer in number.

Such an ultraorthodox view as this obviously won't sit well for most others in society. But at least it is something worth thinking about and an idea from a different perspective that nearly always yields pain-free intercourse for those willing to accept the limitations it brings.

PALSY

Facing the Facts

Bells' palsy, as it is customarily called, is indicated by a paralysis of the muscles on one side of the face. It results from inflammation of the facial nerve, which runs from a tiny hole in the bone between the ear and the jaw. Inflammation of this nerve compresses it inside its bony channel, thus paralyzing the muscles between the forehead and mouth. Those between 30 and 60 seem to be the most susceptible.

My Hungarian grandmother frequently treated older people who suffered from this problem. She would lay warm compresses of yarrow or chamomile or spearmint tea upon the afflicted sides of their faces and then place a dry cloth over it to retain the heat longer. She would change the compress every seven minutes and replace it with another hot one.

PANCREATITIS

What They Do in the Philippines

Filipino folk healers routinely administer the *fresh* juices of guava, papaya, or mango to those suffering from inflammation of the pancreas, always with excellent results. Nonenteric-coated enzyme tablets or capsules are also good for this. (See Product Appendix under ShapeRite for their Enzy-Rite formula to assist with something like this.)

PARALYSIS

Remedy from a Quiet French Town

Of all the hilltop villages in France, none ever so captured my imagination and fancy as did the quiet little town of Vézelay, overlooking the beautiful rolling countryside of the former Duchy of Burgundy. At the village's highest point stands an immense twelfth-century edifice, the historic Basilique de la Sainte Marie Madeleine (St. Mary Magdalene), once one of the most important shrines in the Christian world. I couldn't help but admire the gleaming tiled roofs of the houses and shops of medieval Vézelay as they huddled beneath the church.

Far below, the River Cure wound its way like a silver ribbon through a narrow verdant valley dotted with grazing cattle. Gentle hills, their crests darkly wooded, undulate to the horizon in all directions. Slopes and dales were cloaked with a patchwork of aged vineyards, orchards, and fields hedged with blackthorn and hawthorn.

Jean-Claude Defert, a local farmer whom I met during my short stay in this charming place, told me through a friend of his who spoke some English what his grandmother did for muscle and nerve paralysis. She made a soupy broth of snails, frogs' legs, rabbit meat, mushrooms, and garlic. After letting everything simmer for 30 minutes on low heat to reduce the extra water content by half, she would set it aside to cool. Those paralytic persons still capable of swallowing would drink one to two cups of this *warm* broth five times a day. *Monsieur* Defert indicated that when the liquid had run out, she would fill up the pot again and cook everything a second time. This remedy, he claimed, had helped a number of people from distant places overcome *most* of their paralysis well enough to get around by themselves without further assistance. They would usually continue drinking this broth until satisfactory movement was apparent.

I spoke with some of his neighbors afterwards, who confirmed everything the farmer had told me.

PARKINSON'S DISEASE

American Supplements in Japan

In the latter part of September 1999 I took a ten-day tour of Japan in company with four other Americans. We were there on behalf of an American-based supplements company that sells its line of products mostly in that country (but which are still obtainable stateside for U.S. consumers). My primary task was health education in the four cities we visited. My interpreter was a retired Japanese Air Force general who did the best he could with his somewhat limited command of the English language.

One of our stops was in the city of Osaka, Japan's third largest metropolis and, next to Tokyo, its greatest commercial center. It was created by force expressly for the purposes of commerce by the warlord Toyotomi Hideyoshi (1536–1598), who ordered merchants from neighboring localities to move there "or else" face the consequences of his displeasure. From my hotel room I had a splendid sight of Osaka Castle, completed in 1586. The most impressive thing about it wasn't its stunning beauty or imposing strength but that it was completed in just three years, definitely a major architectural feat for that period. The present building I saw from my window is made of ferroconcrete and was finished in 1931.

One of those attending our group meeting was a middle-aged professor of languages by the name of Kamo Atsutane, who had taken an early retirement on account of Parkinson's disease. We spoke after my talk with the translation being done by a younger person in the audience who had been diligently studying English for a number of years and knew it pretty well. Atsutane-sun (the polite form of Mr. Atsutane) explained what he had been doing of late to find relief for his symptoms.

He had been using a combination of traditional *kampo* medicines and a few supplements from Synergy Worldwide (see Product Appendix). He took 30 small round pills (the equivalent of two to three capsules) of *sanzashi* (Japanese hawthorn berries) and drank one cup of *suika* seed (Japanese watermelon, a close relative to the North American variety) tea every day. These had been prescribed to him by a kampo doctor, who was both a regular physician as well as a practitioner of alternative medicine. The supplements he took with meals were germanium, calcium–magnesium, and a "super-food" formula consisting of numerous fruit, vegetable, seaweed, and herb concentrates. He also used a pure shark-liver-oil concentrate that was very high in alklglycerols from the same source. These, he claimed, helped him very much and he was living proof that they apparently work very well for a condition such as Parkinson's.

PEPTIC ULCER

The Tasmanian Bacterium Tamer

Gastroenterologists everywhere now know, for a fact, that stomach ulcers are caused by an in-dwelling, cork-shaped bacterium known as *Heliobacter pylori*. But it wasn't always so—just a few years ago most doctors still held to the outdated notion that stress and aggravation cause an ulcer. Much of the credit for the change goes to two intrepid Australian investigators, Barry Marshall and J. Robin Warren, who showed that *H. pylori* is, indeed, the likely cause of this serious gut problem. In the beginning, though, most physicians scoffed and considered such a find far-fetched nonsense; but Marshall and Warren tenaciously proved all of them wrong.

An effective remedy for treating 95 percent of the painful symptoms along with the actual cause also comes from "down under." A Tasmanian doctor, Colbert Cruikshank, has his patients drink a glass of diluted canned milk to which have been added five drops of Australian tea-tree oil, twice daily with meals. It not only brings relief but also kills most of the bacteria.

PINKEYE
(See "CONJUNCTIVITIS")

PINWORMS
(See "INTESTINAL PARASITES")

PNEUMONIA
*(See "COMMON COLD," "FLU,"
AND "'WALKING' PNEUMONIA")*

POISON-PLANT CONTACT
(See "RASH")

POISONING

Some Food and Herb Antidotes

Food poisoning is quite common in America today. The Centers for Disease Control in Atlanta estimate that between one and three million Americans suffer from some sort of food poisoning every year. But most aren't too serious, and people can recover from them in a reasonably short length of time.

In December 1998, ironically enough, I suffered from the effects of food poisoning in Orlando, Florida, while attending a large health-food-industry convention. And, no, it wasn't from any of the health food I consumed, but rather it was some tainted salad dressing at a five-star restaurant that eventually did me in. I felt miserable, but with the kind assistance of a taxicab driver I was able to negotiate my way through the aisles of a supermarket and purchase some canned pears, a can opener, and a number of small glass jars of baby-food puree (pears, of course, as well as bananas). Upon being helped back to my room, I asked my driver if he would open some of the cans and unscrew the bottle lids, reflecting the degree of my extreme weakness and physical sickness. I thanked him verbally and also with a generous tip and then slowly ate as many pears as my system would permit. I also consumed some Bio-K+ (a wonderful probiotic from Montreal, Canada), all of which enabled me to enjoy a sound sleep that night and be well enough the next day for a three-hour book signing in the convention hall.

Herbs that work just as well for this include *powdered* slippery elm, fenugreek seed, and marshmallow root. *Powdered* blackboard chalk, milk of magnesia, and activated charcoal (tablets or powder) work great, too, when mixed with a little milk.

POSTNASAL DRIP

A Truck Driver's Hope

A fellow I know by the name of Sidney Wilding, age 31, is a long-distance truck driver working out of Mud Lake, ID (45 miles northwest of Idaho Falls). Sid started driving big rigs with his dad when he was 11 and has been doing it ever since. I hired his rig for $550 in early November 1999 to transport to our family ranch in southern Utah a heavy load of steel shelving, iron tables, oak workbenches, and a used Bobcat skid-steer, all of which I had recently purchased at several "going-out-of-business" sales at very low prices.

In the round-trip ride with him in his Peterbilt (model 378) truck, which was pulling a 48-foot drop-deck flatbed trailer behind loaded to the gills, we chatted on personal health and truck-driving philosophy. Sid mentioned that he had been suffering from postnasal drip and another truck-driver buddy of his suggested spraying a little salt water up each nostril morning and evening. He added a tiny pinch of table salt to a coffee cup of water, stirred with a spoon, and then emptied the contents through a paper funnel into a small plastic spray bottle with a screw-on cap. He said the remedy worked very quickly and gave him considerable relief after that. I told him to stay away from *all* white-sugar products and that that would permanently correct the problem, whereas now he was just treating the symptoms.

Sid spoke a little of his own "truck-driver's philosophy." "Most men and women who drive these big rigs do so because they like to meet and interact with people. We get to go to places we ain't never been before. You yearn for the freedom of the road. Traveling like we do gives us a sense of adventure and spirit. It gets into your blood after a while."

A few of their pet peeves include the following:

- Cars cutting in front of us. They think you can stop on a dime but that's where they're DEAD wrong! When you have 80,000 pounds of heavy freight moving behind you at 70 miles per hour, you just can't hit the brakes like that [snapping his fingers] and expect to stop. That's a sure way of getting killed in a hurry. People who do dumb things like that either must have a death wish or something wrong with their brains.

- Tailgating. No truck driver likes to have a car, pickup truck, or van following too close behind. Not only is it dangerous for those who do it, but it also becomes irritating to the drivers themselves. Why can't people be more courteous when they drive?

- Speeding. This is a real bone of contention for many truck drivers. A lot of drivers out there on the road act as if they're in some kind of a big hurry to get somewhere quickly. Why can't they just slow down, enjoy the scenery, and be cool about things? Then they wouldn't be darting in and out of traffic so much and creating a serious road hazard for themselves and the 18-wheelers they're trying to outmaneuver.

- Image. I've yet to figure out why most of the driving public has such a poor image of truck drivers. I tell you this, if it wasn't for truckers moving people's stuff coast to coast every day, this country would come to an instant standstill. We work our butts off. The living is hard, the hours long, the paperwork unbelievable, and the pay not all that great. You would think we would get more respect than we usually do.

PREMENSTRUAL SYNDROME

Relief for a Truck Dispatcher

A friend of mine from Idaho drives interstate for the flatbed division of Tri-Valley Transportation Co. in Plymouth, Utah. A while back I accompanied him in his tractor-trailer rig to Barric Gold Mine, located some 40 miles distance from Carlisle, Nevada. Along the way I got a chance to nap in the big sleeper located directly behind his cab. It was fairly roomy and had some of the comforts of home (color TV, stereo, nice mattress, clothes closet, a small fridge, and electric hot plate). Once we left the asphalt we traveled about 30 miles on a gravel road that the gold mine kept up and frequently watered down to hold dust to a minimum. My friend Sid had made this same run many times before, hauling out big electric arc welders, generators, and structured materials. This time we were taking them some drilling equipment.

This strip-mining operation covered approximately a thousand acres and retrieved gold from surface pits. A 15-foot-high chain-link fence with rolled razor wire atop it surrounded the compound. Uniformed armed guards greeted us with business-like courtesy at the front gate. We were directed to park in a specific area, where Sid's entire rig was hosed down with hot steam. The same thing happened again before we left a few hours later. This procedure is done to prevent the possible accumulation of gold dust to the truck frame or its tires.

Colossal trucks capable of carrying 40 *tons* at a time were everywhere. I took the time to measure one of their rubber tires and found it to be 12 feet in height. We were not allowed to speak with any of the more than 700 workers but were kept in a restricted area for truckers alone the whole time we were there.

On the way back to Salt Lake City, Sid's radio dispatcher called with another hauling assignment for the following day to somewhere in Wyoming. He told her that I was with him, and she replied, "Oh, you're the herb guy." She then posed a question concerning her premenstrual syndrome and asked what could be done for that. She wrote down what I told her and faithfully promised to follow it. "I'll let Sid know the results," she said.

These were the herbs I suggested: black haw, chaste-tree berry, false unicorn root, and red-raspberry leaves. My Hungarian grandmother, Barbara Liebhardt Heinerman, employed some of them in her treatment of similar symptoms with outstanding success. But each one had to be taken a different way. Two tablespoons of black haw are simmered in two-and-a-half cups of boiling water for 15 minutes, before straining and drinking it warm twice daily. Chaste berry is available either as a fluid extract (15 drops under the tongue twice daily) or in capsules (200 mg. twice daily). The last two herbal teas can be made in larger quantities and work better as a blend than by themselves: Boil one quart of water; add one tablespoon of chaste-tree berry and three tablespoons of red-raspberry leaves; cover, set aside and simmer for 20 minutes; strain and drink two cups daily.

The next time I saw Sid he informed me that the trucking dispatcher to whom I had given these suggestions was doing a lot better. "Apparently your stuff helped her out," he said matter-of-factly.

PROSTATE CANCER/PROSTATITIS

Think Red for Prostate Health

Fruits and vegetables that are crimson colored are of great benefit to the prostate. The recent media attention given red, ripe tomatoes on account of their cancer-fighting lycopene is but one example. But there are others not so well known but just as effective: cranberries and cranberry juice, raspberries, strawberries, currants, red grapes, radishes, apple peel, beets, pink grapefruit, red onions, and watermelon.

These should figure in the diets often of men concerned with the health and well-being of their prostate glands. Such foods not only help to prevent prostate cancer but can actually work in its remission, too, in company with regular medical care. Soy foods, though not of a reddish hue, are of equal medicinal value when it comes to maintaining good prostate health.

PSORIASIS

The Man Who Interviewed Lindbergh

When I was in Torrington, CT in early November, 1999 for a health-related public speaking appearance, I happened to pick up a free copy of an alternative newspaper, *The Litchfield County Times Monthly* from the Yankee Pedlar Hotel where I stayed. In perusing its pages for something interesting to read, I came upon a published interview with an elderly journalist from Norfolk, Connecticut, named Seth Moseley. At the time of the article this gentleman was 90 years of age.

He attributed his longevity and remarkably good health to several things. "One of the reasons I think I've hung on so long physically," he said, "is we walked from the farm two and a half miles to the middle of Norfolk, most of two years, to catch a school bus to Gilbert." Another thing was the care and feeding of animals. "My uncle bought Blackberry River Farm, a beautiful estate of [one] hundred acres. We took care of the horses and cows and other animals on that place. It gave us a real joy and respect for other life forms." He also became an avid reader: "developing my mind so I wouldn't lose it."

The only complaint he had in his late life was the recurrence of psoriasis. "It's a periodic thing but you get used to it after a while." Whenever flareups occur, especially in skin-fold areas where high-strength topical steroids can't be used, relief is found in bathing the skin surface with *cold* stinging nettle tea. It helps ease the misery and isn't reactionary to the system like many of the standard medications are.

As for this brief moment in history, here's what happened. He went to Amherst College and became a reporter for the school newspaper, which he eventually parlayed into a position as a legman or "news runner" for *The New York Evening Journal*. While at Amherst he became close buddies with Dwight Morrow, Jr., the brother of Ann Morrow, who married famed aviator Charles Lindbergh.

He vividly remembers how this friendship got him the "inside scoop" of a lifetime. "The phone rang in my hotel room, around one in the morning in Manhattan. 'Moseley, this is Al Williams, the night editor. I recall at a party or something you saying you were a friend in college of young Dwight Morrow. Well, they've just kidnapped the Lindbergh baby.' I'm half asleep and didn't quite grasp the significance of it.

" 'We understand that young Dwight Morrow is in the house in Hopewell, New Jersey, in the Lindbergh home. He was called home from college . . . Go on out there as soon as you can . . . and see young Morrow and see Lindbergh and talk to them.'

"So I ran out of the hotel, buttoning my fly as I went through the lobby. This is the biggest story in the world, I thought, and so it was. I ran to the train at 34th Street, got on the train, and said to myself, 'I'm ahead of everybody.'

"So I'm sitting next to this guy. He turns to me and says, 'My name is Brett, and I'm with the *World Telegram.*' And I said, 'You've been with them for about 25 years.' He said 'yes.' So I was up against some pretty rough guys. I didn't say anything. I didn't want to tip him off. I got off the train and there were 100 reporters already in town and 200 state police. Everyone [was] milling around the streets in Norfolk."

Well, with a little cunning and stratagem, young Moseley managed to meet Mr. Lindbergh and personally interview him. He was the first one to report to his editor of a ransom note demanding $50,000 and that the kidnapping was a professional job carried out by more than one party. For his daring efforts, he got himself a five-dollar raise, but this "Crime of the Century" case cemented his journalism career for good. He went on to interview such notables as the reclusive Greta Garbo, who refused to speak with any reporter other than Seth Moseley.

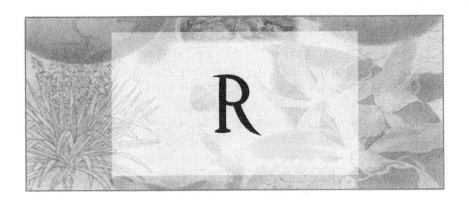

RABIES

When Medical Emergencies Were Self-Treated

There was once a time in our country when certain medical emergencies were self-treated. This necessity usually resulted from a lack of knowledge in the medical profession on how to handle such a problem or the scarcity of doctors in those times or the costliness of the provided care. Today things are certainly much different, and something as serious as a rabid bite from an infected animal or bat is *always* treated in a local hospital.

However, it is worth looking back on some of the things that our early ancestors resorted to when a rabies case cropped up now and again. One method was to make a strong concoction of tobacco tea by gently boiling the leaves for a while until only half the liquid remained. The resulting solution was quite strong due to the intense nicotine present. In a few diaries of those from the southern states, who had good reason to use this formula, it was always reported to be of great benefit.

Belladonna or deadly nightshade was another common standby. This herb was used extensively during the Middle Ages in the practice of witchcraft and magic. Its chief alkaloids, atropine and hyosine, have been used in orthodox medicine for some of the same symptoms ascribed to rabies. It was used as a tea and fluid extract. But due to its poisonous aspects, great care and good judgment always were used whenever any part of the plant was employed. Today, it is still very much a part of homeopathy, although in a safer form, I should add.

RASH

Quarry Opposition

In the latter part of the 1990s, The Church of Jesus Christ of Latter-Day Saints (the Mormons) launched their greatest and most expensive building project ever in downtown Salt Lake City—a huge, amphitheater-like auditorium costing in excess of one quarter of a billion dollars and capable of seating an estimated 26,000 people. At that time no other single building project anywhere in North America required such a vast amount of concrete as this did. The Conference Center, as it came to be called, was faced with large granite tiles retrieved from an old pioneer stone quarry in Little Cottonwood Canyon that still belonged to the LDS Church.

A storm of fierce opposition arose when Church officials made known their intentions of putting their pioneer quarry back into operation. Wealthy non-Mormon residents in the areas surrounding it threatened litigation for fear that the constant commotion of blasting and large trucks going to and from the quarry might endanger lives or depreciate property values. Rock climbers abhorred the thought of these big majestic boulders being torn asunder and hauled away. And environmentalists hated the thought of existing vegetation getting destroyed or animal wildlife being disturbed in any way.

Trouble Results in Classic Rash

A few of the quarry personnel employed specifically to oversee the site during its period of heaviest activity became pretty well stressed-out due to the excessive vandalism and threats. Midnight stalkers would occasionally drain oil from all of the heavy equipment or pour honey, molasses, or sugar into fuel tanks, resulting in costly delays and very expensive repair work. One woman, whose name I won't give, received personal threats on her life as well as those of her children. This soon brought forth a severe rash upon her body, which spread from the neck to both sides of her midsection.

She consulted several dermatologists and was given a number of different prescription ointments and creams to use, but all without much success. Each day during her tenure of employment at the quarry her condition kept getting worse. She had just about given up all hope of finding any relief when I was introduced to her through a mutual friend.

My Recommendations

Sidney Wilding is a long-distance truck driver for Tri-Valley Transportation in Plymouth, UT. His company, along with others, was contracted by the LDS Church to haul huge slabs of granite to a specialty rock company in Idaho Falls, which would then cut them into uniform slabs using a large, diamond-tipped, water-cooled saw. After this the smooth surfaces were given a rough-textured look using hot-steam pressure. I accompanied him to the quarry one time and watched with fascination the method used for separating the granite.

A straight line is measured across the top part of a granite ridge. A series of holes are then made with some type of air-driven machine. Blasting wire about the thickness of a little finger bone is next threaded into each hole, leaving a six-inch tail sticking out above the surface. The holes are filled with liquid blasting putty, and these various wire extensions are then connected to a fuse wire hooked to a blasting cap. Someone shouts, "Fire in the hole!" and then a few seconds later an electronic charge detonates everything. But instead of expecting the kind of loud blast that dynamite always produces, there is more of a muffled "poof" instead. Doing it this way produces very little noise, a minimal amount of dust, and doesn't fracture the rocks so severely. A small group of mountain goats on another ridge higher up the mountain slope looked on curiously but made no real movements to speak of when the charge went off.

Following this little spectacle, Sid introduced me to the woman with the rash. I recommended that she take a high-potency vitamin B-complex (four tablets) and vitamin-E oil (three capsules) daily to help her nerves. For the rash I suggested mixing two tablespoons of liquid glycerine with one-half cup of dairy cream and brushing this on the skin using a narrow, natural-bristle brush. She commenced this at once and within five days saw remarkable progress in the clearing up of this vexing skin affliction.

RED EYES

His Remedy Lives On

As big as the health-food industry is these days, it still is "comfortably small" at the top for the principal players to be known by most everyone connected with it. I had known the late Michael Q. Ford for a couple of years. He was still the leader of the National Nutritional Foods Association (NNFA) and doing what he did best in the natural-products industry—traveling, talking, lobbying, and working—when he suddenly died at age 49 of an aortic aneurysm on the morning of September 23, 1999. One of the industry's most visible figures was gone.

Those of us who knew his negotiating skills, total dedication, and tireless efforts on behalf of natural products silently mourned his passing but would always respect his loyalty and courage. As Senator Tom Harkin (D-Iowa) observed, "Because of this man, the lives of countless Americans are better off."

When Ford and I first met at a past NNFA function, he asked about the books I wrote. Upon being informed that they dealt with folk medicine, food therapy, and general nutrition, he quipped, "Say, Doc, got anything to help my liver?" He made reference, of course, to his inordinate love for single malt Scotch and "blood-rare," thick and juicy steaks. He felt his liver needed a little "botanical overhaul" as he wittingly termed it. I suggested the roots of dandelion, turmeric, and goldenseal.

In turn, he proffered one of his own. Pointing to his eyes, he remarked, "I periodically suffer from red eyes. I think it's probably an allergic reaction to the dirty air of the different cities I frequently have to visit." He then gave me the solution to his problem. "I order some hot water and two bags of chamomile tea at whatever restaurant I'm dining in. I drink the tea but take care to remove the tea bags and slip them in a small plastic zippered bag I carry with me sometimes. When I get back to my hotel room I slip them out of the bag, turn each eyelid back, and slowly squeeze their wet contents into each eye. Then I cover both eyes with a dry, folded hand towel and lie back on my bed for a few minutes to let the tea work. The redness and itching are gone and I'm not bothered anymore after that."

Michael . . . you'll be sorely missed, but your memory lives on in the remedy you left behind during a single meeting with this prolific health writer.

RESPIRATORY-DISTRESS SYNDROME

Help from Hot Salsa

Rudy Chinchilla is a migrant laborer working in the agricultural fields of Northern and Southern California. For some time he had been experiencing breathing difficulties, which a farm doctor finally diagnosed as respiratory-distress syndrome. But the medication he prescribed alleviated the situation only a little bit.

An old *curandero* (Hispanic folk healer) who happened to be traveling with another band of migrant farm workers recommended that Rudy start eating some hot salsa on a regular basis and said that this would eventually cure his problem. He started doing this every day and within a short time his breathing returned to normal.

RESTLESS-LEGS SYNDROME

A Spa Treatment

Tammy L. is a masseuse working out of a Florida health spa in the city of Fort Lauderdale. She is experienced in a relatively new kind of treatment called LaStone Therapy, created by an Arizona massage therapist in August 1998. She informed me while I was in Miami in mid-November 1999 for a health lecture that she uses this quite a bit for people suffering from restless-legs syndrome and claimed it helps them sleep better at night.

LaStone therapy involves the strategic mixture of hot and cold basalt stones. After a customer lies down on her padded leather table, she covers the body with towels, including the eyes. She then places smooth, warm stones all over (and beneath) the person's torso—the legs, chest, abdomen, hands, and back (even putting them between the fingers and toes eventually). After this she commences alternately massaging the individual with her hands and the stones.

She described the sensation of warm stones being massaged into the human body as a series of Vicks VapoRub "scented explosions" but without the eucalyptus smell. While doing this to her clients, she will also serenade them with a number of gentle lullabyes memorized over the years. She believes mental and emotional stress has a great deal to do with jumpy legs and thinks that singing pleasant songs while administering deep-heat massage can help just that much more.

Those unable to find a massage therapist certified in LaStone therapy can still massage their own backs of the legs with a little Ben-Gay ointment while lying down and listening to soft, relaxing music of some kind.

RINGWORM

The Cold Caffeine Treatment

In the early part of November 1999 I was traveling with a friend, Mark Petersen, through parts of Tennessee, Arkansas, Georgia, and Florida for a series of public-health lectures. We drove from Memphis, Tennessee, to Batesville, Arkansas, for one meeting. Along the rural route we were taking we stopped in the little hamlet of Strawberry and got ourselves a bite to eat at the Strawberry Grocery & BBQ. The owner fixed me up with a big BBQ sandwich that included cole slaw, of all things. It sounded strange but tasted downright good!

Knowing we weren't from around those parts, the owner asked our place of origin and the purpose of our business in the Razorback State. Being told I was a doctor of natural medicine and author of numerous health books, the owner volunteered this useful piece of information: Bathe any ringworm infections with *cold* coffee or *cold* cola drink several times daily. Not only would it relieve the itch but it would also clear up the fungal infection.

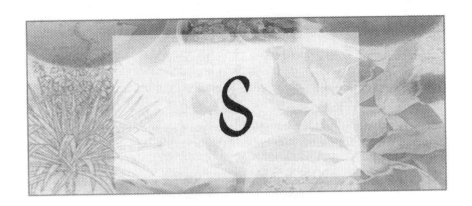

S

SCIATICA NERVE PAIN
(See "Pain")

SHINGLES
(See "Herpes," "Itching," "Rash," "Skin Problems")

SHOCK

An Executioner's Approach

The following material is ABSOLUTELY TRUE! I make this declaration only once in the text, right here! I do so because of an incredible interview I had, quite by accident, with an ordinary-looking fellow who has a highly unusual and almost one-of-a-kind job. His first name is Robert but he asked that I never reveal his last name. We met in Orlando, Florida, at a hotel buffet in early November 1999, just before I flew to Miami for a final public speaking appearance. Robert was of average height, slightly paunchy, somewhat balding, and bespectacled. He was a retired *electrician*, but continued working at another side job when necessity demanded it that also involved electricity, though in a most bizarre way!

We were standing side by side slowly making our way down the food line, loading our plates with whatever seemed tempting and delicious when the conversation started. He said that 22 years ago he saw an ad on television and responded to it. Out of all the male applicants who applied, only he and another fellow made the final selection. They were subjected to several weeks of intense training that included a great deal of psychological counseling.

Both men worked for the Florida State Department of Corrections and had the specific task of putting condemned killers to death. "I get paid $150 for each execution," Robert said matter-of-factly as he put some beet salad on his plate. "The state lets me know ahead when an execution is to take place. We agree on a rendevouz point and after parking my car I'm then taken in a corrections vehicle to the prison." Upon arriving he dons a black hood and robe and then peeks through a one-way glass window into the execution chamber to make sure that everything is ready. The condemned prisoner has already been securely strapped into the old and well-used wooden oak chair known affectionately among the guards as "Ole Sparky." Robert then throws a big circuit switch that sends several thousand volts of live electrical current into the killer's body. Once a doctor has made the final determination of death, Roger then takes off his garb and quietly leaves the facility under heavy guard.

Noticing that each of us was alone, I suggested that we sit together at a table and continue the conversation, to which he agreed. "In the very beginning it was a hard thing to do," he admitted. "No amount of counseling can prepare you for something that requires the taking of human life on a pretty regular basis. This sort of thing can shock the senses, if you know what I mean."

But Robert observed that *how* you look at something tragic or very unpleasant can make all the difference in the world. Right off, he stated that a strong belief in God and a *consistent* practice of religious worship always helps a great deal. "I've gone to church after every execution and find solace and strength in prayer and private worship." A second thing would be attitude: "There are certain elements in our society that, just like bad teeth, need eventual extraction. I'm like a dentist in that sense, only without the Novocain!" He also sees it like "pruning a rose garden." "Sometimes you have to cut away some of the old, ugly ones in order to preserve the rest that's truly beautiful." And finally, "Never, ever dwell on past misfortunes—they'll drive you crazy if you do! Always look forward with a presence of mind, instead of backwards to the behind," he joked in rhyme.

I mentioned high-potency B-complex and vitamin E, as well as calcium and magnesium being good for shock, but he claimed to have never needed any of these. "It's all up here and down here," he finished, while pointing to his head and heart at the same time.

SHORTNESS OF BREATH

Not an Ordinary Place

You won't find row after row of cement-block cages at the Rolling Hills Refuge Wildlife Conservation Center in Salina, Kansas. What you will find, though, is immersion-style viewing and a profound respect for the exotic and endangered animals that reside there.

During a summer visit there I discovered how the exhibits merge so effortlessly with the landscape that I was soon unaware of the barriers separating me from the surrounding wildlife. I had the feeling that I was truly one with the animals. And that is good, because it's precisely what the refuge hopes to accomplish.

The exhibits are large and constructed to duplicate the environment the animals live in when in the wild. For instance, the chimpanzee exhibit has trees to swing on, objects to stimulate their curiosity, and grass growing on the ground. The terrain within the enclosures is designed to permit the animals to escape from the eyes of the viewing public when the attention gets to be too much.

The winter exhibits are also constructed with the health of the animals in mind. Not only do they protect the animals from the elements, but they are designed so that creatures and humans don't inhale the same air.

As of summer 1999 the refuse is home to 73 species of animals. Many, like the pair of South African white rhinos, are endangered. Also calling the refuge home are giraffes, Indian rhinos, bongo, white tigers, chimpanzees, orangutan, Bactrian and Dromedary camels, Amur leopards, lions, snow leopards, Transcaspian urials, kangaroos, and so much more.

This 500-acre facility is an educational nonprofit foundation dedicated to the conservation and propagation of rare and endangered species. It has four primary goals in mind: propagation, education, research, and exhibition. What makes this place different from a zoo is that it has a lot more space so animals don't need to be subjected to public scrutiny for 24 hours a day. Stress due to prolonged contact with humans is greatly minimized. This helps keep them healthy and maximizes their breeding potential. What is learned there about breeding and keeping animals fit is shared by staff members with their colleagues around the world.

What the Snow Leopard Ate

One of the park personnel told me of a rather interesting incident that occurred with one of their snow leopards the previous summer. It had been showing signs of apparent fatigue but without any indication of having exhausted itself through intense physical exercise such as running or climbing. One of the refuge veterinarians made a determination after carefully examining the sedated cat that it was suffering from an unexplained shortness of breath. Since no infection was apparent, no antibiotics were prescribed. While staff members were still trying to figure out what to give it, the leopard itself let nature take its course and come up with a remedy suitable for the problem. Instinctively, the big cat started to chomp on grass just as a cow or horse might do. This was certainly a startling development for refuge personnel, who know that leopards are carnivorous by nature and prefer eating raw, bloody meat to green veggies. However, by the second day the animal was breathing fine again and had regained most of its lost energy.

Sometime later I tested this out on human subjects who suffered from asthma or emphysema. Only instead of having them chew grass, I had them mix wheat- or barley-grass powder with water or juice and drink it that way, morning and evening. They reported that their breathing capacities nearly doubled or tripled and that their lungs seemed to work much better for up to six hours after swallowing a glass of *liquid* grass.

SHOULDER PAIN
(See "PAIN")

SINUS INFECTION
(See "INFECTION")

SKIN CANCER
(See "CANCER")

SMOKING

Kicking the Nicotine Fit for Good

In October 1986 I toured Indonesia for several months, gathering material for future books like this one and doing a little work for the government in helping it to upgrade its own herbal (*jamu*) industry. In one of my many encounters, I met a professional secretary named Josephine Hetarihon, who then resided in the capitol of Jakarta and was 35 years of age. She had been a heavy smoker for many years, but finally managed to quit when she converted to Mormonism. She did it with the aid of carrots and conviction.

Here is her story. "It was on September 26, 1979, that I finally managed to quit smoking. I had been smoking two packs a day of Dunhill [brand] before this. I started smoking when I was in junior high school at the age of 15. A friend suggested that I use carrots to help me quit. It took me about two weeks on this carrot program until I was able to quit smoking altogether. I would eat about two to three carrots a day. I found that the sweet taste of the carrots satisfied me enough so that I didn't crave a cigarette."

SNORING

In Search of "Live" Archaeology

Many years ago an old archaeologist friend of mine (since deceased) had the good fortune of visiting the Wai Wai Indians in a remote part of British Guiana, when those Carib-speaking Aborigines still lived in a fairly uncivilized state. In narrating some of the events connected with this trip for my benefit, he complained that civilized Indians had lost their native hunting prowess and were incapable of silently stalking forest game as they once could do. He spoke of Charlie, one of their expedition guides, who would go out every day with his rifle but return to camp empty-handed most of the time. And when asked what had happened, he would answer rather gloomily, "Me shoot monkey. But him stay in tree, hang by tail."

When provisions began running low, he and his compatriots started looking for an *uncivilized* Wai Wai hunter. They soon found one named Yukuma. And though he was the proud owner of a gun himself, he always left it in his hut and instead took his two bows and stacks of arrows with him whenever he went hunting. He declared that ammunition was scarce and that too many shotgun blasts frightened off the game. My informant and his colleagues glided down a river in two dugouts with Yukuma in one of them and civilized Charlie in the other. As they approached a sandbar where the water ran clear and shallow, Yukuma stood tense in the prow with his long bow ready. Quickly the string twanged and the arrow disappeared. Then the hollow cane shaft reappeared once or twice as the impaled quarry tried vainly to escape to deep water—and a large fish was added to their larder. The native seldom ever missed, my archaeologist friend noted.

He said that at the first glimmer of dawn, when the dripping jungle rang with the melodies of waking birds, Yukuma reached for his bow and arrows and stole quietly away. Then he could soon be heard imitating a bird call by blowing on a leaf cupped between his hands. A few moments later a feathered creature invariably responded. As the sounds continued, his progress could be traced by the others beneath the forest canopy. Soon he would return with the too-talkative bird for breakfast and a monkey to add its rich, sweet flavor to their evening stew.

Bananas Stop Snoring!

The first few nights in the jungle weren't too bad, the old archaeologist declared. But his colleagues didn't appreciate his loud snoring, complaining that it kept them awake most of the time. He was beside himself and didn't know what to do. But when their uncivilized Indian hunter was made aware of the problem, he gave a wide, gracious smile and trotted off into the forest, only to return a few minutes later with some small "finger bananas" (so named because they get no bigger than a man's thumb). He peeled several of these at night and had my archaeologist friend slowly chew on them, being sure to run the mashed fruit pulp over the entire roof and sides of his mouth with his tongue. "It took me 20 minutes to eat two tiny bananas!" he declared. "I felt a little foolish to have to chew these things like a little baby would." But this seemingly strange advice had its desired effect that night and every one thereafter—this archaeologist *never* once snored, much to the delight and happiness of the rest of his company. And only when he missed doing this on a couple of occasions did the snoring return!

SORES

A Prehistoric Makeup Kit

About 45 years ago the only uncivilized people still left in the British Guiana jungle were the Wai Wai Indians. An archaeologist acquaintance of mine, now long-deceased, who visited them on several different occasions, told me quite a bit about them. He produced a color photo of some of them standing beside him: They appeared of stocky build and had light-brown skins glistening with red paint. Clad only in the simplest of breechcloths and aprons and carrying long bows, they wouldn't have seemed out of place at all in Columbus's time save for the strings of glass trade beads girdling necks, legs, and arms.

Every Wai Wai warrior wore bangs and carried a "vanity case" to apply his daily makeup. An ocher paint made from red clay and lime juice was painted in stripes on the cheeks and forehead.

Several archaeologists, including my friend, sustained skin sores along the way. Their native hunter, Yukuma, brought them some of his natural cosmetics, which were painted over the sores with some twigs. The alkaline minerals in the clay and the strong citric acid from the sour fruit helped to kill the infection and dry up the sores within a very short time. In a matter of only a few days nearly all their skin afflictions had disappeared.

SORE THROAT

Citrus Juice and Wild Honey

An old archaeologist friend of mine, whom I greatly respected, shared with me some of his adventures among the Wai Wai Indians of British Guiana way back in 1954. At that time, these Carib-speaking savages were the only uncivilized jungle tribe then remaining in that British possession. He spoke of the differences between civilized and uncivilized tribal members, which has been previously noted.

He related how one of their great hunters, a warrior named Yukuma, had not only an incredible native prowess for getting game, but also an equal capacity for downing food. "One day my colleagues and I decided to keep a record of his consumption," my friend said. "What we noted was incredible even by our own standards of gluttony: one large bird, several pounds of smoked fish, half a huge cake of cassava bread, half a monkey, two long sticks of sugar, six plantains, a small lizard, two large rodents, and large quantities of pepperpot broth! And this was all for just *one day,*" he concluded with emphasis.

One of their number came down with fever, chills, and a nasty cold. Swallowing became difficult when the person's throat became severely inflamed. None of the drugs brought with them seemed to help very much. Yukuma stepped in and offered the wisdom of jungle medicine instead, which was readily and gratefully accepted. He cut open a number of wild limes and squeezed the juice into an empty calabash. He procured some honey from a wild bees' nest nearby and mixed this with the lime juice. He then gave this to the sick person to take sips of. A few hours later the throat pain went away and the fever and chills cleared up of their own accord.

SPIDER BITES
(See "INSECT BITES AND STINGS" AND "POISONING")

SPRAINS
(See "SWELLING")

STOMACHACHE

Sudanese Comfort

Some years ago while in Egypt on folk-medicine research, I accepted an invitation to accompany several Egyptian doctors to the Sudanese capital of Khartoum directly to the south of Cairo, three hours by airplane. We were fortunate to arrive *after* (instead of before) a dreaded *haboob*. This gritty storm called to mind the "black rollers" that swept America's Dust Bowl of the 1930s. The haboob we had barely missed had been blowing up three days previously and coated everything in the city with black desert dust.

One of the best remedies for stomach distress of any kind involves the soaking of two pitted, chopped dates or a couple of diced figs in two cups of boiling water for 15 minutes. The liquid is drunk, and the fruits can be nibbled on as well. Gastric relief comes within minutes and works like a charm every time!

STREP THROAT
(See "SORE THROAT")

STRESS

Whale-Sighting and Other Activities

Stress is a necessary part of all our lives, but good only in measured amounts. It helps drive human ambition to get things done and serves as chemical inspiration for other motivating desires. The problem, though, is that everyone gets too much of it on a fairly frequent basis, which can cause serious health problems over a period of time.

One New York City stockbroker who was being overwhelmed with the unbelievable stress connected with his frenzied schedule had tried all of the conventional approaches but without much success. As he told me a while back, "The B-complex and vitamin-E and calcium–magnesium combo worked for only a short duration. The antistress herbal formula [consisting of skullcap, valerian, and hops] helped for a while but eventually wore off. The weekly half-hour massage treatments provided only temporary but meaningful relief. And the biofeedback therapy only soothed the upper layers of my brain but never really reached deeper into my mind where the real anxiety was. So, after doing all of this for six to eight months and investing a certain amount of valuable time and financial resources, I stopped everything cold turkey and took an assessment of what had been accomplished. To my own disappointment, I found that much, if not all of it, had been only temporary 'Band-Aids' at most and that I was still just as much stressed out about things as before. That's when I concluded that I needed a whole change of focus."

To get this, the harried stockbroker spent a weekend by himself in the Canadian maritime province of New Brunswick, a place filled with both aquatic and terrestrial wonders. He stayed one day in the port city of Saint John and drove a rental car to the Bay of Fundy, an hour's distance away. There he enjoyed watching 40- to 50-foot tides (high enough to submerge a four-story building) constantly pound the steep cliffs and empty beaches. In describing the spectacle to me in exciting tones, he used words such as "dramatic" and "awe-inspiring" to describe what he saw.

After that he drove northeast of Saint John for 45 minutes to the small hamlet of Sussex. He parked his vehicle and rented a mountain bike and took a 20-kilometer, two-hour ride around the town, confirming its place as the covered-bridge capital of the province. His excursion took in not only covered bridges, but also Holstein farms, fishing harbors, and tree-lined hills. "The extra intake of oxygen was just what my body needed," he recalled. "It gave my system an explosion of energy no supplements could ever do. That aerobic workout cleared all of the cobwebs from my mind."

But the real treat lay just ahead. "I returned to Saint John and traded my bike for a boat," he continued. "Whale-watching was the last item on my unscheduled agenda, so I booked in with the Fundy Tide Runners. Captain David Welch navigated a 12-person Zodiac Hurricane some 20 miles out into the Grand Manan Channel. As we skimmed across the waves at 30 miles per hour, this outfitter promised the group that we would spot bald eagles, harbor seals, and, of course, big whales. He certainly delivered on what he said. So did a 25-ton humpback whale, which came close enough to our vessel to show off its magnificent girth with a gigantic splashing full breech that left everyone soaked to the skin. But the adventure was fantastic, and we all laughed and cheered at once when part of the ocean came crashing down as the whale dived deep."

Following this weekend sojourn, my informant was able to return to the hectic routine of busy Wall Street with a renewed sense of purpose. "This trip enabled me to endure the next seven weeks of nerve-wracking stress without much trouble. I then scheduled another weekend visit for myself to the same place and have been making periodic retreats to New Brunswick ever since. It's what I found works best for me in the types of stress to which I'm always exposed."

The purpose in mentioning this individual's story is twofold: It demonstrates that conventional methods of coping with stress such as nutrition, herbs, massage, and psychological therapy may not work for everyone; and that getting out in nature more often to exercise and enjoy its wonderful surroundings is probably going to do more for the body than anything else.

Psychological Counseling from Animals

Many people today seek professional counseling from a mental-health expert to help them cope with the emotional stresses brought on by modern living. This "couch therapy" is always expensive but doesn't work every time.

What does work, though, is animal companionship. I, for one, ought to know. In my life I've had a number of dogs and one cat. My current canine friend is a big cross-mix border-collie–St. Bernard named Sparky, which I obtained as a gift from a Hutterite family, Eli and Anna Kleinsasser, at Fairhaven Colony near Ulm, Montana, in mid-July 1999. He accompanies me most everywhere I go except for long-distance trips. He is the love of my life and brings great joy to my soul.

Even some police chiefs benefit from animal therapy. *The Daily Universe* for Monday, October 11, 1999, interviewed the campus police chief for Brigham Young University in Provo. The last three sentences of this insightful article underscore the tremendous value that animals can be for relieving stresses of all kinds. "[Chief Robert] Kelshaw said he depends on his llamas and other animals to reduce his stress. 'My favorite ones are two males, which I have named Frick and Frack,' he said. 'There is not a psychologist in the world that can do what my animals do [for me],' he said."

STROKE

Quality Food as Prevention

On Friday, October 22, 1999, I attended a lecture at the Baltimore Convention Center to hear nutritionist Rebecca Wood, author of *The New Whole Foods Encyclopedia* (Penguin, 1999) speak to nearly 50 people on the best ways of determining quality foods for stroke prevention and management of other cardiac disorders. Her speech was part of the annual Natural Products Expo East held in Maryland every fall.

"Food is the key to total cardiac care. It is so simple and so fundamental and yet so misunderstood. Three times a day we can savor good food and have quality health," she told the group. "I like to eat good food because I like to feel good. It's such a small effort for such big results."

She then proceeded to outline six essential properties in determining quality foods that would "nourish the body, take care of the heart, and give general health all around." The first is to choose foods that are favorable, with inherent quality. Choose natural and whole food that has been grown without chemicals or genetic engineering, she stated, and you will not only taste, but actually *feel* the difference.

Second is to choose regional foods, Wood said, offering as a primary example a monkey and polar bear. "Can you imagine a polar bear eating bananas, or a monkey eating seal fat? It just doesn't make sense." The same principle applies to humans: It's much more logical to eat foods that are grown in your own region. This, she believes, would help reduce strokes right off the bat.

Eating seasonal foods was her third determinant, while choosing underutilized foods ranked fourth on her list. "The higher a food's commercial value, the more it's been futzed with, or manipulated," she declared. Instead of an ear of corn, go for the underutilized celery root to get more nourishment. The minerals in celery are cardiotonic and promote greater circulation.

Fifth, choose wild foods instead of cultivated. "Wild foods make you feel wild—much more so than any domestic plant would," she noted. Her choices included sea vegetables such as sea palm or kombu, wild rice, wild mushrooms, wild garlic, pine and Brazil nuts, and some fish.

Last, favor intact or whole foods instead of processed. Not only do intact foods have much fuller flavor, she observed, but they offer optimum nutrition and "flow" (a Chinese term referring to digestion).

The following morning at 8:30 A.M. her discussion on whole foods for heart care continued. Root vegetables, dark leafy greens, whole grains, nuts and seeds, berries, and some stone fruits were all good for the cardiovascular system. And herbs such as garlic, onion, sage, thyme, and rosemary, because of their antioxidant properties, keep the heart from becoming diseased or worn out. Other herbs such as cayenne and ginger prevent clotting.

STUFFY NOSE

Stinky Things Clear the Nostrils

The annual Natural Products Expo East convention was held in Baltimore, Maryland, the weekend of October 22–24, 1999. Among the 20,000 attending were three Native Americans from northwest Colombia. Rogelio Mejia, Danilo Villafana, and Margarita Villafana are Tayrona tribal members who live in the highlands of the Sierra Nevada mountains. They were brought to the Expo by Organic Valley and Frontier Organic Products Co-op, purchasers of organic coffee from the Tayrona. It was the first time any of them had ever been outside Colombia.

I had a chance to interview one of them while at the convention. Danilo Villafana told me through an interpreter that he was overwhelmed by Baltimore's many towering buildings and streets choked with cars. He felt a certain sense of hopelessness about Westerners' chances of reversing their headlong plunge into an ecological disaster of Orwellian proportions. He strongly believed that the capitalistic greed of corporate America and elsewhere would destroy planet Earth much sooner than anyone realized.

As we spoke, I noticed he would take a whiff every few minutes from a small leather-skin bag hung about his neck. When I asked him what it was for, he replied, "To help me breathe better." He said that since he and his companions had come to Baltimore, his nose had become stuffy because of the many impurities in the air. He removed the bag from around his neck and untied it so I could inspect its contents. I discovered several pieces of crushed garlic, two broken bay leaves, and some coarsely ground nutmeg. I took a whiff myself and discovered how quickly the strong odor cleared my sinuses.

He claimed that "stinky things clear the nose and keep you from getting sick." He said that he had never had a cold in his life as long as he kept this bag on his person and regularly replenished it with fresh herbs.

SUNBURN

Supplement Sales at $10.4 Billion

The sale of dietary supplements in the United States reached $10.4 billion for the period of July 1998 to June 1999, according to a report from the Bellevue, Washington-based Hartman Group. The study, "Herbs and Supplements: A Year in Review," reports the vitamins and minerals category was responsible for 56 percent of the year's sales while herbs and miscellaneous supplements accounted for the remaining 44 percent.

The report indicates that the industry is continuing to grow. Total sales volume is on the move, and more new customers are exploring alternative health options. In 1999, 71 percent of U.S. households are using dietary-supplements products, a 3 percent increase from 1998, according to the study.

Interestingly, while everyone talks about the Internet, it figures in at less than 1 percent of total sales volume right now for all dietary supplements. What is envisioned for the Internet, however, in terms of dietary supplements is a complement to a lot of the existing industries. The Hartman Group speculates that the Internet is where the next big growth spurt will be for the dietary-supplements industry.

Japanese Sunburn Treatments

Consumer sales for health supplements is also big business in Japan. But it is on the networking side where the real gains are made, as opposed to wholesale–retail. I went to Japan in late September 1999 to do a series of health lectures for a Tokyo-based health-products company that also sells its items in North America (see Synergy Worldwide in Products Appendix for additional information).

I was astonished to learn just how many Japanese people take trace element germanium on a fairly regular basis for improvement of skin condition and energy needs. An average of one capsule twice daily with meals is the standard practice.

And interestingly, the Japanese are big fans of aloe vera. They slather this natural, soothing gel over their skin to help heal sunburns, cuts, scrapes, nicks, gashes, and blisters. Men use it on their faces after shaving, and women like to apply it to their underarms and legs after using the razor in these places for hair removal.

Another unique treatment that the Japanese have come up with is something called Angel Cream. This rich and soothing balm really helps heal even the worst skin irritations, such as contact with poison ivy, for example. The two principal ingredients are borage-seed oil and frankincense-tree extract. These botanicals are especially useful for dry-skin conditions such as eczema or psoriasis, wind- and sunburns, and insect bites. The balm is frequently used on the feet, knees, and elbows to soften hardened skin.

SWEATING EXCESSIVELY

A Typical Japanese Breakfast

On Wednesday, September 22, 1999, I stayed at the fairly new and fancy MielParque Hotel in Nagano, Japan, site of the 1998 Winter Olympics. My traditional Japanese breakfast consisted of a tossed salad, cold cooked rice, several types of cold cooked fish, and accompanying sauces. I had a selection of various cut garden vegetables to choose from when building my "breakfast salad": On top of thin-sliced green lettuce I placed some tomato wedges, thin-sliced onions, thin-sliced red radish, zucchini wedges, shredded carrot, shredded turnip, and shredded daikon radish. I omitted the usual salad dressings and enjoyed the freshness of these crisp vegetables. Many Japanese favor such salads for their morning breakfasts.

Seaweed Reduces Perspiration

While in Nagano I spoke with a ski instructor who helped coach several Japanese skiers to medal victories in the 1998 Games. He said that sweating was a common occurrence during intensive training for those wearing well-insulated ski outfits. While antiperspirants helped to some extent, he favored an even better method. He increased the daily allotment of sea vegetation for those working under his personal guidance. He made sure they had at least two helpings of some kind of cooked seaweed with their meals every day during their training period. He believes that the rich concentration of minerals, including iodine, was a significant factor in reducing overall body perspiration by as much as 65 percent.

SWELLING

Japanese Martial Arts

During a fall 1999 speaking tour of "The Land of the Rising Sun," I investigated the Japanese martial arts, collectively known as *budo*. Three of them are well known abroad: judo, aikido, and karatedo. In judo, there are three phases of training: *kata*, standard forms practiced over and over for as long as one practices judo; *randori*, a free-style exercise in which techniques are applied; and matches, in which points are given for throwing the opponent, pinning him or her, or gaining his or her submission by neck-holds or armlocks. There are many ways, all codified, of doing these.

Aikido, whose origins go back to the eleventh century, shares one principle with judo, that of turning the power and direction of the opponent's attack to one's own advantage. It also has throwing techniques and holds, the latter based entirely on bending or twisting the opponent's arm or leg and applying what are called pain-holds. It is especially well known for developing the ability of a man or woman to thwart the attack of a much larger person, in which respect, speed, and decisiveness are most important.

Speed and decisiveness are also the objectives of training in karatedo, which derives from very closely guarded techniques developed in Okinawa and not publicly introduced to the rest of Japan until 1922. It, too, has *kata*—elaborate but performed gracefully and very rapidly—and these are based on blocking, striking, and kicking, so that it resembles boxing more than wrestling. The only weapons are hands, arms, legs, and feet, but these are so powerful, after long training, that actually making contact with one of the vital points of the human body can be lethal.

Treating Customary Bumps and Bruises

Students of the martial arts—and there are hundreds of thousands of them—are urged to develop physical soundness, agility, and coordination by their instructors. But above everything else, Japanese trainers insist that their students maintain good judgment and be of sound character when practicing any of these arts.

And as anyone who is well acquainted with the martial arts knows, a certain amount of physical suffering is to be expected, regardless of how careful both participants may try to be. One of the popular remedies widely used is a sports-rub liniment. Consisting of aloe vera gel, mountain-spring water, Oriental-mushroom extract, eucalyptus oil, peppermint menthol, and aspirin derivatives, this soothing cream takes away the aches and pains of the numerous bumps and bruises normally encountered in routine martial arts practice. This liniment is also used for aching muscles, sore joints, pulled hamstrings, sprains, cramps, bursitis, backache, and tendinitis. (See Product Appendix under Synergy Worldwide for more information on this Miracle Rub.)

Another popular method is the hot-tub-soak–ice-pack application. The injured martial-arts participant soaks his or her bruised muscles in a tub of hot water for five minutes, then steps out and applies an ice pack to the region for a similar length of time. Back into the hot tub the person goes again, followed by another ice treatment outside the tub. This back-and-forth routine typically lasts 40 minutes but really brings the swelling down.

SYPHILIS
(See "GONORRHEA")

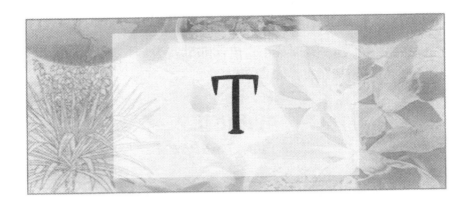

TAPEWORM
(See "INTESTINAL PARASITES")

TEETHING

A Stone-Age Remedy

Some years ago I had the good fortune to accompany several or-
nithologists into the clouded thick forest interior of New Guinea's
central highlands. They went there to study and photograph rare and
exotic birds; I went along to study the primitive ways of prehistoric
tribesmen. Our trip took us first to Lae by airplane on New Guinea's
east coast. From there we flew in a Beechcraft for an hour inland before our pilot landed the aircraft on a flat plateau in a long, narrow
valley.

I looked out my side window and noticed that the cultivated area
below looked prolific and luxuriant. The terrain was spiderwebbed
with ancient trails, deeply scored here and there by wider roads. Flat-
topped promontories capped with casuarina forest and dotted with native gardens stretched between the hills like outflung fingers. We
landed on top of one of these.

Here in the Kubor Range dwelled Stone Age tribes. At that time
Kubor women still preferred adorning their bodies with sequin-like
shells (called tambu), exotic bird feathers, orchids and other colorful
flowers, tree bark, and paint made from crushed seeds, petals, and
roots. Some of the younger women wore hollow reeds or cassowary-

wing quills through their nose septums, making them appear as if they had gigantic handlebar mustaches. Kubor warriors also wore decorative nose quills; both men and women had their nose sides and septums pierced in infancy, and twigs were used to keep the flesh from closing up. Men wore helmets woven from the inner fiber of casuarina bark, skirts made of leaves or grass decorated with numerous shells that made a clacking sound as they walked, armbands of woven orchid fibers, and sandals made of tree bark lined with fresh moss.

A good remedy for reducing gum pain in young babies who start teething is to rub *fresh* pineapple juice over the gums with the forefinger morning and evening. I tested this out back home among friends of mine whose own infants were about to go through this phase of growth. Several of the moms who tried this out on their kids reported that there was hardly any crying as the first teeth slowly made their appearance. If fresh pineapple isn't available, then the juice from canned pineapple slices can be substituted, although there will be additional sugar present. I believe it is the enzymatic action of bromelain that somehow manages to curb gum pain as new teeth grow into place.

TENDINITIS
(See "Swelling")

THUMBSUCKING

Prehistoric Solutions

A long time ago I was invited along by several other scientists on a bird-sighting expedition into the cloud-fringed rain-forest interior of the central New Guinea highlands. Our final points of disembarkation from the aircraft that brought us there was atop a luxuriant green plateau strip that lay between the Bismark and Kubor mountain ranges.

The Kubor tribespeople with whom we stayed were very friendly and exhibited a great deal of kindness and attention to our basic wants and needs. With the assistance of an interpreter, I learned some simple prehistoric solutions to common everyday problems. For instance, infant thumbsucking was prevented by sticking the tiny thumbs into a sliced half of a ripe lime and then turning it sideways several times so as to saturate the skin and nail with adequate juice. It was allowed to dry by itself in the air. Whenever a baby felt inclined to suck his thumb, the bitter taste of the dried lime juice would be there to discourage him from doing so.

Insect bites and stings were routinely treated with a mixture of pig grease—a highly treasured commodity back then—and wood charcoal from the cold embers of a dead fire. I substituted Vaseline for the pig grease and mixed it with a small amount of powdered charcoal. This I daubed on mosquito bites and insect stings and found it worked wonderfully well in reducing the itching and inflammation.

THRUSH
(See "YEAST INFECTION")

TICS AND TWITCHES

Nerve Spasms Stopped

One of the first trips I took across the Pacific to a wild and exotic place happened over a quarter of a century ago. I was given the opportunity to go along with some scientists who were engaged in studying rare birds in tropical New Guinea, and I gladly seized the chance. We spent over a month in the mountainous highlands with Kubor tribespeople. For us it was a return to the Stone-Age past of our very distant ancestors. We learned from these primitive people that a lot could be done with little.

During the time spent there, we subsisted on fish, pig, parrot, snake (green tree python), chicken, sugar cane, bananas (regular size and thumb size), peanuts, onions, various stone fruits similar to plums, and different kinds of squash. The cooked food was either boiled in water, roasted over a spit, or wrapped in plantain leaves and baked in a fire pit with hot coals covering them. After a couple of weeks on this jungle fare, I became aware of the fact that a slight nervous tic that I had had in the right side of my neck for a long time had ceased. I wondered about this and thought it quite remarkable but gave the matter no further attention until I returned home sometime later. Only when the tic resumed did I start seriously thinking about why it had ceased during my stay in New Guinea.

After making some logical deductions, I figured that it had probably been the potassium-rich foods consumed so frequently when boarding with the Kubor natives. I tested out this theory by taking 800 milligrams of potassium every day with meals for a month. Sure enough, the nervous tic stopped. I recommended the same dosage to an older woman, a librarian, who suffered from an eyelid twitch. In four days it stopped. To me this was enough evidence to indicate that potassium is a wonderful nutrient for stopping nerve spasms.

TOE PAIN
(See "GOUT" AND "PAIN")

TONSILLITIS
(See "SORE THROAT")

TOOTHACHE

Where Nose Rubbing Was Once Popular

Sometime back in the early 1970s I flew to the central highlands of New Guinea with some people who were photographing and studying rare and exotic birds. Our group stayed in the thatched grass huts of prehistoric tribes inhabiting the Kubor Range of mountains.

We discovered that New Guinea folk liked to gather weekly in some of these thatched shacks for a sit-down dance called the sing-sing. Like the square dance of frontier days, it was an important social event for all. While older people sat around the sides laughing and chatting, dancers would take places on a low, horseshoe-shaped platform, where they chanted, swayed, and finally rubbed noses in the fashion of their forefathers.

Prior to this event, however, dancers would smear their faces with treasured pig grease and red and yellow paint until colorful bird feathers and decorative shells hung glued in place. Then men and women sat down in rows in flickering firelight. The men swayed and chanted in a nasal singsong. The women, ornaments tinkling, moved in cadence in the opposite direction. Both sexes seemed to go into a trance as the chanting grew louder and bodies swayed faster. Any kind of physical contact was strictly *verboten* except on the noses and faces. However, women could grasp a man's shoulder with one hand if they so desired.

Women brushed noses gently, first with the man on the left, then with the man on the right. Heads rolled in opposite arcs while seemingly hinged at the nose. In this way heavy coats of paint and grease transferred themselves from face to face like inks on newspaper printing-press rollers. The final intensity came when faces were vigorously mashed together, sometimes injuring the physical features and eventually making noses soft and flabby.

Peanut and Onion Relief

One of the most ingenious forms of oral pain relief employed by these Kubor tribespeople was the use of peanut and onion. A few peanuts would be shelled by hand and then crushed into powder on a grinding rock with the aid of a small oval stone that fit nicely into the palm of the hand. Next a wild onion would be peeled and also crushed to a pulp the same way. The powdered peanut and wet-onion mass were then mixed in a gourd with two fingers until a fine paste was formed.

A piece of tree leaf was cut to about the size of a man's thumb. Some of this moist paste was then smeared onto one side of the leaf. It was then placed inside the patient's mouth, pressed firmly against the aching tooth, and left there for several hours. During this time the person didn't speak, laugh, or eat or drink anything. I tried a modified version of this using peeled, crushed garlic, clove, and organic peanut butter on a tiny slice of white bread and found it worked equally well in relieving tooth pain. I believe it is the combination of potassium in the peanuts and sulfur in the onion and garlic that stops the transmission of pain from the brain to the rotten tooth.

TORN LIGAMENT

Dancing Nose to Nose

In the previous entry (toothache) I mentioned a little about the novel nose-rubbing custom that was once a part of the Kubor tribal culture some decades ago. I had accompanied others to the New Guinea central highlands to study folk medicine, while my friends did some bird watching and picture taking. I found the nose rubbing so fascinating that I took extensive notes on it and present here a more detailed account of the same.

It was late in the evening before everyone filed into a long, low thatched building called the sing-sing house. It measured some 20 by 40 feet in size and had along its sides and across its far end a foot-high dais of woven bamboo-like grass.

The darkness within was lightened to some degree by two small fires. As soon as my eyes had adjusted to the blackness, I saw two young girls kneeling across a narrow aisle from each other. Now others trooped in silently and took their places beside them, about two feet apart, tucking their string aprons modestly between their legs and sitting as immobile as carved wooden statues.

Presently, accompanied by a sudden rustling and chattering outside, a line of handsomely decorated men pushed through the hut's small door and encircled the U-shaped formation of girls until each stood behind the partner previously allotted to him. At a signal, the head chieftain sat down with his back to the aisle, a girl facing him on either side. I noted, with some astonishment, that his partners were two attractive and very young maidens; the entire group of girls ranged from about 12 to 17 years of age.

Soon a voice from somewhere in the hut began a singsong chant. Louder and louder it rose as the men chimed in and took up the beat. The women remained mute. Gradually, as the music took hold, girls and men began to sway slightly. The chieftain's partners, firelight flashing on their tawny skins, moved whiplike with the dance's rhythm, ornaments tinkling and swinging across their naked breasts. The women's torsos never touched his, though. But one of them gripped the old fellow's shoulder as if she were squeezing a grapefruit, and her nose rubbed his.

It was this nose rubbing that appeared to produce the ecstasy that seized the dancers. Man and girl would touch noses for an instant, lightly in the beginning of the song. Then the girl, eyes closed in mock pain, would sway ever more rapidly from the man on her left to the one on her right. Nose touched nose for longer and longer periods, until at length the girl rested against one man for as long as five minutes, face frozen, body relaxed, nose pressed against nose with something akin to ferocity.

Yet, for all the intensity that the participants put into the dance, it retained an informal and agreeable air. Children raced around the aisles; old people tossed wood on the fire and chuckled and chattered among themselves; and when each bout had ended the girls broke the tension with a peal of laughter that was at once both mischievous and mirthful.

Mud Pack for Pulled Hamstring

One of our number, while setting up his camera equipment in a tree to photograph some rare and exotic bird species, accidentally slipped from his perch above and almost fell to the ground. However, one foot became entangled in some vines which broke his fall and possibly saved him from more serious injury. As it was, though, his leg suffered a good jerk, resulting in a very painful pulled hamstring.

We helped him out of his awkward upside-down position and placed him on the ground. Some of the tribesmen came around to inspect the difficulty. One of them trotted off to a distant hut but soon returned with an old sorcerer who was skilled in natural healing as well as in the black arts. Our injured companion removed his trousers and this old healer poked and prodded the sore leg until quite satisfied, after enough yelps of pain had been given, that this was the problem area to be dealt with.

He gave instructions for some mud and moss from a nearby stream to be brought forthwith. When the task was completed, he tore up the moss into small bits and mixed it with the mud. He had a hollow gourd brought, out of which he took a generous handful of white powder and threw it into the moss-mud mixture. (I later learned this was pulverized animal bones, quite rich in calcium and magnesium.) He then proceeded to rub this slimy material on our friend's leg until the entire hamstring was adequately covered with it. He let it dry and had the dressing kept in place for several days. The ornithologist then washed away the dried mud and discovered to his delight that all pain and swelling had disappeared.

A similar treatment can be performed on any torn ligament with pretty good results. Instead of mud, use green clay and mix in the amount of water called for on the package. Green clay can be purchased from most health-food stores. In place of moss, use some dried seaweed that has been sufficiently moistened with water. Add one-half cup of calcium–magnesium powder and stir everything until a fine, even paste forms. Be careful of how much water you use—too much will make the mixture sloppy and too little will make it stiff. Apply to the injury much as you would wet plaster of paris when forming a cast. Let it dry and leave it in place for 36 to 48 hours. Remove after the specified time by washing off with warm water. Also, take some calcium–magnesium internally during this time. You will be surprised at just how efficient this heals torn ligaments.

TUBERCULOSIS (TB)

A Nutritional Plan of Action

In the earlier part of this century, tuberculosis (TB) was a common problem for many people. Then antibiotic drugs were invented that helped bring it under control. Now with the appearance of newer, more aggressive strains of drug-resistant TB, those old medications no longer work as they used to.

In order to bring this more virulent TB under control, it is necessary that a full complement of nutrients be taken regularly until such time that the body has been able to manage things on its own. Fish oil (3,000 mg.), omega 3-6-9 fatty-acid complex (two capsules), echinacea–goldenseal combo (two capsules), garlic (one capsule), grapeseed extract (one capsule), and a super antioxidant (two capsules) should be taken each day with meals. (See Product Appendix under Earth's Pharmacy for details.) Wild Turkish oregano (two capsules) and veterinary-strength vitamin E (Rex Wheat Germ Oil, one tablespoon) are also useful. (See Product Appendix under Anthropological Research Center for additional information.)

It is also essential that a person with TB make periodic trips to the mountains, forest, and seashore, where good, clean air that is highly charged with health-giving negative ions can be constantly inhaled. Simple deep-breathing exercises, such as those taught in yoga, should be learned and faithfully practiced. This will do the lungs an immense amount of good.

The diet needs to be altered as well if this current super-TB is ever to be brought under control. No sugar, salt, or fat should be consumed. White-flour products need to be avoided. Stay away from commercially prepared commodities. Foods should be raw, live, and whole as much as possible. Leafy and root vegetables, seaweeds, and some *fresh* fruits such as melons are very nourishing. Good sources of protein include whole grains, nuts, seeds, soy, avocado, and some fish.

The best beverage is water, preferably mineral or spring. And it should always be taken warm, *never cold.* Organic grape and cranberry juices make wonderful and delicious beverages, even when served at room temperature. They, along with tomato juice or low-sodium V-8 or carrot juice, help to detoxify the system and get out much of the TB germs.

A person's strength should be conserved and wisdom used in performing any physical activities that demand a certain amount of energy. Remember that the body is under assault and needs to conserve strength in order to fight this terrible infection. Do everything in moderation, but try to keep active by walking, swimming, and bicycling.

Sometimes a deep, nagging, persistent cough may pass for TB, with humorous consequences. I was on an airplane flight from Orlando, Florida, to Miami in the middle of November 1999. I had been coughing for a spell due to dust in my lungs. A forty-something businesswomen dressed to the nines and with an air of importance about her sat beside me. After a short time she became impatient and lectured me rather sharply on my barking. I apologized with a faint smile and said it was TB, whereupon she promptly got up and moved to another seat further back in the plane without another word.

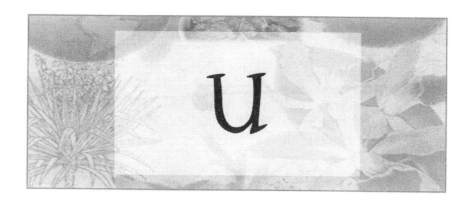

ULCERATIVE COLITIS

Isle of the Unexpected

In the south-central part of Italy on the Bay of Naples lies the city of Naples. It is a major seaport and tourist center. The bay is dominated by the famous volcano, Mount Vesuvius. The city itself is very crowded and noisy, famous for its songs, festivals, and gaiety. I opted for more serene scenery and hopped a boat heading toward the island of Ischia a few miles to the west.

The island has two main features, an old abandoned castle and an inactive volcano. *Isola d'Ischia,* as the locals call it, covers 18 square miles and has approximately 41,000 residents. A Hollywood film company (Warner Bros.) built two old eighteenth-century windjammers for the Burt Lancaster movie, *The Crimson Pirate,* which was filmed there in 1951. Numerous scenes were shot aboard these two replicas, one representing a 28-gun Spanish galleon and the other a pirate's vessel complete with a skull-and-crossbones flag atop her mast. Local residents still spoke fondly of this production many years afterward.

While poking around in one of the local *farmacias,* I came across row after row of patent medicines, herbal pills, and assorted pharmaceuticals lining the walls. I randomly selected one small square, red-colored tin decorated with various plants and took it to the owner in front, who spoke a little English. Not understanding Italian, I inquired as to the purpose of this medicine and an explanation as to some of its contents. The pharmacist described to me symptoms closely akin to those for ulcerative colitis, since he didn't know the exact medical term in English for this colon disease.

The pills, about the size of round BB shot, were made from dried cherries, dried grape skins, dried *nespole* (an apricot-like fruit), and dried black mussel (a common shellfish in those parts). His limited English didn't permit the translation of two remaining ingredients, but I was happy and satisfied with what he had been able to give me. Upon my return to the United States sometime later, I began testing the applications of some of these things in a few people whom I knew to have ulcerative colitis. Only, instead of the pills, I used the fresh articles. Right off the bat, I discovered cherry juice to be too acidic, although it worked great for arthritis and gout. A combination (equal parts) of dark grape juice and apricot puree, however, worked surprisingly well. There was a noticeable reduction in the inflammation of the colon lining and more infrequent episodes of painful, bloody diarrhea. One-half cup of this juice mix was taken with meals twice daily.

ULCERS

Milk on the Hoof

In 1973 I visited Naples, Italy, but found myself drawn more toward the island of Ischia, lying just to the west and in front of the Bay of Naples. I stayed with the Liberato family for the short time I was there. One morning I heard the sound of tinkling bells and small hooves clattering over the pavement. I stuck my head out of my upper-story bedroom window and noticed a goatherder below squat on his haunches, push a pail beneath one of his nanny goats, and start milking for the woman of the house. Milk on the hoof, right at your front door, I mused—now *that's* service supreme.

I went downstairs and enjoyed a repast of fresh goat's milk, homemade goat cheese, and baked bread. My hostess, Carmela Liberato, explained that she was about to make a soup to take next door to an older woman who suffered from severe ulcers. I watched as she cut up chunks of green cabbage and put them into an aluminum pot. Over this she poured some fresh goat's milk and then set the pot on her stove to let the contents cook on medium heat for about 30 minutes. She then strained the liquid into a ceramic pitcher and gave it to her sick neighbor. This was a remedy, she told me, she had learned from her grandmother many years ago. The woman next door drank a cupful of this goat-milk–cabbage soup with every meal. She said it seemed to help her ulcer a lot.

URINARY-TRACT INFECTION
(See "BLADDER INFECTION")

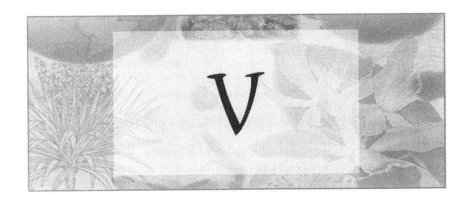

VAGINAL PROBLEMS

Diet and Work Make All the Difference

Italy's third largest city is Naples. It is noisy, overcrowded, and somewhat polluted. But to the immediate west of its famous Bay lies *Isola d'Ischia*, a small paradise unto itself. Here I spent a few glorious days nearly three decades ago, finding not only much folk-medicine information but also a great deal of hospitality to boot.

I got around fairly well, considering I don't speak Italian. Some of the people I stayed with or visited spoke some limited English. And where I needed an interpreter, one of the local Catholic priests who had been educated in America gladly helped me out where he could. Some of the questions I asked were easy, but others were more difficult, especially those few involving delicate health matters that women don't want to talk about.

But I had an ally in my hostess, Carmela Liberato, and her husband, with whom I boarded while there. She seemed to understand the importance of my interviews and wasn't at all offended when I asked highly personal health questions. Now, one of the things that intrigued me was the near *absence* of common vaginal problems, which seem to plague many American women. In company with Carmela, we visited a number of her women friends where I had opportunities to pose questions regarding the health and state of their female organs. Most of the time, such inquiries would draw blank stares or shoulder shrugs. And the accompanying comments would indicate to me that, in most instances, the women had never experienced such problems.

324

So I began investigating the typical island diet and found part of my answer there. Ischia women subsist on a great deal of seafood in the forms of sardines, octopuses, squid, and other types of fish. I went with Carmela to a local fish market one bright, sunny afternoon. Striped umbrellas were set up at various stands shading the brilliantly colored fish. Carmela chatted amiably with one vendor as he weighed great slices of ocean sunfish, a foot across, and we marched off to her house with it dangling on a string.

This species is also called *pesce di luna*, or moonfish, because of its nearly circular shape. Carmela cooked the liver and intestines separately from the rest of the fish. A popular island dish, by the way, is a highly seasoned chowder consisting of fish, mussels, and bits of octopus and squid. One day for lunch Carmela made her husband and me some fried baby-octopus sandwiches accompanied by a few salted, hard-boiled eggs. It took some getting used to eating a piece of meat with tiny, curling tentacles poking out from the sides of two huge chunks of bread, I must admit.

This large variety of seafood provides a great deal of iodine and other trace elements to the female body, which, I believe, are critical for the maintenance of its internal organs and glands. A fair amount of goat's milk and goat's cheese are also consumed, thereby giving these women ample calcium and magnesium.

The women of Ischia also perform a number of daily tasks that involve a good amount of manual labor. The constant stooping, bending, lifting, stretching, and other physical movements of the arms, hips, and legs keeps bones strong, organs sound, and blood flowing constantly to these areas of the body.

I concluded from my observations and notes that the healthful diet and active lifestyle kept these women virtually free of those vaginal problems that women in Europe and North America struggle with so often.

VARICOSE VEINS

An Italian Secret

I've been to Italy on several occasions. The first time was to Naples and its adjoining island of Ischia. Later visits took me to Milan and, of course, to the overpopulated, smog-ridden, crazy capital, Rome, with all of its wonderfully old and architecturally stunning religious edifices.

Each trip was made for health-related purposes. Two were strictly information-gathering visits for future health books and one was to read a paper at an international scientific symposium and to collect data on folk medicine that interested me.

One singular aspect of all these visits was the low incidence of varicose veins among Italian women. Among the elderly, there was an astonishing absence of this, while with women below middle-age, there were infrequent occurrences. How was it, I wondered, that so many Italian women of all ages had managed to avoid getting those swollen, knotted clusters of purple veins on their legs that are so commonly seen in Europe, America, and Canada?

A little mental deduction helped me to figure out this puzzle. The Italian diet consists of large amounts of olive oil, olives, garlic, fish, cheese, grapes, and good, whole-grain bread. The many vitamins and minerals contained in such foods prevented normal veins from becoming inflamed or obstructed in some way. Even something as simple as taking a tablespoon of extra-virgin olive oil every day and chewing one garlic clove can make all the difference in the world. Eating grapes and Italian cheese on a fairly regular basis keeps blood flow normal and uninterrupted.

VOMITING

Juices to Stop It

The inclination to vomit is nature's way of emptying the stomach of contents that are making the body sick and that it wants to reject. However, *repeated* vomiting isn't a good thing and can be prevented by drinking small amounts of certain fruit juices. Juices of pear, guava, mango, and papaya are fairly neutral and won't upset an already disturbed gastrointestinal tract. Instead, they will help soothe and calm a nervous stomach. They may be taken at room temperature or slightly chilled. The ripe fruits are also good to eat when the gut won't accept anything else. Stay away from anything acidic, such as citrus fruits or juices, pineapple, and cherry.

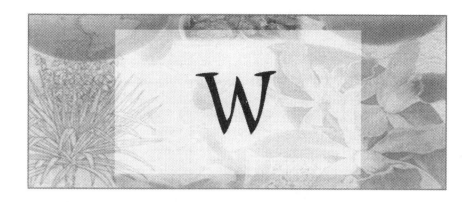

"WALKING" PNEUMONIA

A People of Unknown Origin

The land of the Basques straddles the frontier between southwest France and north-central Spain. This is a region of rugged mountains, rolling hills, and green valleys dotted with straggling villages of white houses roofed with red tile.

Estimates vary on the number of Basques in Europe; it is believed to be somewhere around a million, "give or take a hundred thousand." Nearly two thirds live in the four Spanish provinces of Guipúzcoa, Alava, Navarra, and Vizcaya, while most of the French Basques inhabit the former provinces of Labourd, Basse, Navarre, and Soule.

Basques proudly refer to themselves as Eskual-dunak and their country as Eskual-Herria. Their origin remains unknown and their language seems to have no clear affinity with any other European tongue. Anthropologists believe these people are survivors from an early Stone Age culture of European stock. Moreover, Basques have blood groups similar to those of peoples in other fringe areas of western Europe, such as parts of Ireland, northern Wales, Scotland, and Iceland. This could mean that they are remnants of a once widespread population.

The Basques themselves have an ancient legend, handed down from father to son, that they are descended from Tubal, fifth son of Japheth, who was the son of Noah. Basques believe that their language remained unchanged at the Tower of Babel and that they still speak somewhat the pure language of Adam and Eve.

A Meal to Fight Lung Infection

The condition known as "walking" pneumonia among farmers and ranchers in the American West has its Basque counterpart in Europe. This lung infection is really a cross between a bad case of influenza and what passes for whooping cough (but isn't). The Basque approach is to give the body ample rest and to nourish it with nutritious foods.

A typical meal consumed almost daily during this bout of sickness includes a dish of *piperrada* and fresh citrus juices. The dish, while loaded with a number of antibiotic and antioxidant vegetables and spices, is really quite tasty and nothing more than a glorified omelet. Everything used in its making is *always fresh*. Eggs, tomatoes, green pimentos, bell peppers, onions, garlic, thyme, tarragon, and basil are the ingredients.

This omelet is eaten at least once a day and served with a freshly squeezed juice combination of Spanish oranges and lemons. The omelet is usually cooked in olive oil or sardine oil. A wide variety of health-giving vitamins and minerals are clearly represented here in such a healing meal. Vitamins A, C, and E, along with calcium, iron, magnesium, potassium, selenium, sulfur, zinc, and germanium are present in varying amounts. They definitely give the immune system a tremendous boost with their nutritional power.

WARTS

An Israeli Folk Cure

Way back in December 1981, an American physician, Matthew Midcap, M.D., of Morganstown, West Virginia, happened to be reading that month's issue of the *Journal of Plastic Reconstructive Surgery*. In it was a short article by an Israeli doctor practicing in the city of Safad who related how he treated a 16-year-old girl with painful plantar warts with nothing but ripe banana peels. Within ten days all of her warts were gone.

Dr. Midcap decided to try this on some of his own patients. One of the first was a male Caucasian, 48 years old. He was a prominent banker in Wheeling and loved to play golf. But a cluster of plantar warts on the bottom of one foot, about two inches in diameter, prevented him from enjoying his favorite sport. By the time he came to Dr.

Midcap's office, he had tried all of the conventional medical procedures available for the removal of warts: acid therapy, cryotherapy, surgery, and radiation. But nothing seemed to have a lasting effect, since the warts kept coming back.

Dr. Midcap cut a piece of ripe banana skin and applied the inside portion to the warts and taped them in place. He instructed his patient to replace the banana skin every 14 hours with another one, making sure to always apply the inside face down on the warts. The man did this faithfully for several weeks before returning to the clinic. Dr. Midcap noticed that by then most of the warts were gone and the few that remained were considerably smaller in size and number. A few months after this all warts were gone, and the banker never had recurrence of them. He was able to play more rounds of golf and improve his swing without further foot pain.

Dr. Midcap believed that the same enzymatic action responsible for the browning or ripening of a banana was at work on the warts and actually penetrated the skin deep enough to kill the viruses responsible for them.

WHEEZING
(See "ASTHMA," "EMPHYSEMA" AND "HAY FEVER")

WHOOPING COUGH
(See "COUGH" AND "INFECTION")

WORMS
(See "INTESTINAL PARASITES")

WOUNDS

Ancient Ways

Some years ago an Italian-born and trained pathologist relocated to Boston, Massachusetts, and became a professor of pathology at Harvard Medical School. He later wrote a fascinating medical history, *The Healing Hand* (Cambridge: Harvard University Press, 1975), which covered wound treatment in the ancient world.

Guido Majno, M.D., introduced the subject this way: "A million years ago, as now, a wound implied three major medical problems: mechanical disruption, bleeding, and infection. Nature is prepared to cope with all three; but man can help, even with simple means."

Around 2600 B.C. physicians in southern Mesopotamia, now Iraq, recorded their wound treatments on clay tablets in a unique style of writing known as *cuneiform*. Here is a literal translation of one of them:

> "If a man is sick with a blow on the cheek: pound together fir-turpentine, pine-turpentine, tamarisk, daisy, flower of *Inninnu*. Strain; mix in milk and beer in a small copper pan; spread on skin, bind on him, and he shall recover."

The *asu* or doctor who recommended this knew that *natural* tree-derived turpentine made a terrific disinfectant, while tamarisk and beer help promote healing by drawing the skin and muscle tissue together because of their astringent properties. Milk and daisy and yarrow flowers are anti-inflammatory, as is the copper of the pan in which such is to be combined. The remedy still has practical value even today when *natural* turpentine is used. A California company sells a natural, undiluted, golden-colored liquid pitch derived from the bark of yellow pines for wound treatment in man and beast. (See Product Appendix under Anthropological Research Center.)

The most-used botanical ingredient in Mesopotamian pharmacy was *burashu*, or common juniper berry. It, along with pitted prunes, was "pounded together" in a mortar with a stone pestle, mixed with a little wine or beer and some olive oil, and then placed over the wound as a sort of medical plaster and bound in place with clean strips of cloth. Some years ago on our family ranch in southern Utah I had occasion to use some crushed juniper berries on the palm of my hand, which had been badly lacerated by rusty barbed wire. A wet handkerchief was tied around the hand to keep the berries from sliding off. By next morning the swelling was gone and the wound had closed up.

Ancient physicians usually washed wounds with beer, wine, salt, vinegar, and hot water. Sometimes a rubbing of a mixture that included salt and mustard was done to further disinfect the injury. Surprisingly, Mesopotamian doctors paid attention to the liver at the same time, believing that its state of health directly correlated with successful wound healing. Common liver herbs that were ingested included stinging nettle, watercress, and dandelion flowers and leaves.

The resins from certain trees, such as pine, spruce, and myrrh, were cooked with animal fat and alkali to make strong soaps. Their wonderful detergent effects upon open wounds and sores helped to remove anything that might cause infection. Honey was a common commodity often laid into wounds as a sort of "liquid bandage."

The Old Testament makes reference in the book of Isaiah, 1:6, to general medical treatment for such injuries: ". . . wounds and bruises, and putrifying sores . . . have . . . been closed, . . . bound up, . . . [and] mollified with ointment." Dr. Majno substituted the words "soothing oil" for ointment and pointed out that this was a common dressing in those times. Sesame oil was used in Mesopotamia and olive oil in Palestine. "Oil and grease cannot do much harm on raw flesh, and they also serve the useful purpose of preventing the bandage from sticking to the wound, like today's first-aid creams. Bacteria do not grow in oil. In fact, we tested the survival of staphylococci in sesame oil and found that they were rapidly killed."

Medical papyri from ancient Egypt show a similar level of care and attention given wounds. The Edwin Smith Surgical Papyrus is the most ancient and reliable of these medical texts, being a series of medical notes made by three different surgeons between 2600 and 1650 B.C. Here, for the first time, the word "suture" appears. It is also the only medical text totally devoid of magic and religious superstition. This particular papyrus mentioned two kinds of wounds, those with (infected) and without (sterile) pus.

The Edwin Smith Papyrus recommends the washing of a wound with salt and vinegar and then "binding upon it fresh meat." Dr. Majno commented that "meat, namely muscle, can also act as a clotting agent; crushed tissue in general works very well. An elderly neurosurgeon told me that in his younger days, before safe clotting agents had become available, it was standard practice to check very small hemorrhages on the surface of the brain by applying a tiny bit of muscle taken from the same patient (perfect hemostasis is crucial in brain surgery). This treatment was based on the simple rationale that "flesh mends flesh." Majno noted, "Lots of people still bind a steak over a black eye; the practice is current among boxers."

Wound pain was treated in a remarkable way. Willow-tree leaves and salt were crushed together and applied as a poultice. The salicin content in the leaves was equivalent to powdered aspirin on the wound, thereby reducing both pain and inflammation at once.

While the liver was important in wound care to Mesopotamian doctors, the colon was given special attention by Egyptian physicians. "They apparently took the anus as the center and stronghold of decay," Majno wrote. To them, "the most frightening aspect of the feces was that they contained a very pernicious thing called *ukhedu.* Ukhedu lay there dormant, but might arise and settle anywhere else in the body." The word cannot be literally translated but means something like "rot" or rotten stuff par excellence. "The ukhedu was either male or female, caused disease and pain, and could be killed. It could work its way into the vessels and travel around, setting up disease. In essence, what bacteria can do, it could do. And, of course, ukhedu could turn up in a wound."

That is why they lavished so much attention on the colon. As Majno cleverly stated, "The Egyptians soothed it, refreshed it, smoked it, and somehow even kept it from twisting and slipping." Enemas and laxatives such as aloes and senna were frequently employed to keep the bowels functioning.

Wounds in Verse

The oldest witness of Greek medicine is Homer. During the eighth century B.C. this Greek poet wrote two distinct but complementary epics, the *Iliad* (telling of the fall of Troy) and the *Odyssey* (telling of the wanderings of Odysseus on his adventurous way back to Ithaca).

"There are 147 wounds in the *Iliad*—31 to the head, all lethal," wrote Majno. "The overall mortality rate was 77.6 percent. The single nicety about this bloodshed, besides the poetry, is that for the first time in history one hears of the wounded being carried off the battlefield and tended in barracks, *klisíai,* or in the nearby ships."

Wound care, though, was quite abysmal. "The first attentions that [the wounded] received in the *klisiai* were a seat, lots of story-telling, and a cup of Pramnian wine sprinkled with grated goat cheese and barley meal, served by a beautiful woman." The wine was usually drugged with opium so that the wounded individual couldn't feel the pain from his wounds.

Fresh fig poultices were commonly employed to draw out the pus from wounds and to help reduce the swelling. Fig juice was administered internally and used to wash wounds with. In modern times, figs have been used experimentally to reduce tumors, with some modest success.

The Greek *iatrós* relied on animal fats, tree resin, and minerals for wound treatment. A whitish, greasy ointment, consisting of equal parts of goat grease, swine grease, olive oil, frankincense, and zinc oxide was liberally applied to the injury. Dr. Majno said, "Greasy applications such as this one were kept for clean wounds near healing. They were supposed to make the flesh grow" back.

It was left to the Arabs to introduce fragrant spices and sweet-smelling resins, gums, and balsams for wound treatment. The oils or rose, cinnamon, and cloves, frankincense, myrrh, mastick, and musk were the preferred medicaments of choice. They not only made festering wounds smell better, but also served as effective antibiotics in killing pathogenic bacteria capable of causing serious infections.

The many emperors of ancient China enjoyed reading and listening to good music. Their libraries contained books of poetry, such as the *Shih Ching* of "Book of Odes," at least as old as the *Iliad* and the *Odyssey* and not entirely devoid of medical interest. Such books, as well as compilations by many different philosophers, contain numerous references to wounds of all types and various solutions for taking care of them. External wounds were classified as *yang*, while those inside were considered to be *yin* in nature. Acupuncture was used in the beginning "to let out pus or blood." Over the course of time, however, it became a means of "spiritual drainage" also, releasing "bad energy," while stimulating "the vital energy . . . that fills the cosmos." Wormwood was repeatedly used throughout Chinese medical history in wound management: It could be burned on the skin (moxabustion), poulticed over a wound, or else given internally as a hot, bitter tonic. Wormwood is useful because of its antibacterial and anti-inflammatory properties. It is also one of the best herbs to use for expelling parasites from the system during times of sickness.

The holy books of India contain medical terminology within their ancient religious writings. The strong tradition of *Ayurvedic* medicine stems from these books. The *vaidya* treated arrow wounds in classic Hindu style—first, with a chanted mantra of some sort, second, with dietary prescriptions that *excluded* all animal flesh but included ripe fruits, juicy vegetables, and plenty of water, and finally, with herbal drugs such as turmeric root (the primary ingredient in curry powder), garlic bulb, lotus stems and leaves, onion, and fennel seed.

Roman medicine borrowed from all of the other previous cultures. The physician Galen used ephedra, milkweed, cassia cinnamon, black pepper, garlic, pitted dates, henbane, for the healing of gladiator wounds and the sedation of their pain.

WRINKLES

A Surprise Call

On Thanksgiving Day, Thursday, November 25, 1999, I was relaxing at home with my father, Jacob, and brother, Joseph. We were ready to sit down for a natural turkey dinner with all the trimmings but minus the chemical additives and synthetic hormones. My cross-mix border-collie–St. Bernard dog, Sparky, punctuated the quiet with two sharp barks as the telephone rang. The caller ID showed it was from June Smith.

She introduced herself as a fan of one of my Prentice Hall health titles, *Healing Herbs & Spices,* which she said "contained more information than all of the other herb books put together" in her small collection. She was 38 years of age, lived in Tennessee, and worked full time in an aluminum factory near her home making heads for engine blocks. "But in my spare time I work with herbs to help others get well," she said.

Relax Your Skin with Wrinkle Resolvers

The first part of our lengthy conversation consisted of natural things that are useful for the skin. She brought up the topic of wrinkles herself. "I have *by intuition* [more about that later]," she noted, "come up with three herbs that will actually *relax* [her term] the skin enough to do away with many of them." And while they are amazingly effective for this, these are things that have to be gathered from the outdoors on a regular basis and used in their *fresh* state to work.

"I go outside into the woods a short distance and cut off three cedar twigs about three to six inches long, making sure they're fully green. Then I go down by a creek nearby and harvest about half-a-dozen male ferns, two inches fully grown with no brown in them. Then I gather up about one-and-a-half feet of honeysuckle vine, leaves and everything. I always wear gloves when I do this and put everything in an empty onion sack or small cardboard box.

"When I get back home and am ready to take a warm bath, I crush each of these herbs in my hand and squish them into a ball. This I place inside a cotton handkerchief (or something equivalent) and tie the ends together into a big knot. This keeps the botanicals from floating around in my bath water. I then fill the tub with hot water and place this covered ball of herbs in it. I get the water as hot as I can stand, but not so that it's scalding and would injure the skin. These crushed fresh herbs have about ten minutes to let their natural contents get soaked out by the hot water. Just before stepping into the tub, I'll add a little cold water but only enough to make the heat tolerable.

"I lie back and soak in this herbal bath up to my neck for about 15 minutes or until the water becomes lukewarm. I'll wet a clean washcloth and lay it over my face so that some of these herbs can soak through the pores. When I first did this I was absolutely amazed at just how silky soft my skin became. Wrinkles that were apparent before seemed to almost disappear before my eyes. What I think happens is that the herbs open up the skin's own oil glands, allowing them to lubricate the skin more. I'm not kidding when I say that after a long soak like this, my skin feels as if I just applied baby oil to it.

"It would be nice to patent this, but the drawback is that these herbs must always be gathered and used *fresh*. I'm mentioning this in case you can use it in one of your books somewhere."

I told June that while something like this obviously worked quite well, the ingredients weren't always readily available to everyone. Therefore, the remedy couldn't have wider application. I mentioned several natural products I had seen being used by a number of Japanese women for maintaining soft, wrinkle-free skin. These products included Aloe Magic, Revitalizing Toner, Advanced Face Cream, and Anti-Aging Serum and were distributed by Synergy Worldwide (see Product Appendix). I said that each of them contained various botanicals and other natural ingredients that helped to rehydrate, soften, and nourish the skin so that wrinkles, rashes, and a leathery feel weren't as apparent. Japanese women love beautiful skin and go to great lengths to keep themselves young looking for as long as possible.

June pointed out that her herbal bath soak also helped old surgical scars from being so "puckered looking," as she put it. I added that the Angel Cream and Aloe Magic from Synergy Worldwide accomplished the same thing. In fact, the Total Body Wash that this company sold left the entire body and hair feeling softer, smoother, and silkier. Germanium is a trace element consumed by many Japanese men and women for energy, stamina, vitality, and youthfulness. I told her a little about the Japanese culture in general and how health care is a big part of the consumer consciousness these days.

WRIST PAIN
(See "PAIN")

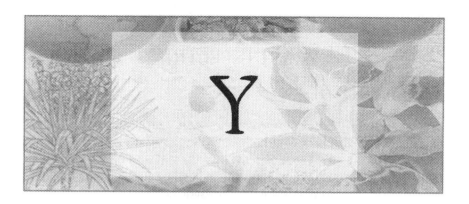

YAWNING EXCESSIVELY

Overcoming Excessive Yawning

I asked June Smith, a Tennessee folk healer, what her own experiences had been in dealing with excessive yawning. She said that it was quite common to see at the foundry she works in. "I'm on the late shift and usually see a number of guys and some of the ladies yawning every so often. You might think I'm nuts, but here are some things I've found to work for me and that have helped some of my coworkers, too. I'll cut me a strip of green bell pepper or a small chip off a raw potato and hold this in my mouth for a while. I don't chew at all, only suck them. They somehow perk the body enough to stop the urge to yawn so much. It really does work.

"You can also use one or two leaves from the saw-briar vine. Just pick, fold, and stick into your mouth and crush a couple of times, then hold next to your cheek like you would do a wad of chewing tobacco. The juice from the leaves mixes with your own saliva and imparts a nice sarsaparilla-mint flavor that revitalizes the system and keeps you wide awake. Fresh peach-tree leaves will do about the same thing. Use one or two leaves in the same way you would saw-briar vine. Vine and tree chlorophyll has a much higher sugar content than the chlorophyll from cereal grasses and is better for revitalizing the body, I think."

YEAST INFECTION

A Soak in Good Scents

During an hourlong telephone conversation, I brought up the subject of candidiasis with June Smith. "I have developed my own treatments for this," she began. "I've had yeast infection off and on for years. I've tried the garlic routine and found it took too long to work. I've also tried various cortisone ointments, but their action doesn't really kick in until six or eight weeks later. That's why I decided to explore some options myself.

"The kind I used to get was similar to jock itch in men. That cedar-twig–honeysuckle-vine parts male-fern-frond combination I spoke of for wrinkles is what works best for me. I also take a handful of the silky down from the ripened seed pods of milk thistle, boneset, or goldenrod and add to these others. I crush everything between my hands and tie them up in a cotton cloth of some kind and add them to the bathtub as the hot water is running. I will then add a few drops of any aromatic herbal oil, such as peppermint, lavender, pennyroyal, or garlic. This mixes nicely with the water before I get into the tub. A little cold water is added so that the hot water doesn't scald the skin. I soak my body for an average of 15 to 20 minutes before getting out. Within a week's time my yeast infection was completely gone. Can you imagine something working so fast like this?"

In Touch with Nature's Cures

From the Tennessee herbalist, June Smith, who gave me so many traditional home remedies, I also learned quite a bit about the healing process. In fact, after we had talked for a while, I specifically asked June to comment on the spiritual connection that one can form with nature. June spoke quite enthusiastically on this topic. "When you're zipping down the highway of life in your fast car or truck with materialistic things on your mind, you don't get much of a chance to notice the weeds off by the side of the road or the small wildlife habitating nearby. People need to get outdoors more often and take some 'back-to-nature' vacations and learn more about the environment around them. Some may interpret this to mean playing or doing recreational kinds of things in the outdoors. But that only complicates the stress they already have. They need to totally divorce themselves from materialism and get out and experience nature firsthand *quietly and thoughtfully*, without a lot of commotion or noisy gadgets or machines to accompany them.

"There is an old theory here in the Cumberlands that if you are addicted to things or people in society or have a bad habit you wish to break, that if you come up here and stand by a tree and stroke its bark and talk to it and ask it to heal you, that some of the spirit life in that tree will permeate your being and slowly effect a change for the better. I know of several city folks who, having heard about this legend, came up this way and jokingly or playfully put it to use. But were they ever surprised some four or six months later at being able to conquer personal addictions such as gambling, smoking, drinking, and even promiscuous sexuality! I know it sounds kind of crazy to city slickers, but the thing *really works* if you do it right and *with sincerity*."

Your Inner Doctor: Intuition

I shared with June some of the contents of this manuscript, which, I noted, was "a year overdue to my publisher and well past deadline time." But I felt grateful to people in the editorial department for their extraordinary patience with me in such unusual tardiness. I mentioned that in the Foreword to this book I had discussed at some length the "healing intuition" feature that has dominated folk medicine so much through space and time. I invited her to give her own spin on this as she saw fit.

"Healing intuition has run in my family background for generations," she said. My paternal great-great-grandmother had it; my maternal great-grandmother enjoyed it, too. And my mother also possesses it, although she doesn't use hers like I do mine. Basically, it's a kind of 'knowing instinct' that you're born and grow up with. If you're pondering on an illness or wondering about a particular health problem, then it seems like you're guided by Something Higher, something definitely spiritual, as to what to do.

"When I'm out wandering in the fields, meadows, and woods around my place, I'll know what to pick for this or that, without having had any foreknowledge concerning the plants being gathered at the time. And if I'm around plants at the time that are *not* supposed to be used, I'll feel a cold sensation in my hand as I reach for them. Or sometimes a kind of humming sensation that comes from the static electricity emitted by an electrical generator when you hold your hand above it. I'll feel one of those kinds of impulses with things I shouldn't be using at the time.

"On other occasions I may suddenly experience a mild headache or stomachache if I'm around plants that are useful but shouldn't be picked at that time or even used for a particular malady I may have intended them for. I'll give you an example of what I mean. During the summer whenever I go blackberry picking in the woods or fields, I simply cannot stand the thought of eating even one of those luscious berries. There is simply no desire whatsoever for them. But during the late fall or winter, when the temperature is much colder and my body can no longer sweat out its poisons, then my system will suddenly crave these berries like mad. I will then load up on them to help flush out those toxins that would have come out through natural perspiration during the summer months.

"Everyone has some kind or degree of 'healing intuition' within them. You may call this medical intuitiveness your own 'inner doctor' if you wish. But it's there in all of us and is very real. What happens, though, with 95 percent of the population is that they get 'out of touch' with this doctor inside them. Their own hectic lives prevent them from ever experiencing it on their own. The crass materialism we see so much of these days is the reason that this inner gift doesn't work for most. And the added stress to people's lives only distances them that much further from their own innate healing abilities.

"Animals are more in touch with their own kind of 'medical intuitiveness' than people are. I've been out in the woods and quietly watched from a distance as a squirrel went straight for a certain tree leaf, nibbled on it, and then spat out the contents into its little paws and rubbed it on a wound or injury suffered from a hunting dog chasing after it. Another time I saw a wild raccoon down by a creek scooping up pawsful of mud and rubbing it over a laceration somewhere on its body encountered from a sharp, manmade object of some kind. These episodes are true. Animals know a heckuva lot more about what to do for themselves in cases of sickness or injury than we do. There's no animal emergency hospital they can go to, unless conveyed there against their wills by well-intentioned but ignorant humans. No! They simply do what comes to them naturally and are pretty well able to take care of themselves in any kind of critical situation."

Finding Medical Intuitiveness

June Smith believes that even though someone may be born with a gift (as she apparently was), that individual must work at developing the gift and maintaining a type of emotional composure and lifestyle that is conducive to it. "There can't be a lot of noise, not much stress, and definitely very little materialistic baggage in one's life if he or she hopes to have this thing grow within them. A person's outlook on life must also be one of hope and joy and a willingness to share with and help others. Compassion of the heart is certainly a big factor here.

"Although the gift has always worked for me in a small, quiet, very personal kind of way, it started to take off when I began working at that aluminum factory in Dixon. I started sensing what was going on medically with my fellow coworkers. Sometimes I would even feel a little of their pain. I would then mention something to them about what I felt, and it was like a big surprise for many of them. Their jaws would drop, their mouths open wide, their eyes get as big as saucers, and they would typically remain speechless for a few seconds before asking, 'How on earth did you know?'

"Some folks in these parts have called me an 'herb witch,' but I've never practiced any form of the wicca religion that I know of. I always pray to God in his holy temple, which is the great outdoors. *That* is my church, and nature is my religion. I don't need to sit in a pew every Sunday with my Bible in one hand and my hymnal in the other to get what I feel outdoors. It was when I started viewing my factory coworkers with *more compassion* that this gift really expanded within me. I believe that *a love for others* is the *true key to success* in everything else in life we do. If we don't have it or fail to display it then we become sore losers in the end and a failure only to ourselves.

"Some say I'm psychic. I don't like that terminology at all. A 'healing intuition' is a more proper term for it. Yes, some sacrifices have to be made if a person ever expects to let this gift become more fully developed. But isn't that what everyone's life is all about? Don't each of us have to make certain choices and decide where we're going and what we want to do with our lives. I think that those who've allowed their medical intuitiveness to become fully expanded have ceased living selfishly. Instead of just living for themselves, they've chosen to live for others. And that is the *key*, I think, to exploring the full range of your own healing intuition. Simplicity, compassion, prayer, and imagination are the things it takes to awaken the 'sleeping doctor' inside yourself."

Those Who Can Guide You

The whole purpose of this book has been to not only bring to readers everywhere reliable remedies that will help them, but also to create a sense of awareness about the medical intuitiveness lying dormant inside them. Both the Foreword and these last few pages contain valuable information that should help in the development of your own 'healing intuition.'

However, those who may wish to have personal guidance on the matter are referred to one of three individuals who can assist them in such endeavors. Two of these are women and, of course, yours truly, the author of this humble work. Each of us has been endowed in our own way with some type of 'medical intuition.' Be advised in advance that *none* of us profess to be medical doctors. One of the other females formerly worked in a state attorney-general's office, while my informant, June, has been a factory worker.

Ms. Smith, who was the major source for most of the information in this last section, agreed to have her location and phone number made public in the event anyone wished to contact her for assistance in developing his or her own healing intuition. Since she works the night shift, the best time to call her is later in the day.

June Smith
(931.582.6253)

The second woman describes herself as a medical intuitive. Although Winter Robinson has never had any formal medical training to speak of, with as little as the name and location she can scan a person's body in her mind and within a few minutes tell the person what's ailing him or her—physically, emotionally, and spiritually. For the last 15 years, she has helped several thousand people for whom conventional medical tests didn't work. She averages almost 300 readings annually. Her clients range from network TV news anchors to politicians and from harried housewives to overworked nurses. Robinson never claims that her diagnoses should be the final answer for her clients. But the data she provides has enabled many of them to decide what tests to ask their regular doctors to perform, which ultimately leads to faster diagnoses. She has written a book on how to use intuition. Unlike June Smith or me, however, Ms. Robinson does charge a fee for her time and services; that is how she makes her living.

Winter Robinson
P.O. Box 484
Bar Mills, ME 04004-0484

Finally, there is the author of this book. Due to a heavy travel schedule every year for lecturing and research purposes that usually takes me all over North America and overseas besides, it is advisable to write instead of calling me.

John Heinerman, Ph.D.
P.O. Box 11471
Salt Lake City, UT 84147

It was clearly the Hand of Providence that guided Ms. Smith to me on Thanksgiving Day (the day on which she was born) and certainly the same wonderful influence that enabled me to learn about Ms. Robinson. And that divine inspiration has also attended me in the preparation of this unique work. If only we look for it more often in our busy lives, it will amaze us at just how often the blessings of Providence have attended us when we've least known it. Greater recognition of this is certainly wanting in all of us.

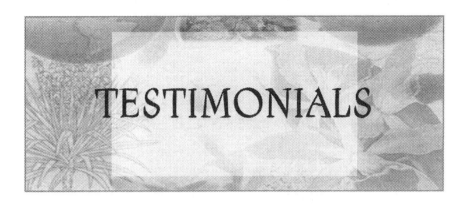

TESTIMONIALS

TESTIMONIALS REGARDING PREVIOUS PUBLICATIONS

I recently obtained your wonderful *Encyclopedia of Juices, Teas and Tonics*. I was very impressed with the simple way in which you communicated your ideas. Clearly, you have a fairly vast amount of information with regard to health issues that I have never seen in print before.
—Judith Jeffers, Long Ground Village, Montserrat, West Indies

I would just like to let you know how much of a difference your books have made to my life. They are informative and structured in such a way as to make them a perfect guide on any health topic. I have totally changed my diet and feel fantastic as a result due to the research that you have done. You are truly special.
—Nitsa Strafkos, Huonville, Tasmania, Australia

I read your book, *Encyclopedia of Juices, Teas and Tonics*. In 1979 I was diagnosed with diabetes and so appreciated the information for healing my condition naturally. Many thanks.
—Maria Rosa Hinojosa De Torres, Villa del Rosario, Zulia, Venezuela

Hello Dr. Heinerman,
I am 26 years old and I live in the Leeward Islands, faced with an active volcano. More than half of the island has been evacuated. However, many of us are holding on. I was really impressed by reading your book, *Heinerman's Encyclopedia of Juices, Teas and Tonics*.
—Patricia Riley, Long Ground Village, Montserrat, British West Indies

I am an Herbalist running a Natural Medicine Clinic here in England, and I've received two of your most brilliant books, *Herbs for Good Health and Science* and *Science of Herbal Medicine,* and I'm very keen to read your book, *The Herbal Pharmacy.* Do you have a distributor here in England? If not, could you tell me who to write to in the U.S.A. to get a copy?

Your view of Herbal Medicine is like a breath of fresh pure air. Thanks for all your kind help and I look forward to hearing from you soon.

—Mr. S. McCoy, Whitstable, Kent, England

I am very happy to know that you have written and published an *Encyclopedia of Anti-Aging Remedies,* which reports nature's secrets for "stalling and reversing" the effects of aging. I think the above publication is a unique one and has a significant relevance in the modern life.

—S. K. Misra, Chief Editor, Indian Journal of Indigenous Medicines, India

I have enjoyed reading your *New Encyclopedia of Fruits and Vegetables.* It's a great book filled with fantastic food information.

—John Colven, Dungog, Australia

I want to express my gratitude to you for being so generous with your knowledge about laryngial paralysis. Now that I have a renewed sense of hope because of you, I can begin to help my dog, Riley. I was almost at the end of my rope of hope when I opened your wonderful book, *Natural Pet Cures* one more time! and said, "the answer's just got to be in here." I had looked at your name many times but didn't think I should bother you. I'm so glad I did. You were so kind and generous with your time and wisdom.

—Amy Winney, Northridge, California

Your book, *Natural Pet Cures* is in my possession and I cannot tell you how much I enjoy reading, underlining, highlighting and also, in some instances using the components. Some of my friends who also believe in natural healing have read, and like me, applied.

—Charles Weiland, West Chester, Pennsylvania

I am an orthomolecular nutritionist and I just finished reading *Dr. Heinerman's Encyclopedia of Nature's Vitamins and Minerals.* I enjoyed it very much and I also learned a few things from it. It is a very good, well-put-version nutrition book.

—Eyal-Moskona Ome, Tel-Aviv, Israel

I have bought your book, *Encyclopedia of Nuts, Berries and Seeds* and have enjoyed it immensely, because I am such a nut and berry lover. I want to make sure that I always find them wild if possible. Again, I thank you for your lovely encyclopedia.

—Dolores Johnsen, Guttenburg, New Jersey

I read and reread your books and always find something new. Your style of writing and describing are particularly easy to read. Your personal comments make the subjects very real.

I've practiced as a Chiropractor and as a Naturopathic Physician for over 45 years, and I practiced with the renowned Dr. Bernard Jensen, whose books are also very descriptive and inspiring. Even when we, as physicians, think we've read and heard everything—new subjects, treatments, and products pop up that flood the literature and airways. Your book, *Nuts, Berries and Seeds* is particularly interesting and valuable to me, and I refer frequently to the book.

I salute you, as a writer, an adventurer and a seeker of health information, and as such, you are a valuable contributor to the health field.

—Dr. S. Jonathan Spector, Sarasota, Florida

I have read your book, *Natural Pet Cures* twice in the past month and am just about to finish *Nature's Super 7 Medicines.* I have two others purchased and waiting to be read.

My husband and I own/are owned by 2 dogs and 80 exotic birds. I have found *Natural Pet Cures* to be very helpful with our 2 girls and have made some changes in their daily diets. What a change we have seen in them. We are absolutely delighted! Our dogs have always loved veggies and fruits—if the birds eat it they have to have some too!

—Pati Hazell, Wichita, Kansas

I phoned your home and requested information from your WON-DERFUL book, *Healing Herbs and Spices.* I have learned so much from this book. Thank you, Thank you for all the easy-to-understand information.
Lavaughn J. Stolba, Cedar Rapids, Iowa

Thank you so much for first having written *Heinerman's Encyclopedia of Healing Herbs,* which provided hope, and for having delivered inspiration to me.
—N.G. Kwee, Lorong, Tia Payou, Singapore

Enjoyed *Natural Pet Cures* a lot. Thanks for writing it.
—Noreen Crouch, Putney, Vermont

I recently bought my second Heinerman book. Now I have two favorite books among my two fairly large bookcases. Don't get the wrong idea, I am not well educated. I left school at 13. I'm also not very well off financially (pensioned). But I like books, plants, and learning things by practical means. I just love your books. I am an old man, in years anyway, but still am pretty lively and only wish I had access to your type of book when my brain was younger and more able to retain what I read.
—Colin MacDonald, Bundaberg, Queensland, Australia

I really appreciate all of your books that I have purchased.
—Sebastian Teh, Hot Springs, North Carolina

I use your *Healing Herbs and Spices* book quite a bit. I enjoy it very much and find it very informative. I have used a few of your suggestions.
—Ann Melcher, Richmond Hill, Ontario, Canada

I have just read *Encyclopedia of Healing Juices, Healing Herbs and Spices, Encyclopedia of Nuts, Berries and Seeds* and *Anti-Aging Remedies,* all in the last three weeks. I bought them all and find them super interesting and helpful. I have much admiration for explorers like you who seek the real wealth of God! Keep up the great work!
—Steve Forbush, Cleveland, Ohio

I have read and enjoyed your books, *Healing Herbs & Spices* and the *Encyclopedia of Nuts, Berries and Seeds* very much. They have become reference books.

—Nell Atkins, Houston, Texas

I possess your book entitled, *Natural Pet Cures,* which you wrote, and have found it to be an excellent source of information.

—Diana Zelnio, Albuquerque, New Mexico

Congratulations on having authored 54 books. Quite impressive!

—Dannye DeLorenzo, Glen Ellen, California

I have your books and am grateful for them. I've about worn your *Miracle Healing Herbs* out, so will need to buy another copy.

—Loretta Reese, Perry, OH

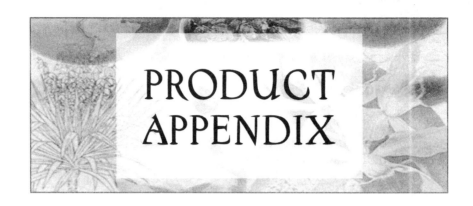

PRODUCT APPENDIX

Anthropological Research Center
P.O. Box 11471
Salt Lake City; UT 84147

The Treatment of Cancer With Herbs, Essex Botanical, Rex Wheat Germ Oil, Liquid yellow pine pitch, *Folk Medicine Journal* (2 years),

Earth's Pharmacy
131 West 500 South
PMB #422
Bountiful, UT 84010

Total Care; Repose; Ginkgo Biloba; Cran Max; St. Johnswort; Echinacea-Goldenseal; Fish Oil; Omega 3-6-9; Garlic; Grape Seed Extract; Super Antioxidant.

North American Herb & Spice Co.
P.O. Box 4885
Buffalo Grove, IL 60089

Wild Turkish Oregano capsules, juice, and oil.

Pines International
P.O. Box 1107
Lawrence, KS 66044

Wheat grass, barley grass, and beet-juice powder.

Rubicon Enterprises Inc.
103-3600 Townline Road
Abbotsford, B.C.
Canada V2T 5W8

Rubicon Health Circlet (made from Canadian tin) for human and animal uses. Intended for promoting vitality and stamina, skin beauty, and disease resistance.

ShapeRite/Dept DRJH
9850 South 300 West
Sandy, UT 84070

Male Formula; Female Formula; Enzy-Rite; Fibre System Plus; Bountiful Harvest; CM Super (calcium–magnesium); MusculoSkeletal Formula; Start+; Inner Sun; Cardio Formula; Immune Formula; Stress Formula; PhytoLax.

Synergy WorldWide
972 North 1430 West
Orem, UT 84057 USA

Euphorbia; Super Food; Body Guard; Germanium Plus; Miracle Rub; Aloe Magic; Revitalizing Toner; Advanced Face Cream; Anti-Aging Serum; Total Body Wash; Angel Cream.

Trace Minerals Research
1990 West 3300 South
Ogden, UT 84401

Arth-X; Complete Calcium Hydrooxyapatite; ConcenTrace; Chromium; Liquimins; Maxi Multi with ConcenTrace; Glucosamine/MSM with ConcenTrace; Noni Juice with ConcenTrace; Flavored ConcenTrace Trace Minerals Drops.

Vita-Mix Corporation
8615 Usher Road
Cleveland, OH 44138-9989

Manufactures top-quality juicer/food processor.

Wakunaga of America Co. Ltd.
23501 Madero
Mission Viejo, CA 92691

Kyolic Aged Garlic Extract; Kyo-Green; Kyo-Dophilus. Bio-K+ Refrigerated live-cultured probiotic.

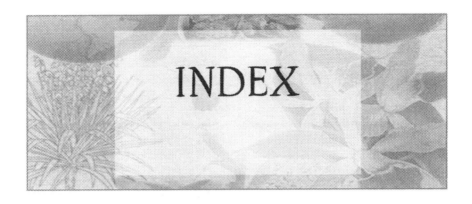

INDEX

A

Abscesses, 1–2
Abdominal cramps, 2–3
and peppermint tea, 250
Abrasions, 3–4
Achromycin, 114
Acidophilus, 219
Acites, *See* Fluid retention
Acne, 4–5
Acorn squash, and cancer, 101
Activated charcoal, and food
poisoning, 282
Active lifestyle, and vaginal problems, 325
Acupressure, and migraines, 252
Acupuncture, and migraines,
252
Addiction, 5–7
Adult anger, dealing with, 10–11
Advanced Face Cream (Synergy
Worldwide), 336
Aerobic exercise, and high blood
pressure, 207
Age spots, 7
Aggressive behavior, 7–11
adult anger, dealing with,
10–11
and cornmeal, 9
and deep-breathing exercises,
11
and diet, 9–10
and lycopodium, 255
and mental diversion, 9

nutritional assistance, 11
and soothing music, 8
and sugar, 9
AIDS, *See* Cancer
Airplane ears, 12–13
Alcohol:
and erection impairment, 218
and menstrual cramping, 248
Alcoholic hangover, 13
Alcohol withdrawal, 155–60
Alfalfa:
and bone healing, 183
and endometriosis, 165–66
Algaes/seaweed, and antiestrogens, 68
Allergies, 14–16
Aloe Magic (Synergy Worldwide),
336
Aloe vera, 113, 154, 308
Alzheimer's disease, 16–22
and fish, 18
and folic acid, 22
and ginkgo biloba, 19–20
and megavitamin therapy,
18–19
and mercury fillings, 20–22
statistics about, 16
and wine, 17–18
Amebiasis, *See* Diarrhea
Amino acids, 31
Anal discomfort, 23–24
and witch hazel, 24
Anaphylactic shock, 16
Anbesol, and herpes, 205

Anemia, 24–26
Aneurysm, 26–28
Angel Cream, 308
Anger, 226–27
  and deep breathing, 227
  and lycopodium, 255
Angina, 28
Animal bites, 29
Animal therapy, and stress,
  304–5
Ankle pain, 29–30
Anorexia nervosa, 30–31
Anti-Aging Serum (Synergy
  Worldwide), 336
Antiestrogens:
  and algaes/seaweed, 68
  and breast cancer, 67–68
Anxiety, 31–34
  and caffeinism, 87–88
Appendicitis, 34–35
Appetite loss, 35–36
Apple-cider vinegar:
  and acne, 5
  and bronchitis, 77
  and cancer, 103
  and crow's feet, 144
Apples, and cancer, 103
Apricots, and cancer, 103
  puree, and ulcerative colitis,
  322
Argemone mexicana, and intestinal
  parasites, 225
Argentum nitricum, and compul-
  sive-obsessive behavior, 255
Arm pain, 36–37
Arnica, and muscle cramps, 257
Aromatherapy, and migraines,
  252
Arthritis, 37–39
  and ayurvedic herbs, 38
  and glucosamine, 38
  and guggul, 38
  and methylsulfonylmethane
  (MSM), 38
  and salai, 38
Artichoke, and cancer, 103
Aspartate, 80

Asthma, 39–40
  and caffeinism, 88–89
Athlete's foot, 40–41
Atrophic vaginitis, 41
Autism, 41–44
  and food sensitivities, 42–43
  and genius, 43–44
  and vitamins, 42
Autoimmune deficiency syndrome (AIDS), *See* Cancer
Aylward's Natural Food (Hackensack, NJ), 46–47
Ayurvedic herbs, for arthritis,
  38

B

Baby-harp-seal oil, and os-
  teoarthritis, 266–67
Back pain, 45
Bacterial vaginosis, 45–46
Bad breath, 46
Bags under the eyes, 47
Baking soda, and jock itch, 232
Banana skins, and warts, 329
Barley tea, and cancer, 101
Bay leaves, and heel pain, 202
B-complex vitamins:
  and aggressive behavior, 11
  and manic depression, 245–46
  and mental illness, 249
  and rashes, 290
  and sexual performance, 219
  and shock, 296
Beans, and cancer, 101
Bed sores, 47–49
Bedwetting, 49–50
Beer:
  and hiccups, 206
  and loss of sexual interest, 242
Bees, and detection of chemical
  odors, 23
Beet root juice/powdered concen-
  trate, and cancer, 100
Beets, and cancer, 103
Belladonna, and rabies, 288
Bells' palsy, 277

Ben Gay and turpentine liniment, 184
Benign prostatic hyperplasia, 50–51
Bermuda Triangle, 211–13
Bilberry, and macular degeneration, 245
Binge and purge syndrome, 78–79
Biofeedback training, and migraines, 252
Bio-K+, 115, 282
Birthing, herbs for, 237–38
Bites:
  animal, 29
  insect, 224–25
Blackboard chalk, powdered, and food poisoning, 282
Black cohosh, and nervousness, 263
Black cumin, and gray hair, 193
Black haw, and premenstrual syndrome, 284–85
Black pepper, and epilsepsy, 166
Bladder infection, 51–53
Bladderwrack:
  and charley horse, 112
  and hot flashes, 248
Bleeding, 54–56
Bleeding gums, 56–57
Blisters, 57–58
  and cranberry juice, 58
Blood clots, 58–60
Blood infection, 221–22
Blood poisoning, 60–62
Blue corn drink, for hallucinations, 195–96
Blue vervain, and nervousness, 263
Body Guard (Synergy Worldwide), 257
Body odor, 62–63
Body piercing, 63–64
  and infection, 63–64
Boiled rice water, and diarrhea, 154–55

Boils, 1–2, 64–65
Bok choy, and cancer, 101
Borage-seed oil, 308
Boron, and mental illness, 249
Bountiful Harvest (ShapeRite), 194
Brain stress, 65
Breast cancer, 66–69
  and antiestrogens, 67–68
  basic plan for combatting, 67
  and fiber, 67
  and red beets, 69
  and soy, 67
Breast pain, 69–72
  and aerobic exercise, 71
  and breast feeding, 70
  common sources of, 69
  herbal therapy, 71–72
  nutritional assistance for, 71
  and PMS, 69–70
Breast swelling, 72–73
Brigham Young's Composition Tea, 187–90
Broccoli:
  and cancer, 103
  and high cholesterol, 207
Broken bones, 73–76
  bone-rebuilding herbs, 75
  emergency treatment, 73–74
  and faith healing, 75–76
  tea for pain relief, 74–75
Bronchitis, 76–77
Brown-rice tea, and cancer, 101
Bruises, 77–78
Brussels sprouts, and high cholesterol, 207
Bulimia, 78–80
Bunions, 80–82
Burdock root:
  and cancer, 101
  and cirrhosis, 124
  and pain, 275
Burns, 82
Bursitis, 83
Buttermilk, and indigestion, 219
Butternut squash, and cancer, 101

C

Cabbage, and high cholesterol, 207
Caffeine, potency of, 89
Caffeinism, 84–89
    alternative solutions, 86–88
    and anxiety, 87–88
    and asthma, 88–89
    caffeine-induced mental disorders, 84–86
    Dandelion Java, 86–87
    and panic disorders, 87–88
    and prayer, 88
Calcium, 31
    and mental illness, 249
Calcium citrate, 80
Calcium fluoride, and muscle-tone loss, 257–58
Calcium magnesium supplement:
    and headaches, 251–52
    and menstrual cramping, 248
    and nail problems, 259
Camel milk, and atrophic vaginitis, 41
Campho-Phenique, and herpes, 205
Cancer, 89–106
    breast, 66–69
    chemotherapy, 92–93
    colon, 97–99, 129–30
    defined, 90
    factors contributing to, 91–92
    history of, 89
    international cancer-recovery program, 95–99
    body, 99–104
    Canada, 102
    China, 103–4
    Great Britain, 102–3
    head/heart, 96
    Hungary, 100
    India, 103
    Japan, 100–104
    Mexico, 103
    nerves/liver, 97
    stomach/colon, 97–99

lung, 242
prostate, 285
radiation, 93
skin, 246
stomach, 97–99
    Treatment of Cancer with Herbs, The, 93–95
Canola oil, and brain stress, 65
Carbuncles, 64–65
Cardiac arrest, 106–7
Carob powder, and Paget's disease, 274
Carpal tunnel syndrome, 107–8
Carrot juice, and macular degeneration, 244–45
Carrots:
    and cancer, 101, 103
    and vision, 191
Cascara de salamo, and appendicitis, 35
Cataracts, 109
Catnip:
    and addiction, 6–7
    and cockroach infestation, 125
    and colic, 128
    and kidney failure/kidney stones, 233–34
    and nervousness, 263
Catnip tea, and nausea, 260
Cauliflower, and cancer, 101, 103
Cayenne pepper:
    and bleeding, 55–56
    and cardiac arrest, 107
    and cold hands/feet, 126
    and the heart, 201
Cedar bark, and painful breathing, 276
Cedar twigs, and wrinkles, 335
Celery, and cancer, 103
Celiac disease, 109–10
Cerebral palsy, 110–11
Chamomile, and aggressive behavior, 11
Chamomile tea:
    and "computer-screen" eyes, 135
    and insomnia, 225

and menstrual difficulties, 249
and palsy, 277
and red eyes, 291–92
Chaparral tea, and melanoma, 246
Chapped hands/lips, 110–11
Charcoal, and food poisoning, 180–82
Charley horse, 111–12
Chasmanthera dependens, and intestinal parasites, 225
Chaste-tree berry, and premenstrual syndrome, 284–85
Chemotherapy, 92–93
Chest pain, 112
and aneurysms, 27
Chicken consumption, and cancer, 105–6
Chickenpox, 112–13
Chickweed, and hepatitis, 203
Chickweed herb, and common colds, 134
Chills, and ginger tea, 250
Chinese cabbage, and cancer, 101
Chives, and cancer, 103
Chlamydia, 113–15
Chlorophyll powder, and bone healing, 183
Choking, 115–20
Heimlich manuever on animals, 119–20
Heimlich manuever on humans:
victim seated, 118
victim standing, 117–18
victim supine, 118–19
history behind the maneuver, 116–17
Choline:
and dementia, 152
and liver, 191
Chromium:
and blood-sugar levels, 251
and sexual performance, 219
Chronic-fatigue syndrome, 121–23
Cirrhosis of the liver, 124–25
Citrus juice:

and lung infection, 328
and sore throat, 301
Cocklebur tea, and abrasions, 3–4
Cockroach infestation, 125
Codex Hammer, 227–28
Coffee:
and hay fever, 197–98
and menstrual cramping, 248
and ringworm, 293
Colas:
and menstrual cramping, 248
and ringworm, 293
Cold caffeine treatment, for ringworm, 293
Cold hands/feet, 126
Colds, 133–34
Cold sores, 126–27
Colic, 128
Colitis, 128–29, 226
ulcerative, 321–22
Collards, and bruises, 78
Colon, and wound care, 332
Colon cancer, 97–99, 129–30
See also Cancer
Colon therapy, and migraines, 252
Color blindness, 130–31
Coltsfoot leaves, and pain, 275
Coma, 131–33
Common cold, 133–34
Complete Calcium Hydrooxyapatite (Trace Minerals Research), 75
Composition Tea, 187–90
Compulsions, 134
Compulsive-obsessive behavior, and argentum nitricum, 255
"Computer-screen" eyes, 134–35
ConcenTrace, 69, 124, 206, 254
Concussion, 136
Congestive heart failure, 136–38
Conjunctivitis, 138
Constipation, 138–39
Contact-lens problems, 139
Copper, and macular degeneration, 245

Copper ore, powdered, and muscle cramps, 257
Corn, and cancer, 103
Cornmeal, and aggressive behavior, 9
Cough, 139–40
Crabs, 140–41
Cracked heel, 141
Cramps:
  abdominal, 2–3
  leg, 111–12
  and menstruation, 248–49
  muscle, 257
Cranberry juice:
  and bladder infection, 53
  and bleeding gums, 56–57
  and blisters, 58
  and hypothermia, 215
  and tuberculosis, 320
CranMax (Earth's Pharmacy), 53, 57
Creole cuisine, 155–60
Crohn's disease, 142–43
Croup, 143
Crow's feet, 143–44
Cuts, 144
Cystic fibrosis, 144–45
Cystitis, *See* Bladder infection
Cysts, 145–46

D

Daikon radish, and cancer, 101
Dandelion:
  and cirrhosis, 124
  and night blindness, 264
  and red eyes, 291
Dandelion-chicory-burdock tea, and cancer, 101
Dandelion greens/flowers:
  and cancer, 101
  and color blindness, 130–31
  and liver, 241–42, 331
Dandelion Java, 86–87
Dandelion root, and liver, 191
Dandelion wine-curried rice cure, for jaundice, 229–30

Dandruff, 147–48
Dates, and stomachache, 302
Da Vinci, Leonardo, 227–28
Deep-breathing exercises, and aggressive behavior, 11
Deep-vein thrombosis, 148–49
Dehydration, 176–77
Delirium, 150
Dementia, 150–52
Dental cavities, 152–53
Depression, 153
  manic, 245–46
Dermatitis, 153–54
Diabetes, 153–54
Diaper rash, 153–54
Diarrhea, 129, 154–55
Difficult urination, 155–60
Dill weed, and cancer, 103
Distilled vinegar, and dandruff, 148
Diverticular disease, 155–60
Diverticulitis, 226
Dizziness, 155–60
Dong quai:
  and endometriosis, 165–66
  and menstrual difficulties, 249
Doryx, 114
Double vision, 155–60
Down syndrome, 155–60
Drug abuse by the elderly, 155–60
Drug addiction, 155–60
Drug and alcohol withdrawal, 155–60
Dry skin, 155–60
Dulse:
  and charley horse, 112
  and hot flashes, 248
Dyslexia, 155–60

E

Ears:
  aches/infections/earwax buildup, 160–64
  airplane, 12–13
  glue, 191–92
  hearing loss, 199

Eating disorders, 164
Echinacea, and impetigo, 217
Echinacea-goldenseal combo, and tuberculosis (TB), 319
Eczema, 164, 308
Eggplant, and cancer, 103
Elbow pain, 164–65
Electrotherapy, and migraines, 252
Emphysema, 165
Encephalitis, 165
Endive:
  and broken bones, 75
  and cancer, 103
Endometriosis, 165–66
Enzy-Rite Formula (ShapeRite), 278
Epilsepsy, 166
Epsom salt baths, and migraines, 252
Epsom salts, 29–30, 182
Erection problems, 166
Erysipelas, 166
Escarole, and cancer, 103
Essential fatty acids (EFAs), 254
Essiac Botanical, and cancer, 102
Eucalyptus drops, and airplane ears, 12–13
Eucalyptus oil, and ingrown toenails, 224
Euphoria (Synergy Worldwide), 219
European allergy recovery program, 14–16
Evening-primrose oil, multiple sclerosis, 256–57
Excessive sweating, 308–9
Excessive yawning, 337
Eyes:
  bags under, 47
  cataracts, 109
  color blindness, 130–31
  "computer-screen", 134–35
  conjunctivitis, 138
  contact-lens problems, 139
  crow's feet, 143–44
  eyestrain, 167
    floaters, 166
    glaucoma, 190–91
    red, 291–92

F

Facial paralysis, 168–69
Fainting, 169
Faith healing, and broken bones, 75–76
False unicorn root, and premenstrual syndrome, 284
Fat Complexer (ShapeRite), 68–69
Fear, 169–71
  overcoming, 171
Feet, cold, 126
Fennel seed, and coughs, 140
Fenugreek, and sexual performance, 219
Fenugreek seed, 81, 83
  and concussion, 136
  and gum inflammation, 193
  and irritable bowel syndrome (IBS), 226
  and Paget's disease, 274
Fenugreek-seed tea, and atrophic vaginitis, 41
Ferns, and wrinkles, 335
Ferrum Phosphate, and mumps, 257
Fever, 172
Fever blisters, 126–27
Feverfew, and migraines, 251
Fiber, 178–79, 248
  and benign prostatic hyperplasia, 51
  and breast cancer, 67
  and high cholesterol, 207
Fibre System Plus (ShapeRite), 129
Fibromyalgia, 172–73
Figs:
  and bedwetting, 50
  and gout, 193
  and high cholesterol, 207
  and stomachache, 302
Finger injuries, 173–74

Fish:
  and Alzheimer's disease, 18
  and brain stress, 65
  and cancer, 101
Fish oil, 254
  and menstrual cramping, 248
  and tuberculosis (TB), 319
Flatulence, 174
Flaxseed oil:
  and brain stress, 65
  and cancer, 103
  and dementia, 152
  and liver, 191
  multiple sclerosis, 256–57
Floates, eyes, 166
Flu, 174–75
Fluid retention, 175–77
Folic acid, and dementia, 22
Food and drug interactions,
  177–80
Food laxatives, 138–39
Food-mood connetion, 9–10
Food poisoning, 180–82
  and pears, 281–82
Food sensitivities, and autism,
  42–43
Foot pain, 182–83
Fractures, 183
Frankincense-tree extract, 308
Frostbite, 183–84

G

Galanin, 268
Gallstones, 185–86
Garlic:
  and colon cancer, 129–30
  and ear problems, 161
  and encephalitis, 165
  and the heart, 201
  and high cholesterol, 207
  and meningitis, 247
  and toothache, 316
  and tuberculosis (TB), 319
  and varicose veins, 325–26
Gastritis, 186–90
Gastroenteritis, 186–90

Gates, Bill, 228
Germanium, 308, 336
Giardiasis, 186–90
Ginger:
  and blood clots, 58–60
  and cardiac arrest, 107
  and migraines, 251
  and sexual performance, 219
Ginger root:
  and the heart, 201
  and menstrual difficulties, 249
Ginger tea, and chills, 250
Ginkgo biloba:
  and alzheimer's disease, 19–20
  and dementia, 152
  and macular degeneration, 245
Ginseng:
  and endometriosis, 165–66
  and sexual performance, 219
Glaucoma, 190–91
Glucosamine, and arthritis, 38
Glue ear, 191–92
Glycerine, and rashes, 290
Goat's milk:
  and atrophic vaginitis, 41
  and colic, 128
  and flu, 175
  and ulcers, 322–23
Goldenseal:
  and blood infection, 221
  and intestinal parasites, 225–
    26
  and jock itch, 232
  and red eyes, 291
Goldenseal root:
  and bacterial vaginosis, 46
  and erysipelas, 166
  and impetigo, 217
Gold, Tracey, 30–31
Gonorrhea, 192–93
Gotu kola, and dementia, 152
Gout, 193
Grape juice:
  and tuberculosis, 320
  and ulcerative colitis, 322
Grapeseed extract, and tuberculosis (TB), 319

Gray hair, 193
Gree clay, for torn ligament, 319
Green cabbage:
  and cancer, 101
  and ulcers, 322–23
Green peppers, and cancer, 103
Guava:
  and heartburn/heatstroke, 201
  and vomiting, 326
Guggul, and arthritis, 38
Guided imagery, and migraines, 252
Gum inflammation, 193

H

Hair loss, 194–216
Hajiki, and hot flashes, 248
Hakka, 142
Hallucinations, 195–96
Hand pain, 196–97
Hands:
  carpal tunnel syndrome, 107–8
  chapped, 110–11
  cold, 126
Hangover, 13, 197
Harriqa, and lung cancer, 242
Hawthorn, and low blood pressure, 242
Hay fever, 197–98
Headaches, 198–99
  and minerals, 251–52
Healing intuition, 339–43
Healthtouch, 180
Hearing loss, 199
Heart attack, 199–201
Heartburn, 201
Heatstroke, 201
Heel pain, 201–2
Heinerman, John, 343
Hemorrhoids, 202
Hepatitis, 203
Herbal steam bath, for acne, 5
Herbal teas:
  and aggressive behavior, 11
  and cancer, 101

Hernia, 203–4
Herpes simplex virus (HSV-1), 126–27, 205–6
Hesperidin bioflavonoids, and macular degeneration, 245
Hiatal hernia, *See* Heartburn; heatstroke
Hiccups, 206
Hiera buena de olor, 36
High-altitude mosquito-borne malaria, 186–90
High blood pressure, 206–7
High cholesterol, 207
Hip pain, 208
Hives, 208
Hoarseness, 208–9
  and aneurysms, 27
Hodgkin's disease, 209–10
Honey:
  and abrasions, 3
  and hypothermia, 215
  wild, and sore throat, 301
Honeysuckle vine, and wrinkles, 335
Hops, and aggressive behavior, 11
Hops tea, and infertility, 223
Horseradish, and high cholesterol, 207
Horsetail:
  and bone healing, 183
  and nail problems, 259
Hot flashes, 210–11, 248
Hot salsa, and respiratory-distress syndrome, 292
Hot-tub-soak-ice-pack applications, and bumps/bruises, 310–11
Hubbard squash, and cancer, 101
Hydrastic canadensis, and intestinal parasites, 225
Hypertension, and aneurysms, 26
Hypoglycemia, 211–13
Hypothermia, 214–15
Hypothyroidism, 216
Hyssop tea, and bacterial vaginosis, 46

I

Ice pack, and herpes, 205
Impetigo, 217
Impotence, 217–19
Indian tobacco, and motion sickness, 256
Indigestion, 219
Infection, 220–22
    bladder, 51–53
    blood, 221–22
    and body piercing, 63–64
    eye, 139
    lung, 327–28
    yeast, 338–39
Infertility, 222–23
Influenza, 174–75
Ingrown toenails, 223–24
Insect bites/stings, 224–25, 314
Insecurity, and lycopodium, 255
Insomnia, 225
Institute for Safe Mediation Practices, 180
Interactions, food and drug, 177–80
International cancer-recovery program, 95–99
Intestinal parasites, 225–26
Iodine, 158
    and Hodgkin's disease, 210
    and vaginal problems, 325
Iron, 31
    and anemia, 25–26
Irritable bowel syndrome (IBS), 128, 142, 226
Irritation, 226–27
Itching, 227–28

J

Jaundice, 229–30
Jet lag, 230–31
Jock itch, 231–32
Juniper berries:
    and pain, 275
    and painful breathing, 276
    and wounds, 330

K

Kale:
    and broken bones, 75
    and cancer, 101
Kampo medicine, 142, 216
    and Parkinson's disease, 280
Kava, and anxiety, 33–34
Kelp:
    and bone healing, 183
    and charley horse, 112
    and hot flashes, 248
    and minerals, 124
Kidney failure/kidney stones, 233–34
Kiwi, and benign prostatic hyperplasia, 51
Knee pain, 234–35
Kohlrabi, and high cholesterol, 207
Kola nut, and lactose intolerance, 240
Kyo-Green, 65, 68
    and cancer, 100
Kyolic Aged Garlic Extract:
    and bacterial vaginosis, 46
    and breast cancer, 68

L

Labor and delivery problems, 236–38
Lacnunga, 47–49
Lactose intolerance, 240
Laminaria, and charley horse, 112
Laryngitis, 208
Lasagen, and cancer, 102
LaStone therapy, 292–93
Lavendar, and aggressive behavior, 11
L-carnitine, and dementia, 152
Leafy green vegetables:
    and brain stress, 65
    and bruises, 78
Learning disabilities, 240
Lecithin, and dementia, 152

Leeks, and high cholesterol, 207
Leg pain, 241
Leukemia, 241
See also Cancer
Lice, 241
Licorice root, and headache,
198–99
Light sensitivity, 241
Lima beans, and cancer, 103
Lime juice, and sore throat, 301
Liniment:
for elbow pain, 164–65
for frostbite, 184
Lips, chapped, 110–11
Liquid Kyolic Garlic, 100
Lithium, and mental illness, 249
Liver, 241–42
cirrhosis of, 124–25
herbs for, 331
Lobelia, and glue ear, 191
Loss of sexual interest, 242
See also Erection problems; Im-
potence
Lotus:
and fainting, 169
and fear, 169–70
and fever, 172
Louisiana Gold Pepper Sauce,
160
Low blood pressure, 242
Lower back pain, 45
Lung cancer, 242
Lupus erythematosus, 242
Lycopene, 285
Lyme disease, 243

M

Mabanga, and lactose intolerance,
240
Macular degeneration, 244–45
Magnesium, 31
and aneurysms, 27–28
and mental illness, 249
Magnesium citrate, 80
Magnesium phosphate, and muscle-tone loss, 257–58

Mahonia aquifolium, and intestinal
parasites, 225
Maitake mushrooms, and cancer,
104
Malaria, 245
Malawi, traditional medicine in,
238–40
Male ferns, and wrinkles, 335
Male Formula (ShapeRite), 51
Mango:
and benign prostatic hyperplasia, 51
and heartburn/heatstroke, 201
and vomiting, 326
Manic depression, 245–46
Marigold flower petals, and macu-
lar degeneration, 244
Marjoram, and hemorrhoids,
202
Marshmallow root:
and emphysema, 165
and food poisoning, 282
and hernia, 204
and irritable bowel syndrome
(IBS), 226
Massage, and migraines, 252
Massage therapy:
for carpal tunnel syndrome,
108
for foot pain, 183
for muscular dystrophy, 258
Measles, 246
Meat, and wounds, 331–32
Medical intuitiveness, 339–43
Meditation, and migraines, 252
Megavitamin therapy, and
Alzheimer's disease, 18–19
Melaleuca oil:
and crabs, 141
and ear problems, 161
Melanoma, 246
Melatonin therapy, and mi-
graines, 252
Meningitis, 247
Menopause, 247–48
hot flashes, 210–11, 248
Menstruation, 248–49

Mental diversion, and aggressive behavior, 9
Mental illness, 249
Mentholatum Deep-Heat Rub, and neck pain, 260
Mercury fillings, and Alzheimer's disease, 20–22
Methylsulfonylmethane (MSM), and arthritis, 38
Mexican-restaurant syndrome, 250
Microcrystalline hydroxyapatite, 80
Migraines, 250–53
and minerals, 251–52
Milk of magnesia, and food poisoning, 282
Minerals, 121–24
Miscarriage, 253–54
Moles, 254
Monodox, 114
Mononucleosis, 254–55
Mood changes, 255
Motherwort, and fibromyalgia, 172–73
Motion sickness, 256
Mountain fever, 186–90
MSG, and migraines, 251
Mud, and insect bites/stings, 224–25
Mud pack, for pulled hamstring, 318–19
Mullein, and glue ear, 191
Mullein leaves:
and common colds, 134
and cough, 140
and ear problems, 161
and lupus erythematosus, 242
and pain, 275
Mullein tea:
and chest pain, 112
and measles, 246
Multiple personalities, 256
Multiple sclerosis, 256–57
Mumps, 257
Muscle cramps, 257
Muscle-tone loss, 257–58

Muscular dystrophy, 258
Musculoskeletal Formula (ShapeRite), 267
Mustard greens:
and bruises, 78
and high cholesterol, 207

N

Nail problems, 259
Nausea:
and catnip tea, 260
and papaya juice, 250
and pear juice, 250
and peppermint tea, 260
and spearmint tea, 260
See also Vomiting
Neck pain, 260–61
Nerve pain, 261–62
Nervousness, 262–63
Nervous stomach, 262
Neuralgia, 263–64
Night blindness, 264
Nightshade, and rabies, 288
Nkalanga, and light sensitivity, 241
Nori, and hot flashes, 248
Nosebleeds, 265
Nut butter:
and brain stress, 65
and cancer, 101
Nuts:
and benign prostatic hyperplasia, 51
and cancer, 101
and minerals, 124

O

Oatmeal:
and bone healing, 183
and concussion, 136
Olive oil, 81, 254
and brain stress, 65
and lung infection, 328
and massage therapy, for carpal tunnel syndrome, 108

and muscular dystrophy, 258
and varicose veins, 325–26
Omega 3-6-9 fatty-acid complex,
 and tuberculosis (TB), 319
Oneida Eating Plan, 269–73
Onions:
 and blood clots, 58–60
 and blood infection, 221
 and blood poisoning, 62
 and cancer, 101, 103
 and flu, 175
 and high cholesterol, 207
 and toothache, 316
Oregano, oil of:
 and asthma, 39–40
 and athlete's foot, 40–41
 and toenail fungus, 41
Oregon grape, and intestinal parasites, 225–26
Osteoarthritis, 266–67
Osteoporosis, 267–68
Overweight, 268–73
 Oneida Eating Plan, 269–73
Oxygen therapy, and cystic fibrosis, 145

P

Paget's disease, 274
Pain, 275
 abdominal, 2–3
 anal, 23–24
 arm, 36–37
 back, upper/lower, 45
 chest, 112
 elbow, 164–65
 foot, 182–83
 hand, 196–97
 heel, 201–2
 hip, 208
 knee, 234–35
 leg, 241
 neck, 260–61
 nerve, 261–62
 wound, 332
Painful breathing, 275–76
Painful intercourse, 276–77

Palsy, 277
Pancreatitis, 278
Panic disorders, and caffeinism,
 87–88
Papaya:
 and benign prostatic hyperplasia, 51
 and heartburn/heatstroke,
 201
 and hoarseness/laryngitis, 209
 and vomiting, 326
Papaya juice, and nausea, 250
Paprika, 110
Paralysis, 278–79
 facial, 168–69
Parkinson's disease, 279–80
Parsley:
 and broken bones, 75
 and cancer, 101, 103
 and gallstones, 185–86
Parsnip, and gallstones, 185–86
Peach-tree leaves, and excessive
 yawning, 337
Peanuts, and toothache, 316
Pear juice:
 and heartburn/heatstroke, 201
 and nausea, 250
 and vomiting, 326
Pears, and food poisoning,
 281–82
Peek, Kim, 43–44
Peppermint:
 and aggressive behavior, 11
 and migraines, 251
Peppermint oil, 36–37
 and bronchitis, 77
Peppermint tea:
 and abdominal cramps, 250
 and colic, 128
 and cystic fibrosis, 145
 and nervousness, 263
Peptic ulcer, 280
Perspiration, and seaweed, 309
Phosphorus, 31
Phytoestrogens, 247–48
Pig grease, and insect
 bites/stings, 314

Pineapple, and boils/carbuncles, 64–65
Pineapple juice, and teething, 311
Pine buds, and coughs, 140
Pine needles, and painful breathing, 276
Pine needle tea, and compulsions, 134
Pinkeye, *See* Conjunctivitis
Pinworms, *See* Intestinal parasites
Pneumonia:
   walking, 327–28
   See also Common cold; Flu
Poisoning, 281–82
Poison-plant contact, *See* Rash
Polynesians, and anxiety, 33–34
Poppy seeds, 3
Postnasal drip, 282–83
Postum, and cancer, 101
Potassium, 31
   and aneurysms, 27–28
   and high blood pressure, 207
   and mental illness, 249
   and tics/twitches, 315
Potatoes, and cancer, 103
Prayer, and caffeinism, 88
Pregnancy Formula, 238
Premenstrual syndrome, 283–85
Product appendix, 347–49
Progressive relaxation, and migraines, 252
Prostate cancer/prostatitis, 285
Prunes, and wounds, 330
Psoriasis, 285–87, 308
Psychiatric cognitive restructuring, 252
Pumpkins:
   and minerals, 124
   and vision, 191

R

Rabies, 288–93
Radiation, 93
Radish:
   and cancer, 103
   and facial paralysis, 168–69

Raisins, and cancer, 103
Rash, 289–90
Red beets, and cancer, 69
Red cabbage, and cancer, 103
Red clover, and endometriosis, 165–66
Red clover tea, and cancer, 102–3
Red eyes, 291–92
Red meat, and cancer, 104–5
Red pepper:
   and cuts, 144
   and erection problems, 166
Red radish:
   and cancer, 101
   and facial paralysis, 168–69
   and high cholesterol, 207
Red-raspberry-leaf tea, and menstrual difficulties, 249
Red-raspberry leaves, and premenstrual syndrome, 284–85
Red Wheat Germ Oil, 115
Reishi, and cancer, 104
Repose herbal blend, 11
Respiratory-distress syndrome, 292
Restless-legs syndrome, 292–93
Revitalizing Toner (Synergy Worldwide), 336
Rex Wheat Germ Oil:
   and manic depression, 246
   and tuberculosis, 319
Rice, and cancer, 103
Ringworm, 293
Robinson, Winter, 342–43
Romaine lettuce:
   and broken bones, 75
   and cancer, 103
Root vegetables, 248
   and angina, 28
   and benign prostatic hyperplasia, 51
   and minerals, 124
Rose petals, and kidney failure/kidney stones, 233–34
Rose vinegar, and cracked heel, 141

Royal jelly, and sexual performance, 219
Rubbing alcohol, and body odor, 63
Rutin, and macular degeneration, 245

S

Sagebrush tea, and acne, 4–5
Salai, and arthritis, 38
Salt Lake City tornado, 54–56
Sanzashi, and Parkinson's disease, 280
Sardine oil, and lung infection, 328
Sarsaparilla, and sexual performance, 219
Saw-briar vine, and excessive yawning, 337
Scallion, and cancer, 103
Scallions:
  and gallstones, 185–86
  and high cholesterol, 207
Scalp message, and hair loss, 195
Sciatica nerve pain, *See* Pain; Nerve pain
Sea vegetables, and cancer, 101
Seaweed:
  and algaes/seedweed, 68
  and charley horse, 111–12
  and Hodgkin's disease, 209–10
  and minerals, 124
  and perspiration, 309
Seeds:
  and benign prostatic hyperplasia, 51
  and cancer, 101
  and minerals, 124
Selenium, and sexual performance, 219
Sesame-seed oil, and atrophic vaginitis, 41
Sesame seeds, and gray hair, 193
Sexually transmitted diseases (STDs), 113–15, 192–93

Shark cartilage, and macular degeneration, 244
Shiitake mushrooms, and cancer, 104
Shilianzi, and fever, 172
Shingles, *See* Herpes simplex virus (HSV-1); Itching; Rashes; Skin problems
Shock, 294–96
Shortness of breath, 296–97
Shoulder pain, *See* Pain
Sinus infection, *See* Infection
Skin:
  aloe vera, 113, 154
  blisters, 57–58
  boils, 1–2
  sores, 300–301
Skin cancer, 246
  See also Cancer
Skoal, and painful breathing, 276
Skullcap:
  and migraines, 251
  and nervousness, 263
Slippery elm, powdered, and food poisoning, 282
Slippery-elm bark, 83
  and hernia, 204
  and irritable bowel syndrome (IBS), 226
Slippery-elm capsules, and bone healing, 183
Smith, June, 334–36, 342
Smoking, 298
Snoring, 299–300
Snuff, and epilsepsy, 166
Soothing music:
  and aggressive behavior, 8
  and depression, 153
  and multiple personalities, 256
Sores, 300–301
Sore throat, 301
Soy:
  and breast cancer, 67
  and colic, 128
Spearmint tea, and palsy, 277
Spider bites, *See* Insect bites/stings; Poisoning

Spinach:
  and bruises, 78
  and cancer, 103
  and macular degeneration,
    244
Sports-rub liniment, 310
Spotted fever, 186–90
Sprains, *See* Swelling
Squash:
  and cancer, 103
  and minerals, 124
  and vision, 191
Stinging nettle:
  and bone healing, 183
  and hepatitis, 203
  and liver, 191, 331
Stomachache, 302
Stomach cancer, 97–99
  See also Cancer
Strep throat, *See* Sore throat
Stress, 302–5
  and animal companionship,
    304–5
  coping with, 302–4
Stretching exercises, and breast
  swelling, 72–73
String beans, and cancer, 103
Stroke, 305–6
  and intact/whole foods, 306
  and natural/whole foods, 305
  and regional foods, 305–6
  and seasonal foods, 306
  and underutilized foods, 306
  and wild foods, 306
Stuffy nose, 306–7
Sugar, and aggressive behavior, 9
Sugary foods, and menstrual
  cramping, 248
Suika seed, and Parkinson's disease, 280
Sulfur, 31
  and high cholesterol, 207
Sunburn, 307–8
Sunflower, and night blindness,
  264
Super Food (Synergy Worldwide),
  257

Sweating excessively, 308–9
Sweet potatoes, and cancer, 103
Swelling, 309–11
Swiss chard:
  and bruises, 78
  and cancer, 101, 103
Syphilis, *See* Gonorrhea

T

Tabacum, and motion sickness,
  256
Tamarind, and liver disease,
  241–42
Tapeworm, *See* Intestinal para-
  sites
Tea-tree, and bronchitis, 77
Tea-tree oil:
  and crabs, 141
  and ear problems, 161
  and peptic ulcer, 280
Teething, 312–13
Tendinitis, *See* Swelling
Thrombosis, deep-vein, 148–49
Thrush, *See* Yeast infection
Thumbsucking, 313–14
Thyme:
  and coughs, 140
  and hemorrhoids, 202
Thyroid hormone therapy, and
  migraines, 252
Tics, 314–15
Tiger Balm liniment rubs, and mi-
  graines, 252
Tincture of witch hazel, and anal
  discomfort, 24
Tobacco tea, and rabies, 288
Toenail fungus, and oil of
  oregano, 41
Toe pain, *See* Gout; Pain
Tomatoes:
  and benign prostatic hyperpla-
  sia, 51
  and cancer, 103
Tonsillitis, *See* Sore throat
Toothache, 315–16
Torn ligament, 317–19

Total Body Wash (Synergy Worldwide), 336
Total Care nutritional packet (Earth's Pharmacy), 11, 69
Trace Minerals Research (Roy, Utah), 75
Truck-driver's philosophy, 282–83
Tuberculosis (TB), 319–20
Turkey tail mushrooms, and cancer, 104
Turmeric, and red eyes, 291
Turmeric root, and cancer, 103
Turnips:
  and cancer, 101
  and gallstones, 185–86
Twitches, 314–15

U

Ulcerative colitis, 321–22
Ulcers, 322–23
Upper back pain, 45
Urinary-tract infection, See Bladder infection
U.S. Pharmacopoeia, 180

V

Vaginal problems, 324–25
Vaginitis, atrophic, 41
Vaginois, bacterial, 45–46
Valerian, and nervousness, 263
Varicose veins, 325–26
Vibramycin, 114
Vibra-Tabs, 114
Vinegar, 2
  and acne, 5
  and heel pain, 202
Violent behavior, and lycopodium, 255
Vitamin A:
  and aggressive behavior, 11
  and eye infection, 139
Vitamin B-6 therapy, carpal tunnel syndrome, 108
Vitamin B-12, and fatigue, 248

Vitamin B, and nervousness, 263
Vitamin B-complex:
  and aggressive behavior, 11
  and manic depression, 245–46
  and mental illness, 249
  and rashes, 290
  and sexual performance, 263
  and shock, 296
Vitamin C:
  and aggressive behavior, 11
  and eye infection, 139
Vitamin E:
  and fever blisters, 127
  and mental illness, 249
  and nervousness, 263
  and rashes, 290
  and shock, 296
  and tuberculosis (TB), 319
Vitamin K, 178
Vitamins, and autism, 42
Vomiting, 326
  See also Nausea

W

"Walking" pneumonia, 327–28
Walnut shells, and kidney failure/kidney stones, 233–34
Warts, 328–29
Water consumption, and anger, 227
Watercress:
  and broken bones, 75
  and bruises, 78
  and cancer, 101, 103
  and high cholesterol, 207
  and liver, 331
Wheezing, See Asthma; Emphysema; Hay fever
White vinegar, and foot pain, 182
White willow bark, and herpes, 205
Whole-grain cereal, and cancer, 101
Whole grains, and minerals, 124
Wholesome foods, and aggressive behavior, 10

Whooping cough, *See* Cough; Infection
Wicca, 58–60
Wild honey, and sore throat, 301
Wild Turkish oregano, and tuberculosis (TB), 319
Willow tree leaves, and wound pain, 332
Wine, and Alzheimer's disease, 17–18
Wine vinegar, and crow's feet, 144
Wintergreen, and glue ear, 191
Witch hazel:
   and anal discomfort, 24
   and herpes, 205
Wood charcoal, and insect bites/stings, 314
Worms, *See* Intestinal parasites
Wormwood, and hypothermia, 215
Wormwood powder, and intestinal parasites, 225–26
Wounds, 330–34
   in verse, 332–34
Wrinkles, 334–36

X

Xabila, 154

Y

Yarrow:
   and cough, 140
   and glue ear, 191
   and measles, 246
   and palsy, 277
Yawning excessively, 337
Yeast infection, 338–39
Yellow dock, and cirrhosis, 124
Yimucao, and fibromyalgia, 172–73
Yoga, and migraines, 252
Yogurt, and indigestion, 219
Yohimbine, and sexual performance, 219
Yucca powder, and blood infection, 221

Z

Zinc:
   and fever blisters, 127
   and sexual performance, 219
Zinc sulfate, and macular degeneration, 245
Zithromax, 114
Zucchini, and cancer, 103
Zu'rur, and low blood pressure, 242